SPEAKING OF NURSING

READERS' COMMENTS

Reading this book was moving, informative, affirming and inspirational. ... It speaks of nursing in a way that makes its work and its wonder accessible to all. For nurses in general, studying or not, this is the kind of book we give each other as a gift.
—Professor Mary Chiarella, RN, LLB (Hons), PhD, is Chief Nursing Officer, New South Wales Health, Sydney, Australia.

Diers' core preoccupation has always been the practice and work of nurses. Her mission is to illuminate the complexity of that work and to help people understand what is it nurses know and do. That's why this book should be core reading for nurses and nursing students wherever they work, learn, or teach.
—Suzanne Gordon is a journalist who writes about nursing and health care. She is author of *Life Support: Three Nurses on the Front Lines* and co-author of *From Silence to Voice: What Nurses Know and Must Communicate to the Public.*

The collection of essays she has produced that begin in the 1960s and span more than four decades provides a colorful, challenging, controversial, and futuristic perspective on the evolution of clinical nursing research, advanced practice nursing, and nursing's engagement in policy debate.
—Linda H. Aiken, RN, PhD, FAAN is The Claire M. Fagin Leadership Professor of Nursing, Director, Center for Health Outcomes and Policy, University of Pennsylvania.

All nurses should read this work; all nurses should ensure that those who challenge the need for nurses and needing education read this. It truly shows the power of the words of nursing.
—Frances Hughes, RN, DN, FCON, ANZCMHN, Commandant-Col RNZNC is Chief Advisor, Nursing, Ministry of Health, Wellington, New Zealand.

Her prose is delicious—smart, funny, succinct and in-your-face. The practical wisdom she offers is accessible and unpretentious. It hasn't aged a bit over the years encompassed by this book. When she writes about nursing, she gets it right. Every time.
—Veneta Masson, RN, MA is a family nurse practitioner (*Ninth Street Notebook— Voice of a Nurse in the City*) and poet (*Rehab at the Florida Avenue Grill*).

SPEAKING OF NURSING...

NARRATIVES OF PRACTICE, RESEARCH, POLICY AND THE PROFESSION

Donna Diers, RN, PhD, FAAN

Annie W. Goodrich Professor Emerita
Yale University School of Nursing
New Haven, Connecticut USA

Adjunct Professor
Faculty of Nursing, Midwifery and Health
University of Technology—Sydney
Sydney, Australia

JONES AND BARTLETT PUBLISHERS

Sudbury, Massachusetts

BOSTON   TORONTO   LONDON   SINGAPORE

World Headquarters
Jones and Bartlett Publishers
40 Tall Pine Drive
Sudbury, MA 01776
978-443-5000
info@jbpub.com
www.jbpub.com

Jones and Bartlett Publishers Canada
2406 Nikanna Road
Mississauga, ON L5C 2W6
CANADA

Jones and Bartlett Publishers International
Barb House, Barb Mews
London W6 7PA
UK

Library of Congress Cataloging-in-Publication Data

Diers, Donna.
   Speaking of nursing : narratives of practice, research, policy, and
the profession / Donna Diers.
      p. ; cm.
   ISBN 0-7637-4854-4 (pbk.)
   Includes index.
1. Nursing—Research. 2. Nursing—Miscellanea.
   [DNLM: 1. Nursing—Collected Works. 2. Nursing Research—Collected
Works. WY 9 D563s 2004] I. Title.
   RT81.5.D533 2004
   610.73'072—dc22   2003025939

Production Credits
Sponsoring Editor: Penny M. Glynn
Production Manager: Amy Rose
Associate Production Editor: Jenny L. McIsaac
Editorial Assistant: Amy Sibley
Marketing Manager: Joy Stark-Vancs
Marketing Associate: Elizabeth Waterfall
Manufacturing Buyer: Amy Bacus
Cover Design: Anda Aquino
Composition: Interactive Composition Corporation
Printing and Binding: Malloy, Inc.
Cover Printing: Malloy, Inc.

Printed in the United States of America
08 07 06 05 04   10 9 8 7 6 5 4 3 2 1

For Jim and Jan
and
Ted and Kerrie
and
Nate and Ella

my dears

TABLE OF CONTENTS

Acknowledgements   ix

Forewords
   American Foreword   x
   Australian Foreword   xiv

Introduction   1

Clinical Nursing Research
   Clinical Nursing Research   7
   Patient-Centered Mental Health Nursing Research   13
   Application of Research to Nursing Practice   23
   The Role of Continuing Education in Promoting
      Research in Practice   29
   Generations in Nursing Research   40
   Practicing Research—Researching Practice   51
   Richness in Practice, Diversity in Research   65
   Clinical Scholarship   79
   Editorials   90
   Second Thoughts   94

Advanced Practice Nursing
   Advanced Practice Nursing   99
   Research and Nurse Practitioners:
      Lessons from Nursing's Past   101
   Nurses in Primary Care: The New Gatekeepers   113
   Nurse Practitioners: Skirmishes, Strategies, Successes 120
   Nurse Practitioners: Letter to the Editor   139
   Between Science and Humanity: Nursing Reclaims Its Role 141
   Second Thoughts   149

Nursing, Policy, and Leadership
   Nursing, Policy, and Leadership   153
   To Profess—To Be a Professional   155
   Lessons on Leadership   165
   The Emperor Has No Clothes   175

Beyond Chicken Little   193
Nursing and Shortages   214
Whoa!   243
Between Practice and Policy   247
Second Thoughts   262

Writing Nursing

Writing Nursing   267
Why Write, Why Publish?   269
The Role of the Editor   279
Colonizing: A Measurement of the Development
    of a Profession   286
Congratulations! You're the Worst!   293
Editorials   294
The Adventure of Thought and the Adventure of Action   298
Finding Nursing   308
The Power of Narrative   323
Knowing What I Know Now, Would I Do It Again?   335
Second Thoughts   337

Index   339

ACKNOWLEDGEMENTS

A book that covers 40 years or so has had a lot of influences.

Annie Warburton Goodrich's collection of speeches, *The Social and Ethical Significance of Nursing,* was the inspiration. Miss Goodrich was the first Dean of the Yale University School of Nursing (from 1923) and when, many years later, I succeeded her in that position, I came to understand through her words something about speaking about nursing.

Helen Varney Burst, great friend and colleague, took on the task, twice, of summarizing my professional life as I retired from the deanery and then from the faculty of the Yale School of Nursing. She saw most of my speaking oeuvre and thought there was something in my unpublished writing that might say things I hadn't already said in print. She connected me with Jones and Bartlett Publishers and Penny Glynn, Sponsoring Editor, a nurse who knows advanced practice and policy.

The special experience of completing a PhD by Publication at the University of Technology, Sydney, Australia in 2002 made me take my published work and professional life and make sense of it. Dean Jill White of the Faculty of Nursing, Midwifery and Health (and isn't that just the best, most encompassing label?) opened that opportunity and then she pushed me to make the contexts and themes more public. Since the work that went into the dissertation was already published, I couldn't see the point until I began to think about unpublished speeches I had given, and why and how.

When it came time to put the thing together, Donna Epps at the Yale School of Nursing and Jeffrey Campbell at Yale's Reprographics and Imaging Service leapt in to make scanning technology work, to my vast relief. Katie Bauer found my archived speeches. At Jones and Bartlett, Jenny McIsaac turned into a special support.

I learned fairly early on that I am a much better advocate for and speaker about nursing than I am a clinical nurse. To do the work of speaking of and for nursing has meant always seeking and keeping conversations flowing with those who do the work, so that I know what nursing is at "the coal face," as the Australians say.

Thank you all, my unnamed army.

AMERICAN FOREWORD

I cannot recall when and how Donna Diers first came to my attention. Perhaps that's because she's always been part of my professional life. Her first publication was in 1963, three years before I began my undergraduate studies in nursing at West Virginia University. The *American Journal of Nursing (AJN)*, *Nursing Outlook*, and *Nursing Research* were required reading and continue to be part of my regular professional reading—and all three include her writing. Over the years I came to look forward to reading what she published in these and other journals, marveled over her brilliant and witty editorials in *Image— Journal of Nursing Scholarship*, and seized every opportunity to hear her speak, knowing that my thinking would be jarred in curious but affirming ways.

There are three encounters with Donna that remain fixed in my memory and that illustrate some points that are evident in this wonderful collection of her writing and speeches. In 1983, Susan Talbott and I were convinced that nurses needed to be more involved in shaping health policy and politics. We set out to edit what became the *Political Action Handbook for Nurses,* published in 1985. As we identified topics and potential authors, we were certain that we wanted to invite Donna to contribute a chapter that would define and describe policy and politics. I was to contact Donna. We had never met, but I knew of her work and held her in high esteem. I was a lowly instructor of nursing in New York City, though I had been active in nursing organizations and nursing politics in the city and state. I was thoroughly intimidated by this assignment.

I made the call sitting in my apartment kitchen, where I could have privacy to mourn what I was sure would be a rejection of my presumptuous invitation. I described the vision for the book, its framework, and what we wanted her to write. She hesitated briefly, and then said, "I'll tell you what—I'll write the chapter if you'll tell me about what's going on in nursing in New York. I'm to give a speech there soon and would be grateful for any inside perspectives you can provide."

I'm not sure that I helped Donna whatsoever to think about what she would say, but I was grateful for the trade-off. She wrote an excellent chapter that required little editing. I don't recall how we lost her participation in the second edition of the book (eventually renamed *Policy and Politics in Nursing and Health Care*), but we had the foresight to invite her to write what turned out to be a clear and clever discussion of research as a policy and political tool for the third and fourth editions. In all cases, my colleague editors and I just smiled after we read her submissions. Not only were they on point and thought-provoking, they were absolutely entertaining to read—which is characteristic of what you will read here. She has a way with words that leaves me in awe and unnerved at the task of writing this foreword.

Donna has a self-described passion for nursing that is evident in what she writes and says. She loves being a nurse, recognizes the fullness of the profession and its opportunities, and enjoys the work and company of other nurses. I was a bit of an upstart, but she must have seen a nurse who shared her passion for nursing and wanted to make a contribution to its development. Seeing and supporting the potential—whether in the person or the profession—that is what she does.

My second story about Donna occurred when she was editor of *Image*. I submitted a manuscript on grassroots organizing for political action in nursing. She sent me the reviews with an encouraging letter requesting I revise the manuscript. I did so and resubmitted it. Again, I received a letter from Donna telling me that the manuscript was still not quite right, and encouraging me to continue to develop it. By this time, I was sick of the manuscript and had the smarts to invite two other nurse colleagues (Barbara Backer and C. Alicia Georges) to join me in revising it. My colleagues brought fresh perspectives to the paper and we even retitled it: "Towards a Feminist Model for the Political Empowerment of Nurses." We submitted the re-revision. I cheered when I received the next letter from Donna that told me that she was accepting this version. (I have saved that letter). The article was a hit, reprinted in three other journals and cited in numerous other publications.

Donna's skill as an editor and analytic thinker enabled her to see the potential in what I was writing and to encourage me to keep developing the ideas in the paper. I have taken this lesson with me to *AJN,* sometimes encouraging authors when I probably should not, but always looking for the potential in the authors and the manuscripts they submit. Although we have not discussed this, I think Donna wanted to encourage my feminist analysis of nursing's political work. As is evident in this book, she has a feminist frame for nursing and health care that challenges our assumptions about who we are as nurses and how the world sees us. Her frame also challenges feminists to examine why they have not paid attention to nursing's struggles and successes.

My final "Donna story" happened in 1999 shortly after I assumed the position of Editor-in-Chief of *AJN*. I had never been an editor of a journal before and knew that I needed some wise counsel. I considered Donna to have been one of the best editors in nursing, although she was no longer editor of *Image*. I called her and asked if I could meet with her to talk about the journal and being an editor. "Of course," she said. I spent the better part of a day at the Yale School of Nursing asking her a laundry list of questions about my new job. She generously shared her publishing and editing insights. At the end of the day, I made my second audacious invitation: would she support my vision for the journal by joining the editorial board? "Of course," she said once again.

I returned home convinced that I would be able to transform *AJN* into a highly regarded, lively, sophisticated, relevant journal that could lead the profession and provide nursing perspectives to the broader health care and public communities. I now realize that my confidence in being able to transform *AJN* arose largely from the influence of Donna Diers—both through the encouragement and support I received at that meeting, and through her words of wisdom, wit, and clarity about nursing practice, research, leadership, policy, and writing that I had heard and read over almost 40 years. Although I was never a student at Yale, she taught me how to think about nursing.

For nurses and others who have not had the pleasure of reading and hearing her words, *Speaking of Nursing ...* will be a treat. For people like me who have read many of her works, here are more, including speeches and writings for Australian nurses with whom she has been associated for over 20 years. And her commentaries about these speeches and writings provide context that is both informing and amusing, making the works even more insightful and entertaining than they were the first time around. One speech I remembered from being present when she first delivered it was the Jessie M. Scott Lecture at the 1986 convention of the American Nurses Association. In reading that speech here, I was enthralled with the story Donna tells about Jessie Scott to set up the piece. It's one of those inside stories that puts a new twist on the lecture. And what a delight to read the speech that made a major foundation's staff uncomfortable, as Donna said "out loud what many of us where thinking behind the scenes—that primary care is and always has been nursing."

For Donna Diers, practice is the profession's *raison d'etre*. Research is for practice. Leadership is for practice. Policy needs to be support practice. Education ought to connect better with practice. So, early on she challenged the profession's predominance of research that was irrelevant to practice noting "the biggest and best source [of research problems] is *nursing practice itself*." Her words are instructive today, as some schools of nursing are promoting the direct BSN-to-PhD as a means for increasing the supply of faculty without regard to the need for the next generation of nurses to be taught by expert clinicians or for developing research that is informed by practice.

Who but Donna Diers could have pulled off being a spokesperson for nursing research without having a doctorate (her PhD is a recent accomplishment)? She was an early proponent of "research that matters," research conducted by clinicians as well as trained researchers, continuing education credits for conducting research, and teaching research early in the undergraduate curriculum, rather than as an afterthought in the senior year. She repeatedly challenged researchers to study nursing practice and nursing's contribution to health care delivery. Her writing published here provides readers with a history of nursing research and exquisite examples of how clinical research could and does make a difference in nursing care delivery and patients' lives. I'm convinced that Donna Diers was a leading force in prodding the profession to its current position of producing important clinical and health services research that is being published in the best nursing, medical, and health care journals. She knew the profession was capable of generating serious, relevant science and so she provoked and cajoled until we got the message.

Most importantly, Donna speaks with clarity and passion about nursing and its place as the core of health care. She is a visionary and provocateur of the first order. When I laid down this book, I felt wiser and emboldened by Donna's courage to speak the truth—whether denouncing the imprecision of the language of nursing diagnoses, or encouraging nurses to refuse to accept unsafe working conditions, or reminding us what leadership is really about, or challenging advanced practice nurses to recognize that their battles with medicine and the health care system were political and arose from the success and primacy of their work. She admonishes us to resist the shroud of an oppressed group: "the problems with nursing ... are *not nursing's problems* ... What is seriously wrong is that we—nurses and nursing—have changed a lot over the years and the world has yet to catch up with us." She even challenges the notion that the profession is too divided to move forward on the important issues of our times, noting that we are all bound together in our commitment to excellence in nursing practice. Her descriptions of what this work is about are awesome—but she would argue that it's the work that's awesome, not her telling of it. Her words give us a renewed appreciation for the work nurses do and restores our hope for nursing's future.

This collection of writing and speeches will be considered an important record of nursing's development, particularly over the last 40 years. It chronicles many of the profession's challenges and celebrates its progress. Her writing and speeches are grounded in historic context, as she reflects on the works of notables such as Florence Nightingale, Annie Goodrich, and Virginia Henderson, and shows their relevance for today's nurses. It is 'must' reading for all nurses and those who want or ought to understand better what nursing is about.

Donna Diers has thrown the mantle of leadership out to all nurses that we may follow her lead in thinking about, advocating for, and speaking of nursing in all its glorious complexity. At the end of the book, she notes in a funny, self-deprecating way that public speaking as a leader is not always easy and certainly has not been for her. "I think of myself as actually quite quiet, timid and chicken. But with the responsibility to use a leadership position or role in the service of advancing nursing, I morph into *Tyrannosaurus Rex.*"

And so she roared and I hope will roar for many a day.

Diana J. Mason, RN, PhD, FAAN
Editor-in-Chief
American Journal of Nursing
New York, NY

AUSTRALIAN FOREWORD

Early in my nursing academic career in Australia I came across the words of Donna Diers. Donna managed to say elegantly the things that I struggled to articulate about nursing. She became a literary heroine of mine and over the years the most oft-quoted of all nurse writers in my papers, speeches and teaching.

This literary association began with "Nursing as Metaphor"* as I struggled to find words to explain nursing to non-nurses in the new University environment for nursing in Australia. Quickly the association moved to clinical scholarship, as I wrestled with the lack of relevance to practice of so much of the early Australian nursing research. Donna's constant emphasis on the need to move the focus of research from the worker to the work struck a strong chord. When policy became my passion it should have come as no surprise that Donna's words were there, accessible, pithy, intelligent and interestingly at a tangent to the contemporary nursing discourse. I loved it, but have been challenged to imagine an area of nursing one could traverse that Donna had not already thought about, talked about, and written about.

This book is a wonderful addition to the library of anyone interested in health care. It is at the same time both a fascinating read and a wonderful scholarly publication, aching to be a postgraduate text.

It is rare for such access to be granted to the thinking behind the published works of great authors. This volume captures many of the unpublished speeches given by Professor Diers and thus enables us to track several decades of thought development in our profession. We see the development of the ideas that were transformed into germinal works. We see also Donna's joy in words and wordsmithing evident throughout the speeches and the commentaries.

There is a privilege in the intimacy granted to the reader here. This is twofold. Firstly, Donna locates the work historically, giving us a glimpse of where and when the speech was given and who the major players were, who were part of the intellectual conversation at the time. This is a gift but for me the greater gift is the manner in which this is done. Donna speaks in the introduction of her family tradition of reading out loud together on Christmas Eve. The tone Donna achieves in the introductions to her speeches feels just like

*Fagin, C.M. & Diers, D. (1983). Nursing as metaphor. *New England Journal of Medicine, 309*(2), 191–192.

that, like a fireside chat among friends, the inside story told lyrically and with good humour.

I am eternally grateful to the people and circumstances that brought Donna to Australia. It occasioned the beginning of her love affair with our country and for me enabled the development of a treasured friendship and episodes of the most splendid intellectual tussling about nursing and nursing practice, which have been among my greatest privileges and pleasures.

In her October 2003 speech at the *Health Affairs* narrative writing conference Donna opens by saying:

> This has got to be the scariest speaking engagement I have ever accepted. You've got my writing idols here and you want me to speak to *them*?

Well "ditto", Donna—writing idol.

This book is a collection of extraordinary speaking/writing. It is a significant contribution to nursing scholarship and a brilliant companion to the digest of Professor Donna Diers' published works. Throughout the book Donna makes visible the processes of finding clinical scholarship, of doing relevant practice focused research and of the politics of policy influence. It provides a fine example of the way in which "issues occasion research and fuel leadership, informing and confronting policy"(from the Introduction).

Put succinctly, it is *"Speaking of nursing ..."*

Professor Jill White, RN, RM, MEd
Dean
Faculty of Nursing, Midwifery and Health
University of Technology—Sydney
Sydney, Australia

INTRODUCTION

Nursing is two things: the care of the sick (or the potentially sick) and the tending of the entire environment within which care happens.

That nursing's first charge is the care of the sick is unremarkable. Calling attention to the second of nursing's charges—tending the care environment—positions nursing at the center of the health care delivery system. "Environment" is a metaphor. The health service delivery system does not exist in a vacuum. Health policy and politics shape the quality and quantity of nursing's service.

While others have toiled to define the parameters of the discipline or solidified professional, organizational, educational and political strategies, my target has been the practice of the profession—unlocking knowledge about nursing practice. That knowledge *values* nursing. Nursing comes to *own* the work, and to *claim* deserved and public *credit*. Nursing becomes visible—a player on clinical, operational, and policy stages.

The theatre metaphor is deliberate. Nursing is a secret world, hidden behind the more publicly accessible performances of physicians and administrators. Behind the proscenium, nursing is stage management, even choreography. In this secret world is a rich language and understanding of human experience, not only of the patients we are mandated to serve, but of the range of human contacts with colleagues in all disciplines. Nurses know how the world of health service delivery works.

For 40 years or so I have been speaking of nursing, out loud and in print.

I didn't intend to become a public speaker and in the first years, standing before an audience scared me witless. That never goes away, though it becomes manageable either through the wonders of modern chemistry or the confidence born of experience.

I did intend to use writing, if not actually to become a Writer, from the time I first knew in junior high school I could get good at this. I was one of those unpopular students chosen by spinster English teachers whose names I can still remember, to read my compositions to the class. I learned how to write for speaking and to be funny.

By the time I finished high school in Sheridan, Wyoming, I had been Editor of the newspaper, a columnist ("Cactus Donna," don't ask) and I had won several local and state writing prizes.

My parents were both readers. Dad tilted more to non-fiction, especially history, and Mother to practically anything. A Christmas present for my father was books. Dad was a great public speaker, funny, erudite, engaging, and generous, with a big bass voice. He was bit of an actor as well, in local plays and musicals. Mother was also a ham and a World Class Organizer. She told my father and me we should take typing lessons if we wanted to write, which we did at the local community college, best advice I've ever had. She got me a typewriter—old Royal—oh, how I loved the sound of the striking keys! I dropped out of the typing course before I learned the number line on the keyboard so I still have to look to find the % or $ or @. My dentist subscribed to *The New Yorker* and I devoured the magazine in his waiting room and his living room, as I babysat his terrible daughters.

I was always a reader. In summer, my brother Jim (4 years younger) and I, along with our friends would ride our bicycles down the hill where we lived into the valley where the public library was. The maximum number to check out was seven, and I did it every week—the Oz books (I think there are 27 of them) was one series. I would sometimes read to my brother and his friends in our backyard. I even made up stories and I saw them as reading what was written in my head, though I never wrote them down.

Jim turned into an English teacher and an expert on southwest USA writing, including detective fiction. We talk a lot about writing and reading. Our Christmas ritual—Jim, my more-than-sister-in-law Jan, and I—is to read some selection of seasonal writing to each other after our Christmas Eve dinner. Sometimes it's children's books, sometimes classics, and we search for the right ones all year long. Once we read all of Dickens' *Christmas Carol* after dinner and were astonished at how short it is, and how powerful the writing.

The majority of this book comes from previously unpublished work. Converting the spoken to the written publishable word drains the original of some of its passion and humor. I have tried to preserve the sense of the spoken word here. I have also included in whole or in part some essays that began life as speeches and were published later. Some of my favorite written pieces published in obscure or forgotten places are included. They were the speeches nobody asked me to give.

The process of cutting hour-long speeches to fit produces text that is more crisp than the spoken version was. Examples are particularly sacrificed. I have used ellipses (...) to indicate where major chunks have been cut but I have not identified small editorial cuts. Anachronisms and contemporary non-PC turns of phrase have been preserved, the nurse as "she," the patient as "he" among them. I've corrected the more egregious abuses of the language, blushing at every one.

Where speeches were never intended to be published, I did not capture references in the detail one should do. The rule I adopted here was that if a citation referred to data-based material, then I have supplied it. Where I have cited my own discursive writing, I have let the words stand (sometimes redundantly, though I've tried to cut repetition to the bone) on their own.

I personally converted longer pieces to shorter, no editor did it.

The work covers the period from the late 1960s to the present. I was lucky enough to have been present at the creation of clinical nursing research, of the nurse practitioner movement, of nursing's growing sense of its place in policy, and the contemporary search for ways of valuing our work as narrative. To say nothing of having lived and loved and participated in the awakening of our consciousness to civil rights, and the issues of women in society and the move of nursing into the University.

The contexts of the speaking occasions explain a lot of why the words come out the way they do. The contexts had to include where I was in my professional life at the time and where nursing was, so this has turned out to be more autobiographical than I originally intended.

I have actually written a small bio that began:

> Once upon a time, I got into an elevator in Texas to get to an amphitheatre where I was going to give a speech. There was a poster on the back wall of the elevator advertising my appearance. Someone had written next to my name, "Who she?" And somebody else had written, "Flamboyant! Controversial!"
>
> Who me?
>
> This shy person from Wyoming?[1]

The themes from that paragraph sound throughout this book.

The form for putting this material together as a book came from my very special experience in completing a PhD by Publication in 2002 at the University of Technology, Sydney, Australia. Some of the text that weaves the sections here together comes from my dissertation. In supplying the contexts I have told stories I've never told elsewhere.

Four themes organize the work: (1) clinical nursing research, (2) advanced practice nursing (nurse practitioners in the main), (3) policy and leadership, and (4) writing nursing.

The themes overlap in time and content. Nursing research provides a foundation for nursing's intellectual and policy strivings, advanced practice nursing being an example. Nurse practitioner issues occasion research and fuel leadership, informing and confronting policy. Writing nursing, well, that's what this book is about.

The title is a deliberate double entendre.

"Speaking of nursing..." Say it off-handedly, by-the-way, about-to-tell-a-story.

"Speaking of nursing..." Speak of issues and triumphs and failures made visible, brought to consciousness, made visible by speaking and writing.

ENDNOTE

1. In Schorr, T.M., & Zimmerman, A. (1988). *Making Choices, Taking Chances—Nurse Leaders Tell Their Stories* (pp. 78–84). St. Louis: C.V. Mosby.

CLINICAL NURSING RESEARCH

CLINICAL NURSING RESEARCH

This work began in the late 1960s at Yale University School of Nursing. That was a time when nursing in the USA was moving rapidly into universities with the requirement to ground the discipline in research and to develop a recognizable nursing science. The oldest nursing research journal in the world, *Nursing Research*, began publication only in 1952.

I came to Yale first to work in its Psychiatric Institute in 1960, 6 weeks or so after I finished my BSN. In 1962, I became a graduate student, in 1964, a faculty member. I knew the actors here.

In a monumental exercise of scholarship, Virginia Henderson and her research team at Yale University had catalogued **all** of the studies in nursing from 1900 to 1960 in a four-volume series, the *Nursing Studies Index.*[1] Henderson[2] and Simmons and Henderson[3] summarized their review, concluding forcefully that the bulk of research in the field to that date had been about "the workers rather than the work." Miss Henderson's editorial plea, "Research in nursing practice—when?"[4] became the anchor for developing clinical nursing research—studies of nursing practice—especially at Yale but also elsewhere. Dumas and Leonard[5] at Yale reported what is generally recognized as the first randomized controlled clinical trial (RCCT) in the discipline, testing the effects of nursing preoperative preparation on stress expressed as post-operative vomiting in the recovery room. This study was tiny by contemporary standards—51 patients in all, in three replications. But it set the methodologic standard and broke through conventional wisdom that had said nursing was too complicated (or too "soft") to be subject to the standard scientific test.

Because there were few nurses with doctoral preparation, schools of nursing sought social scientists, some funded under government programs to help develop research capacity. In most schools of nursing, this tended to produce a version of nursing science that was "applied sociology" or "applied psychology" or "applied anthropology," using the clinical setting as the laboratory for whatever the science was. Some social scientists found this an exciting collaboration and they developed programs of research with budding nurse scientists.[6]

At Yale, Professor Robert Leonard did not take the route social scientists at other universities did and impose his sociological theories on nursing. He believed that the proper role of the social scientist in nursing was to provide methodological options that could be selected, as appropriate, for the study of patient care problems.[7] That meant nursing faculty were free to examine nursing practice in as much detail as could be mustered without being tied to conceptual lenses from other disciplines.

To examine the question of what the best kind of evidence is to support nursing practice, it is necessary to stipulate what nursing *is.*

"If we do not know what nursing is, how can we teach it, or practice it, or train researchers to study it? Obviously we do the first two, and we even license people as 'nurses', with some kind of standard to differentiate us from 'un-nurses'[8] ...Before one does any research in nursing practice, he [sic] must believe that nursing is important. Otherwise it makes no sense to study it. If nursing has nothing to offer patients, why bother to test different nursing approaches for their effects on patients? And there does seem to be more than a little doubt both in and outside the nursing profession that nursing has anything significant to contribute."[9]

The underlying question—to what purpose is definition needed—is rarely asked. "A definition of nursing might be, and as a matter of fact is, very different depending on whether the definitional requirement is in the law, in professional organizations' political turf statements, in nursing theory, in the public media, in job descriptions, or in conversations over dinner with one's family."[10]

The move of nursing in the USA into universities, and the nearly simultaneous creation of master's level specialty curricula, seemed to make the discipline lose its definitional compass. If nurses were no longer to be "handmaidens to the physician" in the hospital school tradition, what were we? In the 1960s, nursing turned to science, especially social science, to save us, to provide new definitional space.

The young journal, *Nursing Research*, published a series of articles about the relationship of social science to nursing in 1963. One of the articles, by a social scientist, whinged:[11] "Nursing...is a highly diversified field and...these diversities in nursing are in the constant throes of change and redefinition—often resulting in uncertainty and confusion, disagreements and tensions about the field of nursing, its content, and the role of those practicing it."[12]

This social scientist felt as if she and her science were being called upon to fix nursing's definitional problem. The first publication I ever wrote (with others) was a response to this comment as a letter to the Editor arguing that this was neither the proper construction of the problem nor the proper role for social science.[13] Instead, we proposed that the matter of discipline definition be left to the discipline to work out. The role of social science should be to inform *particular* research problems, when the problem lies within the social science domain. If the problem is not a "social science" problem, then the theories and methods of social science have nothing to offer. We suggested that theories and methods were to be found or selected among; they did not come embossed with a disciplinary paradigm.

Focusing on the relationship of social science to research, rather than on interpreting discipline discourse made clear the role of the social scientist in nursing research. We tilted the balance from the nurse being the "helper" in social science research to nurses being able to direct research and collaborate with others who might bring their theories and methods to the project. "Once the nurse has decided what effects she wants to obtain or thinks she does obtain by her practice, the behavioral scientist can help as a consultant on methodology and in the measurement of the effects of practice."[14]

This was a departure from the way in which nursing practice and the sciences or social sciences had been viewed. In this view, nursing was no longer simply "applied science," "borrowing" theory from other disciplines, although there were heated arguments about whether nursing could ever be a "real" science, especially if the focus was practice. As the notions of "nursing theory" and "nursing science" began to evolve the applied/basic argument faded away.

If nursing was not to be saved by borrowing social science then it was going to have to develop its own science.

Apart from hortatory intended to convince the discipline to think differently about nursing research and infrastructure development, it was going to be necessary to create new ways of thinking about the association of research to practice. If we could not depend on social science for problem definition (although we might well count on social science for methods and procedures), we were going to have to invent our own ways to translate clinical nursing practice problems into research problems.

My effort was to equip nurses to see their practice issues as potentially solvable through research. That has to begin where nurses begin: the gripes, complaints, observations, curiosities of expert practice.

> A "problem" is something that seems wrong. It is a difference between two states of affairs, a discrepancy between the way things are and the way they ought to be, or between two sets of facts, or [between] what one knows and what one needs to know to eliminate the problem. A problem makes itself known as a feeling of discomfort...a gripe...[N]ot all problems are going to be researchable (and some will not even need research). The quality that makes a discrepancy a potential research problem is that it is a *difference that matters*. ... What makes a difference matter is its consequence in patient care. The appropriate focus for clinical research is the systematic study of problems in patient care.[15]

If the source for nursing research wisdom was going to be nursing practice, then nurse researchers were going to have to pay attention to their colleagues in practice (if practicing nurses themselves weren't doing the research). The notion that all practicing nurses could also do research was attractive, but ultimately naïve.

Research requires emotional space for contemplation. The researcher must have the patience to plod through the detail of research design and analysis. Practice requires acute observation and swift action. Expert practitioners make the muscular leaps of insight that characterize expertise. That capacity can identify the truly important research problems. The habits of mind of the researcher and the expert practitioner are not necessarily the same, which is why respectful collaboration is a more desired strategy to bring practice and research together.

In addition, the infra- and superstructures of nursing education, practice and research would need to devise mechanisms to support practice-based knowledge development. I suggested three initiatives: (1) that nursing masters and doctoral programs turn to develop their science out of practice, out of *nursing,* rather than social science, (2) that clinical institutions create positions for researchers in practice,[16] and (3) that the criteria for funding research projects used by the federal government and other funding sources "raise the standards for relevance [to practice], not relax the requirements for scientific rigor."[17] Incentives in service settings for research and in academe for practice in the form of promotion, salary increases and publicity were proposed.

These were radical proposals to a discipline striving for upward mobility by leaving the practice environment. The effect of concentrating nursing's research in practice at Yale during this period—to begin the development of a science of practice that made sense to practitioners—has been acknowledged by others who have reviewed the history of nursing research.[18] These ideas now seem prescient for there is still work to be done on all of these initiatives.

ENDNOTES

1. Henderson, V. (1964–1969). *Nursing Studies Index.* Philadelphia: Lippincott.

2. Henderson, V. (1956). An overview of nursing research. *Nursing Research, 6*(2), 61–71.

3. Simmons, L., & Henderson, V. (1964). *Nursing Research.* New York: Appleton-Century-Crofts.

4. Henderson, V. (1956). Research in nursing practice: when? *Nursing Research, 4*(3), 99.

5. Dumas, R.G., & Leonard, R.C. (1963). The effect of nursing on the incidence of post-operative vomiting. *Nursing Research, 12*(1), 12–15.

6. Symposium: Research—How will nursing define it? (1967). *Nursing Research, 16*(2), 1008–129. Glaser, B.G., & Strauss, A.L. (1965). *Awareness of Dying.* Chicago: Aldine.

7. Leonard, R.C. (1957). Developing research in a practice-oriented discipline. *American Journal of Nursing, 67*(7), 1472–1475.

8. Diers, D. (1970). This I believe...about nursing research. *Nursing Outlook, 18*(11), 50–54, p. 52.

9. *Ibid.*, p. 51.

10. Diers, D. (2001). What is nursing? In J. McCloskey Dochterman & H.K. Grace (Eds.), *Current Issues in Nursing, 6th ed.,* (pp. 5–13). St Louis: Mosby, p. 51.

11. "Whinge" is a particularly expressive verb, used in the UK, Australia, and New Zealand especially for political commentary. It means "complain", but with a needy edge, somewhere short of "snivel". It is not in USA dictionaries, more is the pity.

12. Sheldon, E.B. (1963). The use of behavioral sciences in nursing: An opinion. *Nursing Research, 12*(3), 150–152, p. 150.

13. Ellison, M., Diers, D., & Leonard, R.C. (1965). The use of behavioral science in nursing: Further comment. *Nursing Research, 14*(1), 71–72.

14. *Ibid.*, p. 71.

15. Diers, D. (1971). Finding clinical problems for study. *Journal of Nursing Administration, 1*(6), 15–18, p. 15.

16. Several such positions were eventually created in the USA but the model was independently developed more fully in Australia in "Clinical Chair" positions which place Professors actually *in* the clinical settings.

17. Diers, 1970, *ibid.*, p. 54.

18. Gortner, S.R., & Nahm, H. (1977). Overview of Nursing Research in the United States. *Nursing Research, 26*(1), 10–33.

Patient-Centered Mental Health Nursing Research

This paper was the first really big speech I ever gave. It was delivered at the Walter Reed Army Institute of Research in a short course on Mental Health Concepts in Nursing, April 25, 1969 in Bethesda, MD. This was a time when psychiatric nursing was much more generic than it is now, and when the intellectual work centered on understanding the nurse-patient relationship. The invitation to give this speech came from the late Harriet Werley, RN, PhD, the first Director of the Nursing Research branch of WRAIR—WRAIN. (Pronounce the acronyms to get the point). Col. Werley was one of the early nurses in the military with doctoral preparation. She later went on to found the journal Research in Nursing and Health *and the* Annual Review of Nursing Research *and she was a pioneer in nursing informatics, honored especially for her work in creating the Nursing Minimum Data Set. She was a visible presence, always pushing nursing forward, until her death on October 14, 2002. And she was a generous colleague, particularly interested in making opportunities for the young ones coming up. Many of us benefited from her attention. She played that role for me on more than one occasion, but this was the first.*

Clinical nursing research was just beginning to gain some credibility and she wanted the Army to notice. At that time, there was so little published clinical nursing research that I relied upon unpublished Master's Theses at Yale. I was five years out of my own master's study, an Assistant Professor, 29 years old, and terrified by this occasion.

Patient-centered research in nursing is relatively new and regrettably relatively infrequent even today. Investigators still elect to study the *workers,* that is, nurses, rather than the *work* of nursing.[1] While it may be fascinating to discover that psychiatric nurses are intelligent, creative, and cynical, while maternity nurses are warm, religious, and idealistic, it escapes me how such information is related to the care of patients. And the improvement of patient care is the goal for nursing research. Research which is unrelated to that end simply siphons off energy from nursing, and nurses have plenty to do already. ...

The issue of whether nurses should do research, and if so what kind, occupies a lot of time for us academic types. I would rather not use up the time arguing the relative merits of clinical versus non-clinical research. Rather, I'd like to talk about some patient-centered research in nursing, describe how it has been done and what it means, and let you decide for yourselves whether this kind of research makes sense.

Since we have to begin somewhere, I thought it might be useful if we start with some real data. Then we'll all have the same frame of reference at least, and we can begin to look at how one builds up to a clinical nursing study.

> [Here, I asked a member of the audience (set up in advance) to participate in two brief role-plays, in both of which the audience member as patient had asked for something for pain. I played the nurse. In one role-play, the nurse was focused entirely on the task of giving the medication. In the other, the nurse explored the patient's complaint of pain and the circumstances surrounding the pain.]

What were we trying to show here?

First, to call attention to the fact that interaction in itself is a treatment.[2]

We can't disregard the effect of even the most casual conversation (as the first situation was) but we can maximize the effect of a deliberative kind of interaction, as the second situation showed. But if interaction is considered a treatment, then it has to meet the criteria any other treatment does: it must be specific to the patient's condition, its effects must be measurable, and it must be teachable.

We tried to present these two situations so that they were as different from each other as possible—so that we would have a natural comparison. If you're trying to isolate the characteristics of some data, it's always easier if you can have two chunks of data that differ along the dimension you're interested in.

So how did the two situations differ? I'll tell you how we wanted them to, and you can check that out with your own perceptions.

The interactions differed in their patient-centeredness. In the first, the nurse had a task to get done—give the patient what he had asked for, fulfill that "need." Yet the task can never really be separated from the patient. In the first situation, the nurse was being "patient centered" in that she was focused on the patient, even if it was on a superficial level. She recognized his humanity even by so trivial a means as asking about his pain. She accorded him the dignity of human being status at a very basic level. Yet it should have been obvious that there was something wrong with that situation, something incomplete. While the nurse was at least treating the patient as human, she was not attending to his "real" situation. He tried to tell her; she didn't listen.

Now what happened in the second interaction that makes it different from the first? The nurse tried to be more in tune with the patient, and allow his behavior to guide her actions. As a result, both the patient and the nurse revealed more of themselves.

No doubt you all have your own ways of defining what you saw. Your descriptions might be similar or very different both from mine and from each other's—and that's exactly the point. If you're trying to define something as elusive as patient-centered nursing, you need to first start with some data, as we did, then think about what you've seen and heard, maybe refer to the literature and eventually come up with a stance, a point of view, or hopefully, a definition of the phenomenon. Right now all we have are our many different perceptions.

This is the area in which my research has been concentrated. The research began with something very much like the role-playing experience you just saw. I had the hunch that there were certain ways of interacting with patients that were more patient-centered than other ways, that helped the patient more or were more effective. The problem was to figure out a way to find out what those were.

I needed some real data, some verbatim recordings of what nurses and patients normally say to one another. ... Arrangements were made with a large VA hospital for me to follow the nurses on one ward around with a small tape recorder and record everything they said to patients. The staff were told that I was just interested in what does go on between nurse and patient, because we had very little of this "real" data. Patients gave their signed permissions to be recorded, and no one was identified by name. I wore a uniform and cap and made it clear that although I was not there to give nursing care, I would pitch in when it seemed necessary.

Out of this experience I obtained some 200 tape recordings of interactions. Some were very brief, a sentence or two, some were several pages long when transcribed. ...I had the assistance of a fellow graduate student, a sociologist. We read and reread the data and talked about it at great length. As he was not a nurse, he could respond to things I missed, and I could tell him if the categories he suggested didn't make nursing sense. ...

Eventually we came up with a concept called "orientation," defined as the set or perceptual stance...one person uses to categorize another. Within orientation there are three dimensions: orientation to the person as a *feeling* person, as a *thinking* person or as a *being-doing person.* ...

Using these categories, it is possible to compare interactions. That's just what we did to see if the categories were sensitive. The technical term for this is "construct validity" and what it means is that given a supposed difference between two groups of interactions, will the categories pick it up? We took the data and divided it up in various ways—interactions with old vs. young patients, those with alcoholics, with aphasics, with mentally ill patients, and those with patients nurses liked and patients they disliked. In all cases, there were differences between the groups of interactions. Just as one example, interactions with mentally ill patients were less feeling oriented and less frequent than interactions with other patients. ...

One can now propose a definition of patient-centered nursing. *Patient centered nursing refers to nursing care in which the nurse is oriented to the patient as a physical being, a rational, knowledgeable being, and a being capable of experiencing emotion.* The patient-centered nurse relates to the patient on all three dimensions—the experiential, the cognitive, and the emotional.

This may seem like an excessive amount of work to go through to come up with something that's just common sense, but that's often the way it is in research. Common sense is all too uncommon. ...

But so what? There has been a lot written about the importance of patient-centered nursing and why nurses should try to be patient-centered, but most of what's written is administrative, or theoretical, or inspirational. So do we really know that patient-centered nursing does any good at all? If not, then there is the danger that patient-centeredness, cultivated in practice, will turn into just another ritual.

The *best* though not the *only* way to answer the question of whether patient-centeredness makes any difference is to set up an experiment and try it out. ...

At the same time I developed the Nurse Orientation System, a colleague was interested in the effect of nursing on pain. We decided to collaborate. She would use my system to define her nursing approaches, and I would use her data to test the effect of such definitions on certain patient variables.[3] We designed three approaches. The first one specified that the nurse would be oriented to the patient as a feeling, thinking, *and* doing person. The second approach specified that the nurse would treat the patient as a thinking and doing person, but would limit the feeling orientation. In the third approach, the nurse would be oriented to the patient as only a being-doing person. ...

The results came out just as predicted. Patients who were nursed with the feeling-thinking-doing approach did better than either of the other two groups. The average decline in pulse-respiration rates was greater; the average improvement in pain was higher.

The study had one great gaping hole: the length of the interactions was unequal among the groups. The study was repeated the following year. The same nurse did the nursing...but this time she standardized the length of time spent with all patients. Again the results came out the same way: patients nursed with the feeling-thinking-doing approach had greater relief from pain, and larger decreases in pulse and respiration rates. ...

But every study has its problems and the trouble with this one was, could another nurse get the same results? ...

So we designed another study only this time another nurse did the nursing. And again the results tend to support the hypothesis. This time there were some confounding factors. There was a great deal more variation in patient response to the three nursing approaches. This made us wonder if there are certain kinds of patients for whom certain approaches will work better than others. For example, some patients simply didn't want to talk about their feelings, or had no conscious feelings to be discussed. Other patients, who fell by random assignment into the doing approach, had such obvious feeling needs that the nurse was hard pressed to stick to the study design. ...

There are lots of ways to define nursing treatments. In fact, there are about as many ways as there are nurses interested in trying to define them. ...A small group of investigators at the Yale School of Nursing has tried to determine the differences between effective and ineffective interactions. Most of the studies have used data from clinical experiments so that the judgment of "effectiveness" could be made on the basis of improvement in patient welfare. ...

This series of studies can be summarized as follows: In *effective* interactions, nurses discuss or elicit feelings more; there was more attention to the patient in the immediate situation; there was less change of focus off the immediate; there was more use of perceptions, thoughts about the patient, more support and recognition of the patient and less concentration on factual information, fewer commands and more questions, and less expression of authority.[4] ...

The implication of all of this is that the more the nurse truly involves herself in what the patient experiences and the more she listens to and supports the patient, the more effective the interaction is likely to be. Or, put another way, the more patient-centered the nurse is, the better.

But patient-centered research in nursing can't be confined just to these kinds of interaction studies. In fact, to do such a study is extremely tedious for what sometimes seems like very little profitable or even new information. Similarly, nursing can't wait until all the tiny little particles of nurse-patient interaction have been defined before going on to see how patient care can be improved. ...

There have been a number of studies that have tested the effect of nursing using fairly loose definitions mostly based on Ida Orlando's work on the dynamic nurse-patient relationship.[5] Orlando suggested that there were three phases to the nurse-patient conversation: exploration, clarification, and validation. She proposed that the nurse must first find out, through exploration, what the patient's need is, then do whatever is necessary to meet that need, then validate with the patient that the need has indeed been met. Orlando suggests a process by which the nurse does this: first she observes or perceives; she gets the data. Then she shares this perception, along with whatever thoughts or feelings accompany it, with the patient, telling her, "I see (or think or feel) this, am I wrong?". The patient responds in some way, which becomes the next piece of data for the nurse. But the nurse herself enters into the interaction. She doesn't just question the patient—"Are you worried?", "Are you hot?". Instead, she may say something like, "The way you're perspiring makes me think you're hot. Am I wrong?" She always leaves it open to the patient to confirm or deny her perceptions or thoughts or feelings, but she also gives the patient some data to work on. She tries to find out how the patient is experiencing *his* situation. But at the same time she uses *her* experiencing of it to help the patient test the reality of his. ... The nurse does not take it for granted that the first thing the patient says he wants is really what he wants or needs. ... Two very interesting studies have suggested that more than half the time the patient's original presenting behavior, be it a request of the nurse personally, or a call over the intercom, bears little relationship to what the patient really has on his mind.[6] ...

If you're going to test the effect of his process on patients, you need a situation in which patients are probably having similar kinds of experiences. One of the situations where patients might need some help from the nurse is pre-operative preparation. ...

Rhetaugh Dumas was the first to recognize that this situation might be a good one to see if a nurse could reduce the patient's anxiety before surgery and help him have a better experience. She selected a group of patients having gynecological surgery. She knew from previous work that this group of patients has a relatively high rate of post-operative vomiting. Mrs. Dumas gave the nursing care the morning of surgery, beginning at least an hour before the patients were scheduled to be called to the operating room.

Mrs. Dumas used Orlando's nursing process. ... Both in a small pilot study and in the study itself, the patients who received the experimental nursing had a lower incidence of vomiting in the recovery room. In the pilot study, 50% of the control patients vomited; none of the experimental patients did. In the regular study, 60% of the control patients vomited; only 30% of the experimental cases did. ...

The study was important not only for the findings—the fact that nursing could be effective in this situation—but also because it was the first clinical experiment of this type done. It showed that it was possible to do this kind of research in nursing, that it was possible to use the real-life practice situation, where patients are experiencing real problems and where the nurse is at least physically available to help the patients with their problems.[7] ...

No matter whether patient-centered nursing is operationally defined by categories...a script or a theory, these experimental tests have demonstrated over and over that the inspirational exhortations about patient-centered nursing can be justified in fact: patient-centered nursing *does work*.

That is important in itself, but what may be equally important is that these studies show how really meaningful nursing research can be done, in the context of practice, with fairly specific implications for improving patient care. And that's what *nursing* research is all about.

Research always begins with a problem. And a problem is a feeling of discomfort with things as they are—the perception of a difference between two states of affairs. The difference may be just between what we know now and what we need to know in order to give better patient care; or it may be between two opposing sets of facts; or it may be, and most often is, between things as they are now and as they ought to be. But one other quality makes of a difference between things a "problem." The discrepancy between things as they are now and as they ought to be has to be a *difference that matters*.

So what makes of a discrepancy a difference that matters?

This has to be, in part, a matter of individual judgment, for part of what makes a problem a problem is one's own individual interest in it. That interest has to be present, because a lot of the work of research is sheer tedium and an interesting problem will help carry you through that phase. The goals and ideals of the profession can also help tell what problems are likely to be important. As nurses, we know the kinds of things that should be done for patients, and we are professionally committed to relieving suffering and helping people cope. If we find there are situations in which suffering isn't being relieved, or we're not being as helpful as we could be, that may be an indication that there is a problem that needs some work done on it. Other qualities that make a problem a problem are its size, its long-standingness, its criticalness or immediacy, and the size of the gap between what needs to be known and what is, or what is and what ought to be. ...

Given that problems prompt research, where do the problems come from?

The biggest and best source is *nursing practice* itself. The nurse in practice is in the very best position to know what needs to be done, what is not getting done, and more important, he or she knows at least intuitively some ways to approach the study of nursing practice problems.

For example, a few weeks ago I worked as a staff nurse on a medical-surgical unit. My major purpose was to refresh my skills preparatory to doing some more research. But I was assigned a few patients per day and could ask to be assigned to certain patients I became interested in. This ward was having a short run on laminectomies...and I was intrigued with this discrepancy: that these patients seemed to be having more pain, and requesting more pain medication than would be expected from the extent of their surgery. In addition, they were very compulsive about the medication, making sure to ask for it every 3 or 4 hours, however the order was written. Even the relief they obtained...seemed out of proportion to the dosage that had been given.

Being a psychiatric nurse by training and inclination, I began to wonder about all these differences. I asked to be assigned to one of these patients one morning. He was 2 days post-op, able to sit up in a chair to eat, but still having what he called "spasms," in his back. He really looked like he was in pain; he would catch his breath, splint his back, crinkle up his forehead and pant until the pain passed. I worked with him for a couple of hours one morning, helping him with his bath and breakfast, helping him shave, changing the bed and doing all the other morning care things. I tried to be sensitive to what he was presenting, the questions he had about his pain, the fear he felt of moving, which excited the spasms, the anger he felt at his doctor who would whip in, ask him how he was, and whisk out without telling him anything, the depression he felt that he'd had surgery that he thought would cure his back pain and he was still having it. At the end of the morning, he had not requested pain medication at all, and in fact he did not receive another dose until late that afternoon. This was the longest he had gone without it.

I began to wonder what it was, if anything, that nursing had done for this man. Certainly I had paid a lot of attention to him, helped him feel physically refreshed. Was it that? Was it just casual conversation? Time? Or did it have anything to do with nursing at all?

This is how clinical research begins. Because the problem is a nursing problem, the approach to it would be different from that of a physiologist, a psychologist, a medical sociologist, all of whom might have a legitimate interest in the subject of pain. The physiologist might ask, "How is the pain experienced—what nerve pathways are involved? Are there certain substances in human inflammatory processes that are in themselves irritants and cause pain?" A psychologist might ask, "What are the dynamics of pain? To what life experiences does the patient relate his pain problem? What are the secondary gains of the regression that accompanies physical illness and hospitalization?" A sociologist might ask, "Are there differences between or among ethnic groups or subcultures in the incidence of interpretation of pain?"[8] The nursing question is "What can the nurse to do relieve pain?" Of the things that are within the nurse's control or to which she has access (equipment, procedures, people, knowledge, skill, interest, and so forth), which will relieve pain most, fastest, best?

Now, how does one get from the initial observations in practice to a research study?

The first few steps have already been suggested. First, one identifies the problem, the discrepancy. You try to get a conceptual handle on the phenomenon. For example, if the problem has to do with the concept "pain," how are you going to define that? And further, if the problem has to do with nursing and pain, how are you going to define "nursing"? Often in the course of analyzing a clinical problem, it becomes clear that there is some background information that will be needed before you can launch into studies at higher levels of inquiry. For instance, in the problem here it might be important to examine the personality characteristics of patients having laminectomies, in order to design a nursing approach that would fit these kinds of patients. Or it might be necessary to do some epidemiological research first to find out the extent of the problem. ...

The decision on whether to do this kind of background research is really fairly arbitrary and depends on how much knowledge is really needed to proceed to a research study testing the effect of nursing on pain. At the current stage of nursing knowledge, it is even legitimate to go directly to an experimental test of nursing, see how it works out, then get some ideas of what other information would be required to continue to test the hypothesis.

But the important thing here isn't how rigorous a study one can do. ... Rather the question is how to do the kind of research that will contribute something to *nursing*. The most intricate measurements in the world are of no use if it is impossible to install them or use them in the natural, normal practice of nursing, or if it is impossible to correlate them with some measures nurses *can* use. ...

[Here I described a number of nursing studies of facial expression, postural attitude, kinesics, and other forms of non-verbal behavior.]

There are many other sources of data on patient behavior. Tone of voice, for example, or flushing or pallor, occurrence and amount of perspiration, eye contact, muscle tension, and so on. The problem in nursing research is lack of good measurements, not lack of good things to measure. Any nurse knows, intuitively, how to tell when a patient feels better or worse, even if such knowledge is pretty much unconscious. Research is one way to bring such intuitive insights, such "unconscious intelligence," out into the open so others can have access to it too.

In fact, I'd like to develop this idea in some detail as a grand finish to this paper.

The word "research" to many nurses conjures up a picture of the cold, inhuman, living computer of a scientist in a dirty lab coat, divorced from the world of people and feelings. Althought that picture is not so far from reality in some fields, it is in nursing. Research in nursing, to be of any real value in solving nursing problems, or contributing to the building of nursing knowledge, has to be intimately tied to practice—in its search for problems, in its design and conduct, in its measurements, and in its feedback of findings. ...

There are not many examples in the nursing literature of how research can be done in an on-going clinical situation. Most of the nursing research being done now is by graduate students. However, the study reported by Kathryn Healy in the *AJN* is a particularly provocative one.[9]

Mrs. Healy and her staff wanted to find out if preoperative instruction really makes a difference to patients—"Is it worth the time and effort?" Mrs. Healy and her staff wrote up a nursing procedure for admitting the patient and for instructing him in coughing, turning, deep breathing, exercising the legs, and so on. Then, over a 4-month period, the staff nurses and LPNs followed the procedure with 181 patients. Another group of 140 patients were given the same care, reassurance, and explanation, but without explicit detail, and without the specific instructions and follow-up practice in postoperative exercises.

They found that 75% of the patients given the special preparation were discharged 3 to 4 days prior to their expected discharge date. In contrast, only 3 of the 140 patients not given the special preparation were discharged early. The experimental patients were able to come off narcotics earlier, and there were fewer complications from surgery in that group.

The experiment stimulated auxiliary personnel to desire greater knowledge about preoperative care and specific conditions. They seemed to have found the fascination of knowing how and why something is done. ...They no longer looked on the evening shift as the "cleanup" shift.

When one sees studies like this one, one gets less depressed about the state of nursing knowledge and nursing research. Although a lot, or maybe most, of nursing practice is not based on scientific knowledge, but on folklore and tradition, nurses *do* know their own practice. Otherwise, how could we do it and teach it? What is needed is just the sort of thing Mrs. Healy and others are doing—trying to substantiate that the knowledge one has is the right, or best, knowledge. Or, put another way, that nursing really can have the desired effect on patients.

The essence of nursing practice is patient care, no matter how far away from it some nurses get into administration, education, supervision, or research. It's not very hard to develop research from practice problems if one is self-conscious about it, and if one sees that research doesn't have to be just the ivory-tower distraction it so often seems. It is possible, it's necessary, and it's essential that nurses who have the responsibility of patient care, who are in the best positions to know what needs studying and how best to study it, get busy with actually doing some research. Or at the very least, using in practice what others have found.

I'll end this by tossing the ball back to you. We began this morning with some real data. On Monday morning you will all be out there in that real world with all that knowledge and information and experience. So study it; document it; think about it; write about it; and please, come and share it with me when you're finished.

ENDNOTES

1. Henderson, V. (1956). Research in nursing practice: when? *Nursing Research, 4*(3), 99.

2. Bursten, B., & Diers, D. (1964). Pseudo-patient-centered orientation. *Nursing Forum, 3*(2), 38–50.

3. McBride, A.B. (1967). Nursing approach, pain and relief: An exploratory experiment. *Nursing Research, 16*(4), 337–341.

4. This summary refers to the following unpublished Master's Theses at the Yale School of Nursing: Joyce Cameron (1961); Sheila Taylor (1962); Ada Sue Hinshaw (1963); Julina P. Rhymes (1962); Helen Varney (1963).

5. Orlando, I.J. (1961). *The Dynamic Nurse-Patient Relationship.* New York: GP Putnam's Sons.

6. Dye, M.C. (1963). Clarifying patients' communications. *American Journal of Nursing, 63*(8), 56–59; Hogan, M. (1966). Relationships between patients' needs and requests made via the intercom system. Unpublished Master's Thesis, Yale School of Nursing.

7. Dumas, R.G., & Leonard, R.C. (1963). The effect of nursing on the incidence on postoperative vomiting: A clinical experiment. *Nursing Research, 12*(1), 12–15.

8. Discussion abstracted from Wald, F., & Leonard, R.C. (1964). Towards nursing practice theory. *Nursing Research, 13*(4), 309–313.

9. Healy, K.H. (1968). Does preoperative instruction make a difference? *American Journal of Nursing, 68*(1), 62–67.

APPLICATION OF RESEARCH
TO NURSING PRACTICE

This paper was published in Image *in 1972 (5[2], 7–11, reprinted with permission). It was originally an address to the New York University School of Nursing's chapter of Sigma Theta Tau, nursing's honor society. This was a time when Martha Rogers, Head of the Department of Nursing at NYU, was enjoying considerable high-profile attention in nursing for her notions of nursing theory and the nursing profession.*

I could not have represented ideas more different from Martha's and it was a bit of a mystery to me why I had been asked to speak. I was given the title for the speech and I seized gleefully (and stridently, as it turns out) the opportunity to try to turn the rhetoric about the place of research in nursing around. This speech is overtly political. I wasn't really trying to be contrary—or maybe I was—but I remember vividly what I wore: black pants and a black crocheted vest a friend had made for me. This was long before wearing pants in academic events was normal. NYU's campus is in Greenwich Village. The women's movement was upon us. I was also feeling my oats. The Research Program I chaired at Yale was getting some good attention, I'd been sought for a visiting professorship in Canada, I'd been funded for research of my own, and I was on a roll—without a doctorate. And I was angry at the slow progress of developing nursing clinical research.

Nell Watts, the steadfast Executive Director of Sigma Theta Tau, was in the audience and encouraged me to submit the paper for publication in the society's struggling journal, Image. *That brief meeting forged a connection that lasted many years, as I eventually became the Editor of* Image.

Think of the word "application," or even its verb, "apply." In nursing practice, you apply an ointment to a rash; you apply a dressing to a wound; you may even apply a principle or a concept as in applying the principle of asepsis to reverse isolation. All of these uses of the word "apply" seem to mean spreading something foreign or strange on. The analogies fit the way we often think about the application of research to nursing practice.

We do seem to think of research as something foreign, something to be applied. In the same way that an ointment will wear off and have to be reapplied, or a dressing will have to be changed, there seems to be a temporary connotation to the way research in nursing is often discussed.

But "apply" also means to "put to use for some practical purpose, to employ diligently and with close attention." Nursing practice can use the *discipline* of research (in both senses of the word); it can use the *process* of research and, most conventionally, it can use the *findings* or results of research. ...

Although there is a good deal of lip service given to the notion that nursing is a professional practice, not a vocation—that it is scientific, not just intuitive, that it is rational, not merely reactive—it's hard to find the evidence that any of these are true. Look at some frightening statistics:

Lucille Notter pointed out in her editorial in the May-June issue of *Nursing Research* last year that applications for project grants to both the American Nursing Foundation and the Division of Nursing of the National Institutes of Health have dwindled alarmingly.[1] Further confirmation comes in the list of current grants supported by the Division.[2] There are only 39 project grants being supported as of December, 1971. Remember that there are nearly a million nurses in the United States, 676 at last count with doctorates. Of the 39 project grants, 16 were not research grants at all. They were conference grants, or research development projects. Of the remaining 23 studies listed, only 9 could be called nursing practice studies judging from their titles. The American Nurse's Foundation lists five projects supported in 1970–71. Only one of them is a patient care study. ...

The review of nurses with earned doctoral degrees published in *Nursing Research* last year was illuminating, and chilling. Of the 676 nurses surveyed, only 21 indicated any real activity in research, though another 171 said research was "one of my position responsibilities." The authors calculate that these 192 people represent .04% of the population of employed nurses in the United States.[3]

The other sense of the word "discipline" is orderly conduct. Nursing has been enamored with something called "problem solving." We teach that instead of teaching the so-called scientific method, and that's supposed to guarantee a "research orientation" or "research attitude." We get into arguments in professional organizations about whether you can legitimately teach research to undergraduates, and if you do, shouldn't you really confine it to their senior year, as an honors elective? Whenever we have visitors to the Research Program at Yale, one question that is often asked is don't we think it is really awfully hard on students to require them to take both a heavy research course and a heavy theory construction course in the first semester of their first year [of graduate study]. The implication is that if students find the material hard, perhaps we ought not to teach it. Be kind to students, because, poor things, they're not up to thinking. ...

The article in the first issue of the new magazine *MS* on why women fear success is right to the point.[4] If we expect little of students, it's because we expect them to be capable of little. We fool around teaching them problem solving, but we don't teach them to *do research*. They get a watered down version of logic and methods of inquiry, just as in years past, nursing students got watered down versions of chemistry, biology, and so on—not because that's all nurses needed to know to practice but more probably because that's all nursing educations thought nursing students could learn. ...

Research is even more critically needed now that we are moving into new practice territory. One of the first battles that will have to be fought is whether nurses can be effective in expanded roles—an empirical research problem. But when we continue the model of nursing education and practice of doing, doing, doing—expanding functions at ever increasing speed, will we also expand our ability to base expanded practice in tested theory, to develop prescriptions for better care through systematic study, and most important, will we evaluate these new practices as they emerge? As long as we continue to make that artificial separation between nursing-as-doing and research-as-thinking, neither the practices of the profession nor the profession itself will grow.

The first application of research to nursing is to put research *in* nursing, not just apply it on. To make another medical analogy, research shouldn't be just grafted on, only to slough off again, but should be transplanted inside the body of nursing. And to continue the analogy, the success of the transplant will depend on the ability of the host to not reject this foreign body. That means we are going to have to stop some of the immunological arguments: whether research has a capital R or a small r, whether it can be done without a doctoral degree, whether it's necessary to teach in an undergraduate curriculum, whether non-nurses can do meaningful nursing studies.

Discussing the use of the research process in nursing is much easier. The research process is those steps that make up systematic empirical inquiry, including analyzing and stating the problem, posing the research questions and hypotheses, designing ways to collect the information needed, developing and implementing measurements and instruments, collecting data, processing and analyzing it, and interpreting the findings.

The first step in any study is to define the problem. What problem solving leaves out that the research process includes is finding out not only the practical difficulty that feels like it's wrong, but determining what the abstract class of problems is that one's practical problem belongs to.

One of the things that characterizes the ideal of nursing practice is the notion of individualized patient care. As an ideal, that is great; what is often missed is the transfer of learning that comes when instances of a given phenomena are seen as related, instead of individual idiosyncrasies of patients.

Only when one can conceptually relate incidents can one bring to bear on them theory, which is by definition abstract.

A student told me this story. She was working on a surgical service one evening. The nurses were having a problem with one patient who kept following them around asking for pain medication. The nurses had defined this instance as a problem, meaning that they wanted to get this patient off their backs. The student saw this case as an instance of a larger class of events and began to work with the patient to find out what his experience was. Pretty soon the patient was assured that someone would listen to him and that he could get the medication he needed, and he began to stay in his room or visit other patients instead of bugging the nurses. ...

It takes a certain kind of thinking to find the theoretical essence of problems. That kind of thinking is the beginning of the research process, but the thinking process alone can be used in nursing practice. In the example, the nurses defined their problem as "the patient is bothering us." That's not a class of events, that's one particular instance. To put that instance into a larger category of like instances is to move the problem from the merely practice to the possibly researchable. To move it to the abstract also makes available other knowledge—literature, theories, previous studies, and so forth—that are not available so long as the problem remains merely a patient peculiarity. Finally, to move a problem to an abstraction makes possible transfer of learning from one instance to another, because the abstraction provides the rubber cement between events.

[Here I used a number of other research terms, translated into practice application: reliability, validity, stratified sampling, experimental verification.]

There is another aspect of the research process that could have interesting implications for nursing practice immediately: the ethical standards of research for protection of rights of subjects. It is ironic to note what researchers have to go through to guarantee their subjects, especially patients, the rights to informed consent and privacy, where no such precautions are taken in practice. A researcher will make sure that her interview with a patient about how he feels about impending surgery will not be overheard by anyone. Ten minutes later, two nurses standing outside the patient's door will discuss the most intimate details of the operation within his hearing. (Doctors, of course, are much worse offenders.) Researchers will carefully explain experiments, procedures, give the patient a chance to refuse to participate, even get signed consent from patients when nothing untoward is going to be done to them. Nurses can and do painful, embarrassing, and dangerous procedures to patients without a word of explanation. ...

The application of research findings to nursing practice might seem a straightforward activity, but it seems to have three problems—finding the findings, finding the good findings, and implementing.

According to the Editor, *Nursing Research* still gets many more manuscripts having to do with education in nursing, or studies of nurses than studies of patient care.[5] Yet there is a whole underground of patient care research that, taken as a whole, could be revolutionary. There are nurses who are studying patient care problems as they practice nursing, without fanfare or publicity, which is sad. Bringing research findings into public seems to frighten nurses. ... Even master's theses and doctoral dissertations die unmourned on the library shelves.

Publication is just one end of the problem. At the other end is the dearth of patient care studies. We simply must reverse the order of things. We cannot legitimately figure out what to teach, or how to organize services until and unless we know what in nursing effects patients and how. It is ludicrous that we pour thousands of man and woman hours into curriculum revision when there is so little hard evidence on which to plan a teaching program that will produce desired effects with patients. We have got to stop arguing about definitions of nursing and start evaluating its practices. If we don't, and right now, nursing is going to be squeezed out between the physicians associates on the one end and the increasingly better trained paraprofessional health workers on the other.

Finding the good findings means having some standard for judging good research. Some of the standards are conventional methodological ones: reliability, validity, objectivity, appropriately rigorous design, pertinent statistics, and so on. In addition to the more conventional standards, the *nursing significance* of the study should be evaluated.

What evidence is there that a problem is conceived as a nursing problem? What does it matter to nursing if the problem is solved? Or if it's ignored? Is the study done in a way that approximates practice? Could the conduct of the study be detrimental or destructive from a nursing standpoint? Is the research concerned with the solution of a nursing problem, or merely with the collection of data? In addition to considering reliability and validity of measures, does the researcher consider the appropriateness and usefulness of procedures for nursing practice? If the study is only remotely related to actual nursing practice problems, are the intermediate steps to bring the findings closer to use in practice spelled out? And finally, what evidence is there that the economics of research—the time, energy, money, interest, commitment, and so on—were worth it?

It would be a rare study that could live up to such criteria. But assuming there are relevant studies, how will their recommendations be implemented? People who know the research have to be in a position to put it to use. But people who know the research now are siphoned off into education and administration with little contact with patient care. Those who stay close to patient care have an enormous job of attitude changing on their hands, mobilizing whole staffs to change or modify their practice by basing it in research, especially when the research may suggest better patient care will result only from more work on their part.

In wistful moments, I yearn for a time when all nurses will have research education—not training—so that research and nursing will always be mentioned in the same breath.

You of Sigma Theta Tau are in the catbird seat. Your membership in the society guarantees that you are leaders in your schools. Your organization has an explicit commitment to nursing research. You are the intellectual elite. I challenge you to help nursing expand its meaning to encompass research as a natural part of the definition. I've written before that I don't believe science will save us, but I do believe that the saving of nursing, if it isn't already too late, will come in the radical improvement of nursing practice.[6] That is the mission of nursing research, that's the only reason for advocating it and "application" is simply not enough.

ENDNOTES

1. Notter, L. (1971). Research in nursing—A critical need. *Nursing Research, 20*(3), 195.

2. Current Research Project Grants, Division of Nursing, PHS, NIH. DHEW Publication NIH 72-88, 1971.

3. Taylor, S.D. et al. (1971). Nurses with earned doctoral degrees. *Nursing Research, 20*(5), 415–427.

4. Gornick, V. (1972). Why women fear success. *MS, 1*(1), 37–43, January.

5. Notter, L. (1972). Report of the Editor. *Nursing Research, 21*(1), 3.

6. Diers, D. (1970). This I believe—about nursing research. *Nursing Outlook, 18*(11), 50–54.

THE ROLE OF CONTINUING EDUCATION IN PROMOTING RESEARCH IN PRACTICE

This speech developed themes that were later to appear in my late lamented nursing research book, Research in Nursing Practice.[1] *(It didn't sell.) The opportunity to address an audience in a much better position to support clinical nursing research than a faculty audience might be was not to be ignored. Continuing Education folks (now called Nursing Education in hospitals, CNE—clinical nurse educators) develop nursing practices and keep them up to speed. But they are largely ignored by faculties of schools of nursing as not being "real" educators. I don't know that I knew that then, but I surely do now. This speech was delivered at the National Conference on Continuing Education in Nursing in Austin, Texas, October 13, 1976. It was published nearly intact in the* Journal of Continuing Education in Nursing *(8[3], 54–62, 1977, used with permission). The picture that ran with this article shows a toothy, impossibly young woman (I was a Dean but not yet a Professor) with an awfully long neck. The teeth and the neck are still there, a bit the worse for wear.*

I was trying so hard to connect with these clinicians and as I read this now, it is awfully patronizing, the sin of the academic. Earnest as my efforts were, heart in the right place and all, this speech was still not collegial. Interestingly, this piece may read as more contemporaneous in countries such as the UK and Australia where a role called "Clinical Chair" has evolved. We have no equivalent role in the USA. Clinical Chairs are university professors who are located in clinical settings, hospitals, long term care facilities, and the prison system. Their work is professional development including research development that benefits the institution or agency.

The fact that the conference planners have chosen to link the words "continuing education" and "research" in the title of this presentation is of more than passing interest. Indeed, as I hope to develop, this farsighted title-mongering is a radical, perhaps even historic move. Without getting too pretentious about it, and without trying to fathom what was in the minds of those who wrote the title, it may have the effect of moving the cause of the intellectual life of nursing ahead by a quantum jump.

First, let me limit the tendency to drift into sweeping generalities and put some boundaries around what nursing practice research is. Research in nursing practice is the systematic study of problems in patient care. Problems for such research arise out of the clinical setting, from real-life patient situations and are, for the most part, studied in the real-life clinical situations. The ultimate purpose for research in nursing practice is to develop better information on which the care of patients can be based, through answering important questions about the nature and effect of nursing on patients.

Problems for nursing practice research, in contrast to other research in and about nursing, arise from discrepancies found in the clinical situation. The discrepancies are differences between the way things are now and the way they ought to be, or between what one knows now and what one needs to know, or between two opposing sets of facts. What makes problems and discrepancies into research topics is that they are *differences that matter*—matter to the improvement of patient care. The test of whether something matters is to ask the question, "What would it look like if the discrepancy were removed?"

The clinical world is full of discrepancies, just waiting to reach out and grab you. But not all of them matter, or matter enough to call for the energy and discipline that research to solve the problem involves. The mere existence of a perceptible difference does not automatically make a discrepancy into a research problem.

Some differences that seem to matter on first inspection turn out not to matter when further pursued. For example, suppose a pediatric nurse practitioner who works in a newborn nursery notices that a very large proportion of the patients she meets postpartum do not return to the clinic for their well-baby care. This looks, on the surface, like a nice discrepancy—nice in the sense that there's a real problem here, with real potential consequences for the health of mother and baby. But suppose that this PNP looks a little further into the situation and discovers that while her patients do not come back to her clinic, they go somewhere else for their postpartum care—a local neighborhood health center, a private physician, well-child conferences of the visiting nurse service, or other clinics. Her nice, neat discrepancy turns out not to be one at all, and while she can be happy that the patients apparently are getting care, she's short one research problem.

Discrepancies for clinical nursing research arise out of a feeling that something is wrong, an irritation, a wish either to change things, or to know something more about a situation. For example, a nurse graduate student was herself hospitalized for diagnostic surgery. She found herself very anxious preoperatively and unable to bring herself to use the intercom to call a nurse just to come talk with her. After she recovered from the surgery, she began to wonder whether patients are intimidated by the intercom in asking for what they really want or need. Here, the student's experience and her own discomfort stimulated a research problem.

Sometimes, discrepancies come out as a hunch, an itch to see if something will work. Here, the difference that matters is between what one knows now and what one needs to know. For instance in one hospital, several patient care units have recently shifted from team nursing to primary nursing. The discharge planning nurse, who knew that the shifts were happening, and which units, began to notice what she thought was a pattern: the referrals she was getting and the requests for consultation on discharge planning from the primary nursing units were qualitatively and quantitatively different from those on the other units. She suspected that since primary nurses get to know their patients a good deal better than team nurses do, they would put more thought into discharge planning and it would show in the referrals her office retrieved. ...

One final example: Sometimes discrepancies in practice come with emotion and erupt as bitter criticism. The nurses working in a plastic surgery unit stimulated one study when they felt totally unable to deal with what they saw as the anger and hostility of patients who had had massive mutilative surgery. To the nurses, it seemed as if the patients had not been adequately informed about what was going to happen and they could get furious at the physicians for not doing their job and dumping all the reactions on nursing. With some effort, this situation was translated into the less emotional research question: what do patients know about their surgery, how do they know it, and what is the relationship between knowledge of information and recovery from surgery? ...

This kind of research is only recently developed in nursing. As you may know, studies of the workers rather than the work predominated until the early 1960's; then studies of curriculum and administrative questions ruled. ...

There are some interesting parallels in both the past and present of nursing research and continuing education in nursing.

Nursing practice research grew out of the realization that nursing education as the repository of scholarship in the field had moved rather too far away from its sources in nursing practice. There were some articulate spokespersons who said that it was folly to put one's efforts into devising complicated curricular structures or administrative maneuvers until and unless one knew first, *what* in patient care worked.[2] There were others who recognized that the knowledge on which the practice of nursing is built has to be knowledge about that practice, not necessarily knowledge borrowed from other disciplines.[3] ...

It has seemed to me that the roots of continuing education in nursing developed from some of the same concerns. While in the politics of continuing education the theme of protecting the safety of the public through assuring them competent, up-to-date practitioners was sounded, that theme is essentially the same as the research tune—improving the quality of nursing care by increasing the knowledge of its practitioners. And in the continuing education arena, there were rather important assumptions made that nurses need to learn more, not only to keep up, but to develop their practice. And behind that assumption is the even more important one that nurses *can* learn, and continue to learn, that nursing is more than mere technical competence. Indeed, continuing education has made a crucial distinction between inservice education, done primarily for orientation to new equipment or drugs or procedures, and continuing education, done to expand the mind of the professional nurse and thus expand her practice.

So both nursing research and continuing education have put their commitments on the line, and in parallel ways: that nursing is intellectual work which constantly needs refreshment, enrichment, and development, and that such development is in the service of providing better and better care to those whom society has mandated us to serve.

And it should be pointed out that both in research and in continuing education, there is a nearly explicit realization that as a woman's profession, nursing has not been given and has not taken the credit for the heavy brain work that is involved. Nurses as women are not supposed to think, at least not abstractly, which both research and "continuing education" in its broadest sense connote. And nurses as women are not supposed to be able to deal with the complexities of statistical analysis or mathematical models, or the philosophy of science as research requires, or physiological chemistry, or psychopharmacology, or the electrical conductive system of the heat as continuing education provides.

There are parallels also in the putative future of both continuing education and clinical nursing research that boggle the mind, and make of the title of this paper the visionary statement it is.

Both continuing education and nursing practice research are nontraditional. "Education" is supposed to mean degrees or diplomas, granted by some institution with granting powers, properly surveyed and quality controlled and generally relatively structured and boxed in. Similarly, nursing research, or more commonly, research in nursing is supposed to be, almost by definition, remote from the practice of the profession, because it is by becoming remote that we raise our status. It used to be common in nursing research polemical literature to see espoused a total lack of reliance on nursing as the source or delta for research ideas. Great flowery statements were once the fugue—that nursing research should deal only with the testing of social/psychological concepts, or the application of theory devised for other purposes, or that all nursing theory was, was theory of man.

But now nursing practice research and continuing education ideas have brought us back to where we should be in the first place: worrying about how to improve nursing care. And joining these two forces has quite incredible potential for changing the face of the profession as a learned discipline.

Because continuing education deals entirely with already prepared practitioners, it is free to concentrate its efforts differently than traditional education, which is largely geared to preparing people for entry into practice, even entry into advanced practice.

There are two ways to think about research and two ways to think about a continuing education. One can think about using research in practice and one can think about doing research in practice. Similarly, one can think about the purpose of continuing education being eradication of obsolescence in practice or one can think of it as upgrading knowledge and skill by providing essentially new content.

To make use of knowledge gained from research in practice, one must first have some sense of how to decide what research knowledge is good knowledge. Research in any field contains excellent, seminal work, and work of highly questionable quality. Even that which is "okay" research on the surface may prove upon deeper inspection to be so full of bias and invalidity as to be useless. I remember well one study I used to assign to our graduate students. This study compared the use of nurses and physicians as triage officers for fractures in the emergency room setting. The results indicated that nurses were terrific at triage, making the correct decisions for referral and x-ray, and reducing waiting time in the ER. But when one looked at the sample, one discovered that of the nurse group, no one has less than 27 months of ER experience. One looked a little closer and discovered that the physician staffing in the ER consisted of interns just out of medical school.

One's political heart turned over to see those nice results go down the drain but it is simply not fair to compare experienced ER nurses with newly minted MDs, no matter how favorable the comparison is. It might be, by the way, that nurses make lovely triage officers and that the major impact of the study was to convert people to that way of thinking. But it is a misuse of research to make simply biased political points sound less biased by highfalutin' research jargon and impressive statistics when the design of the study itself is so poor.

So it seems to me that it might be well of continuing education to consider offering classes or other work in how to read research, dealing with some of the basic principles of good study design, control, and reporting. Then, and perhaps only then, one can think about ways to teach nurses what is new in patient care and what the nursing research literature says. We need not foist any more garbage on our colleagues than is already there for them to find themselves! ...

To do justice to research knowledge, it would probably be necessary to concentrate in continuing education on relatively small chunks of information. That is, one could suggest holding a continuing education course on "pain," for example, in which one could go into some depth on the theories and findings of studies in this area, rather than trying for more global combinations of topics which breeze over things so superficially that neither the content itself is absorbed, nor is the audience usually inspired to continue study in the area on their own.

There is another way continuing education can help get research knowledge into practice, and that's through the function of "translation." Here, I'm not talking about simply translating from the research jargon to the practice situation. Indeed, in the kinds of sessions I just talked about, I would use the original source material—the studies themselves—rather than reports written for the non-technical audience, and the responsibility would be on both the instructor and the student to make sense of it. There's no reason to think nurses don't want to stretch their brains to read highly complex material.

The kind of translation I'm thinking about here is the translating of knowledge that is not specifically nursing into knowledge for nursing practice. There is a great deal in the psychological, sociological, psychiatric, medical, and other literature that has direct implications for nursing. The complicated biopsychological studies of stress, for example, can be related easily and usefully to the care of patients in predictably stressful situations, such as intensive care or even just general surgery.

Similarly, the psychological studies of helplessness in animals may be useful in understanding the reactions of people confronted with situations over which they have no control, such as hospitalization, accident, rape, etc. Some quite exciting continuing education experiences could involve discussions of this kind of material to tease out the clinical implications, as well as more orthodox sessions intended simply to acquaint nurses with other sources of knowledge.

It is a continuing frustration to me that it sometimes seems as if nursing, like automobile manufacturing, functions under a conscious program of "planned obsolescence," training for situations that are outdated the minute after graduation.[4] So very little nursing research is encountered in formal nursing education programs and it seems unfair to suggest that continuing education must be used to plug up the holes. But in fact, that is what's needed, and the rapidity with which new knowledge is evolving in nursing, medical science, and the social sciences means that continuing education will probably always find itself in the position of this kind of knowledge updating.

So far I've talked about continuing education's role in promoting research through use of the research knowledge. Even more important, and more interesting perhaps, is the role continuing education may have in directly promoting the conduct of patient care research.

But here we have a two-fold problem: there isn't enough nursing practice research going on, and organized continuing education is not enough involved in promoting it. Taking the first part of the problem first, the next question is, "Why isn't there more nursing practice research?"

First, there aren't enough people trained to do it (obvious implication there, for continuing education to leap into the breach). But there are some cautions immediately. Doing nursing practice research isn't like doing any old research. The kind of "teaching" that's needed must include some of the tools of research, the methods or conventions for assuring objectivity and reliability and validity, but more important and harder to accomplish is teaching people how to discover nursing practice problems for research and how to develop them into doable studies. What's so hard about that? At the bottom line, nurses are not by and large trained to analyze patient care situations in the way that analyzing them for research requires. All too often, nurses treat each potential irritation, criticism, or discrepancy as if it were isolated and unique, rather than as if it were an instance of a larger problem. The nature of research is such that discrete and specific problems are investigated in such a way that the information gained says something about more abstract issues. There is a constant interplay between the very concrete data and the very abstract concept, and this is a skill and way of thinking that is not bred into traditional nursing education programs, the graduates of which then become prospective continuing education students.

The analytic approach to nursing practice requires another psychological shift for many nurses—from protecting one's self from criticism, to actively criticizing one's practice, and one's information base so as to define holes in it that could be plugged with further education or research.

So one way continuing education might promote research in nursing practice is to develop continuing education experiences that deal with issues of research *process* rather than issues of content. ...Specific instances of real life situations would be discussed and developed, using inference to available theory, other cases of the same kind, the increasingly microscopic examination of the elements of a situation in order to tease out all the subtleties, and the increasingly complicated potential explanations, using more and more abstractions.

Such a process depends heavily on the "clinical wisdom" of the nurses involved, in making their intuition, their "unconscious intelligence" available for public perusal and hopefully, empirical investigation.

If continuing education were to develop ways to help nurses learn this kind of process, immediately we would need to look at the other half of our problem statement, that is, some modifications in the way continuing education is viewed. Continuing education has some real and important problems inherent in the notion of education which is not required for degree credit, and thus which does not have in it necessarily the kinds of quality control that more traditional education has. In the case of possibly offering the kind of analytic training I mentioned before, the difficulty for continuing education is that for it to work, there almost have to be some requirements for production. Nurses, like all human beings, are great sitters-around-and-talk people but unless there is a push for some obvious product, the talk will lead nowhere, and will not even be taken seriously as the very complicated method it is. In traditional education, students can be required to write papers, or present seminars, or otherwise demonstrate that they've learned what they are supposed to. In teaching the analytic process of research, mere class attendance or even contribution to the discussion are not sufficient to assure that any "education" has taken place. So any continuing education offerings to promote research through developing the thinking powers of nurses must have some kind of built-in expectations for performance, and that may be counterproductive to interesting nurses in research, or enrolling them in a program.

Which leads to the next piece of the analysis of our problem of the relationship between continuing education and research in nursing practice: another reason why there isn't enough nursing practice research going on is that it isn't rewarded.

Nursing research is hard work. That alone makes many nurses shy away from developing their talent through research, and that coupled with a lack of basic analytic tools may make research a frightening and off-putting thing for the practicing nurse to contemplate. But continuing education is in a prime position to make dramatic changes in that situation, and by doing so, contribute significantly to the power of research to improve the practice of the profession.

Suppose it were the case that conducting a research project were defined as deserving continuing education units (CEU). Suppose further that states developed some criteria that rewarded nursing practice research with more units than other kinds of research. In theory, it would not be difficult to work out such an arrangement, and even to grant variable CEUs for the various parts of a research project. Suppose it were determined that a formal statement of a research problem, with the accompanying formal analysis of the practice problem and the initial conceptualization were worth, say 5 CEUs. Then suppose that plus a review of literature were worth 10. And suppose a full-fledged research proposal were worth 20, and a fully developed and conducted and reported study were worth 40 or 50 CEUs.

I submit that a nurse's education is "continued" far more fully from such personal involvement in systematic study than the equivalent of contact hours of sitting in courses or programs, especially when the study is a study of nursing practice that automatically sends the nurse to the nursing research literature and to related literature in other fields.

In Connecticut, and I am sure elsewhere, CEUs can be earned by teaching, by publishing or presenting papers among other things. Why not doing research as well?

Another reason why nursing practice research isn't done all that much and why continuing education may be helpful is that there is an unfortunate tendency in nursing to think that only those with doctorates can do "research" with a capital "R," or that research training should occur only in conventional educational institutions and only after basic nursing. My position is that the best nursing practice research will come out of those who are closest to that practice, not necessarily those who have removed themselves through years of course work in another discipline or whose administrative or educational position has not permitted involvement in the real world of patient care. Further, there is nothing so mysterious about research methods or statistics that means it has to be hidden away in the elite ivory tower.

It is possible to do quite useful nursing research with the application of intelligence, some basic knowledge about design and logic, a *lot* of knowledge about clinical practice, and the motivation to attack problems systematically and without bias. Sure, there are frills of design and fancy theoretical notions, and they are important, but not the overriding concern in conducting studies of problems in patient care.

If a continuing education program were to make a real push toward educating a defined group of nurses to conduct studies, it can be done, and it would be beautiful to see. Continuing education simply must take on some of the responsibility for preparing people to do studies, especially since such small percentages of nurses go on for higher education that prepares them for research. Research, at least in the sense of analytic, systematic processes of inquiry, if not in actual study design, should be part of *every* nurse's armamentarium.

Yet another reason why there is so little nursing practice research done by nurses in practice is that there is some feeling that researchers are so ethereal and unreal that nurses don't even want to have contact with them, much less with their output. There's a certain amount of truth in that, but simply griping about it doesn't do anything. Rather, nurses in practice should take every opportunity and continuing education should find a way to reward it, to participate in research conducted by others. That's the only way to assure that the research has any applicability to the real world, and that the topics studied and the methods used have the potential for improving the quality of care.

For example, there is a very important study in the literature comparing the practice of family nurse practitioners and physicians in Canada.[5] In fact, there are rather a lot of studies of the practice of nurse practitioners floating around, but I know of very few in which the nurse practitioner herself was a co-investigator or consultant to the project, and therefore in a position to make sure that the project said something of interest to nurses. In the famous study I mentioned, the entire focus is on the medical care of patients, the extent to which non-physician primary care nurses can deliver care which is as safe as that of physicians in this setting. While that may be an important problem, conceiving the study that way seriously limits its impact. There is no attempt in the study, for example, to measure those things nurses in primary care do that are not medical practice, the teaching, counseling, referring that are traditionally the province of nursing. Had they been included, it might have been the case that while nurses could be demonstrated to give quality medical care, using physician practice as the standard, physicians give rotten nursing care. The point is that primary care is more than simply the practice of orthodox medicine, it is also care based on the needs of patients, some of which are not "medical" at all. A study that attacks only a piece of the problem contributes only a piece of the information to solve the problem.

My other favorite example of this kind of inadequacy of study that stems from not involving nursing is a study done some years ago of postpartum blues. It was done by several male psychiatrists, who were astonished to find out that their operational definition of "blues," crying in the early postpartum period, would not work. They state wistfully at the end of their paper that they came up with essentially no conclusions because women apparently cry for reasons other than depression, and some show depression in ways other than crying. Any nurse could have told them that!

Involvement of nurses in studies conducted by others is also a way to attack the potential obsolescence of nursing where nurses are not exposed all that much to other disciplines. It can be highly instructive to work with a team of physicians or social scientists and to realize that they have some of the same kinds of intra-professional, conceptual, political, territorial problems we chastise ourselves for having. And that kind of "continuing education" is extremely valuable in preparing people for increasing levels of interdisciplinary responsibility.

I have not dealt much in this paper with continuing education at the postmaster's or postdoctoral levels. Clearly, however, some of the suggestions here would be equally appropriate, if not more so, to people whose educational background should have included a more defined concentration on research. Among the more depressing statistics I know about nursing is the one that indicates that in a national sample, only an infinitesimal percentage of nurses with doctoral degrees were doing any research after the doctorate.[6] If research were rewarded by continuing education units or an equivalent means, perhaps people would be stimulated to stay with it.

Political arguments and other such ephemeral considerations aside, there is now in these times an even more powerful argument for nursing's involvement in research, and the efforts of all of us to support the increasing pressure on the health professionals to document the effects of our services. Quality assurance programs are part of that, as is the new PSRO (Professional Standards Review Organization) system for nursing being developed. These activities are, if done right, *research,* and they should require the same rigorous standards of thought and design that conventional research does. Therefore, continuing education which addresses quality assurance or peer review should do more than simply define the terms and describe the programs; it should help us work together to define the standards of practice (which is in itself a research activity) on which we will base measures of performance (which is also a research activity). Since quality assurance is so much on the minds of nurses, at least those employed in institutional health services, it provides a wonderful excuse and motivation for getting nurses involved in research-type activities.

I said earlier that nursing research is hard work. It is, and that means rather powerful motivations have to be brought to bear to involve nurses in it. Formal rewards are one thing; enlightened self-interest is another. I would suggest to you, without being overly dramatic about it, that unless continuing education and nursing practice research get together (along with research and orthodox nursing education) we stand a distinct chance of never being able to establish nursing as the true profession we believe we have. And we will do women and nurses a disservice if we do not confront consciously our anti-intellectual heritage in nursing and find all possible ways to bring research and continuing education into partnership to reinforce and demonstrate that nursing is, in Annie Goodrich's words, "the adventure of thought and the adventure of action."

Dean Goodrich goes on to say: "...to effectively interpret the truly great role that has been assigned [the nurse], neither a liberal education nor a high degree of technical skill will suffice. She must also be master of two tongues— the tongue of science and that of the people."[7]

I couldn't have said it better myself.

ENDNOTES

1. Diers, D. (1979). *Research in Nursing Practice.* Philadelphia: Lippincott.

2. Leonard, R.C. (1967). Developing research in a practice oriented discipline. *American Journal of Nursing, 67*(12), 1472–1475.

3. Wald, F., & Leonard, R.C. (1964). Toward nursing practice theory. *Nursing Research, 13*(6), 309–314.

4. Kramer, M. (1974). *Reality Shock.* St Louis, CV Mosby.

5. Spitzer, W.O. et al. (1974). The Burlington randomized trial of the nurse practitioner. *New England Journal of Medicine, 290*(2), 251–256.

6. Abdellah, F.G. (1970). A review of nursing research 1955–1968, Part 1. *Nursing Research, 19*(1), 6–17.

7. Goodrich, A.W. (1933). *The Social and Ethical Significance of Nursing.* New York: Macmillan (p. 14).

GENERATIONS IN NURSING RESEARCH

Graduation speeches and alumnae/i events are wonderful occasions to go lyrical. These are sentimental occasions where the point of the speaker is to make the audience feel good about themselves and their accomplishments. Everybody is happy; there's no agenda to do anything about anything.

*There is a difference in speaking style in this piece, now much more colloquial, but also now what I felt to be a level of comfort in speaking **for** the profession. This speech was given at the 25th Anniversary celebration of the School of Nursing of the University of Florida, in 1981. The writing here will read somewhat repetitive, but if read out loud, the repetition will make sense. For these kinds of speeches, a certain drumming style is in order.*

This was a chance to look back over the 25 years of the assignment, and I had fun with the historical analysis. Because it was not an occasion of scholarship, references are not supplied. This was never going to be published. Good thing, too, because the themes here are developed better later.

The University of Florida School of Nursing was distinguished from its very beginning by its commitment to the marriage of education and service under its first Dean, Dorothy Smith. There was a connection between what we were trying to do at Yale and what Dorothy was doing in Florida.

*Somewhere in the **AJN** there is a lovely story about how the students in the first class of the University of Florida's School of Nursing designed their cap. (Remember caps?) As I recall it, one of the students turned her shoe over, put it on her head and it looked really good. I thought the Florida cap was one of the better ones.*

I loved that story because I was in the first and, as it turned out, next-to-the-last class to graduate from my BSN program at the University of Denver. Our cap was the same as the diploma program that had preceded us: a T-shaped affair when flat (we used to use liquid starch to paste them to a flat surface to dry. When I went back to the dorm for our own 25th anniversary and stayed in the same room I had lived in, there were still the marks of my caps on the wood of the closet doors). When folded, it was a traditional Metro-Goldwyn-Mayer cap, buy it in any uniform shop. We got a special blue velvet ribbon that went across the right hand corner of the folded cap: one for the junior year, two for the senior year. At graduation, a full velvet ribbon across the whole front of the cap, precisely 3/8 inch from the edge. I still have my cap and whoever has to dispose of my effects will have to pitch it. This is a piece of nursing visibility that may have been overdone at the time, but the notion of recognition through symbols is important and I can't throw it away.

After all, there's the black or blue suit for business types and God forbid there are cowboy boots underneath. Or the suit is the wrong cut with a too-bright tie, or the too-short skirt. The dress code in business in health care organizations now is far more vicious than our old nursing outfits were. They may have looked silly and been clinically irrelevant (caps fell off in bedpans— yuck!). But wearing the uniform and cap made me feel tall and strong and clean and competent.

The references here are to Rozella Schlotfeldt, then the distinguished Dean of the School of Nursing at Case Western Reserve University, and one my idols and mentors, and Linda Aiken, another idol, and an early graduate from the University of Florida School of Nursing.

A 25th Anniversary Celebration is a time to look both backwards and forward—at where we've been and where we're going. To have the assignment to look back over the last 25 years is to be stunned by the changes and progress one can see in nurses and nursing.

Twenty-five years ago, your speaker tomorrow, Rozella Scholtfeldt, had not yet become Dean of the Frances Payne Bolton School of Nursing of Case Western Reserve University. The developments there that made it the premier school of nursing in the United States were yet to happen. Twenty-five years ago, this morning's speaker, Linda Aiken, was a sophomore in high school and there was then no Robert Wood Johnson Foundation. There *was,* however, a shortage of nurses. Twenty-five years ago, your dean was finishing her nursing degree and 25 years ago her distinguished predecessor, Dorothy Smith, was just beginning to accomplish the miracles of leadership of education and service that lead us here today. Twenty-five years ago, I was a freshman in college, worrying about being tapped for a social sorority as I dissected a pregnant cat in anatomy class. I had yet to take care of a patient, much less read any nursing research. All of which could make me feel very smug until I remember Tom Lehrer's wonderful humbling line: "When Mozart was my age, he had been dead for ten years."

The title of this presentation, "Generations in Nursing Research," was chosen deliberately to have a double message. While a generation in terms of studying families is thought in this country to be between 25 and 30 years, in nursing research I suspect we hit a new generation about every 5 years. It takes about 5 years for nurses to "grow up" in their professional field through their own undergraduate and graduate preparation or through a doctoral program.

Thus, 25 years of nursing research represents at least 5 generations of nurses, each one taking a slightly different perspective and each building on the work of the earlier ones. The second message buried in the title of this presentation has to do with the derivation of the word "generation." It comes from the Latin *genera* meaning type or kind (actually plural, types or kinds) and one of the themes I will develop in this paper is precisely that: the types or kinds of nursing research which might be concentrated upon in the future.

Our professional journal, *Nursing Research*, began in June of 1952. When I reviewed the four issues published 25 years ago, the journal was 4 years old. In 1956, then, this is what nursing research, at least as represented by our then only refereed research journal, included.

There were 16 major articles. By far, the largest single category of articles had to do with nurses (seven articles). These papers dealt with staffing, with the activities of nurses on a psychiatric ward, with studies of occupational values or personality structure, studies of the numbers of nurses in a particular geographic area, and a wonderful study of the success of commercial school graduates in nursing education programs. There were three articles on curriculum or curriculum evaluation, one article on the role of the school nurse, two articles on research methods, one time-motion study, one satisfaction-with-care study, and one article which could be legitimately classified as clinical nursing research, which had to do with the feeding of premature babies. One might conclude that nursing in 1956 was obsessed with who nurses were and what made them tick. That would not be a surprising conclusion, for in those days, advanced programs in nursing were just beginning and there may well have been concern about how nursing manpower would ever develop an intellectual field or a conceptual practice base.

Even more interesting than the articles themselves were the news items.

There was a story to the effect that Virginia Henderson and Leo Simmons had just been funded to start their study which, as you know, became the benchmark for the development of nursing research. They reviewed all of the nursing research from 1900 to 1959 and eventually published a book and four volumes of an annotated index to nursing research. Their book, *Nursing Research*, blew the first trumpets for studies of clinical nursing practice, a theme elaborated by Miss Henderson in several articles and editorials within the last 25 years, the latest in 1977 when she was nearly 80 years young. ...

The editor of the journal *Nursing Research* in 1956 was Edith Patton Lewis, who went on to become editor of *Nursing Outlook* and who revolutionized it as she was then establishing standards for the research journal of the American Journal of Nursing Company.

To show just how far we've come, not only in research but in another field, there was a book review by Virginia Henderson in 1956 of Greenblatt and Brown's famous book, *From Custodial to Therapeutic Care in Mental Hospitals,* a volume that was instrumental in starting the direction of advanced psychiatric nursing training and practice—only 25 years ago.

There was an editorial in 1956 by Helen Bunge, then Chairman of the Editorial Board for the journal, crying out for nurses to *use* research in their practice and chastising nurse researchers who do not study problems of interest to practitioners or whose reports of research are not useful to the practicing clinician. That theme has characterized any number of editorials by any number of editors of *Nursing Research* since that time and it bears stating as much today as it did 25 years ago.

Finally, there were several reports in the 1956 volume of *Nursing Research* of the first year that nursing research grants were ever funded within the Division of Nursing of the United States Public Health Service. In the first year of funding, $500,000 had been allocated to the support of nursing research grants. (It may amuse you to note that the current allocation before the latest Reagan budget cuts is only a ten-fold increase: 5 million dollars). Twenty projects were funded in that first year. They dealt with curriculum research and with determining the needs of discharged patients for public health nursing service in the home. One study was intended to develop criteria for the hospital bed, that is, the design of the bed. (I've never seen a report of that study and it would be fun to track down.) Several studies which later became famous and instrumental in the early history of nursing research were funded in that first year—David Fox's study of stress in nursing, which eventually produced his textbook on research in nursing, Peter Kong-Ming New's study of the relationship between nurse staffing and nurse-patient interaction, a study about the career selection into nursing, and finally, Myrtle Kitchell Aydelotte and Marie Tener's groundbreaking study on the relationship between nurse staffing and delivery of service. You may recall the results of this latter study; it showed that no matter how many nurses were added to a nursing staff, the amount of nursing care did not particularly increase, as nurses found other ways to use their time. Parenthetically, it amuses me to note that those who advocate Primary Nursing have not reached back into our history to retrieve that old study for it is my impression that had Primary Nursing been the way of organizing care in those days, the results of the study would have been quite different.

In those days, not so very long ago, there was but one textbook on nursing research, Loretta Heidgerken's. Indeed, the author of the second big nursing research text, Faye Abdellah, was just publishing her doctoral dissertation in 1956.

How very far we've come! It is simply no longer the case that research in nursing is something tacked on, added, or maybe not even considered, in nursing curricula. For there was a time when it was thought that research was antithetical to nursing since nursing was, after all, an art and a calling. Such reasoning today seems sentimentally Victorian. There was a time when it was thought that it was impossible to study nursing practice directly, so complicated was the clinical situation that it defied rigorous methodology. Dumas and Leonard's study, done in 1961 and published in 1963, is given credit for destroying that illusion. Twenty-five years ago there were no ANA Clinical Sessions in which nurses could present their research subject to the critique of their colleagues. (And a quick perusal of the early critiques makes one happy to see the change from brutal *ad feminam* criticism to the very high quality of intellectual and scholarly debate we now see in the WICHEN series, Communicating Nursing Research, and in reports of the ANA Council of Nurse Researchers.) Twenty-five years ago, the debates in nursing research, which we now know and love, had not started—whether one must have a doctorate to do research, whether there is a difference between theory-based research and research to develop theory, whether one ought to do exploratory studies before one even attempts clinical experiments, whether quasi-experimental designs are superior, given clinical considerations, to classical experimental designs. In some ways, one might wish to return to those earlier times for a great debate about what constitutes nursing theory and, for that matter, nursing, with which we are now achingly familiar, had not yet begun. In those days, we knew what nursing was; it's what nurses did.

On the occasion of a different 25th anniversary, the 25th year of the publication of *Nursing Research* in 1977, Susan Gortner and Helen Nahm published a magnificent overview of nursing research since the early 1900s. They conclude that a major characteristic of research efforts in nursing in the mid-1970s was responsibility and accountability for health care. They go on to say:

> Questions regarding the authenticity of the base of knowledge underlying nursing practice, the efficacy of the art of practice, optimal structures for care, measurement of care and application of research findings are being addressed. The growth of practice related research ... appears to be gaining momentum because of the interest in augmenting the knowledge base and because of increased numbers of investigators.[1]

Subsequent articles in the 25th anniversary series reviewed research in medical/surgical nursing, community health nursing, maternal-child nursing, psychiatric nursing, and nursing gerontology. Introducing these reviews was Virginia Henderson again, in a superb editorial. As is her wont, she pins nursing research to the wall with her observations. She says:

> While I ... rejoice and ... applaud our progress and our present emphasis on "sound research" ... I also hope that future health related research has humane goals. I hope that the hypotheses it tests are worth testing, that nurse researchers are more interested in improving practice than in academic respectability.[2]

Miss Henderson calls for vision of the kind shown by Frederick LeBoyer, Sister Kenney, and the pseudonymous "Dr. Bob," founder of Alcoholics

Anonymous, all of whom invented and eventually tested new approaches to improving the lot of suffering humanity.

Miss Henderson goes on:

> It does seem to me that nurses are still loath to take responsibility for designing the methods they use, for undertaking studies that, if the findings were applied, might revolutionize practice. They are, perhaps, less comfortable in collaborating with physiologists and physicians than with social scientists, less likely to expect or ask for a colleague relationship if they work with physicians on questions of health care.[3]

Indeed, we have come a long way, baby. That nurses should become involved in research is no longer even a question. That nurses should do research which may eventually improve practice is now a maxim. That nurses should be taught research from the beginning of their professional education is a contemporary standard. That nurses should make public their research both to educate colleagues and to change the public image of nursing is a new cry. And that nurses should find pride in the accomplishments of our professional group in building an increasingly solid basis for practice, while at the same time expanding the limits of human service, is increasingly our agenda.

As we move or are drawn (depending on how you look at it) into the 1980s it may be well to reflect on Miss Henderson's point and raise certain other themes. In contrast to other times in the history of nursing research, I do not believe we are at any crisis or crossroad. Nursing and nursing research are far too healthy for those kinds of analogies to Armageddon. Federal funding may well disappear for nursing research and cuts in programmatic expenditures may force schools of nursing to re-think their emphasis and priorities in clinical training and research. Yet I am firmly convinced that the progress made in nursing research, indeed, the progress made in raising nursing's intellectual consciousness, has come too far to be eroded by something as simple as money. In times of predicted austerity, it is easy to think that the solution to survival is to set arbitrary priorities and assume they will be followed. In nursing research, I believe we are far too diverse in interests, in autonomy, and in development of professional assertiveness to think that any priorities, even if articulated, would be followed. In fact, one of the most exciting things about contemporary nursing research is the many directions it is taking as we feel our intellectual oats.

But it is useful on occasions such as this to pause for a moment and make sure the ground is solid under us. That is, what is it that nursing research is supposed to be for, what is it supposed to do for us, given the predictable troubles ahead, how can we make sure it does that?

The conventional answer to the question, what is research good for, is that it helps establish the base for practice. Would that that were true. For it is fairly clear that in nursing, research has followed rather than lead developments in nursing theory or even changes in practice. The major examples of nursing theory development in the past 25 years arose out of serious thinking, but not necessarily out of research. One could cite here Martha Rogers, Dorothea Orem, the nursing diagnosis thrust, Imogene King, Betty Neuman, or any number of other theorists. While research has now accumulated to test various pieces of these theories, the theories did not grow out of original research in the beginning.

Even major changes in practice cannot always be tied to a research base. Primary Nursing, for example, grew out of some studies of the role of the ward manager but not out of what we would understand to be a clinical research base. The development of the nurse practitioner role in primary care, certainly one of the themes for the future, did not grow out of research either, but out of Lee Ford and Henry Silver's observation that nurses were not practicing to the level at which they might be capable and in which they could relieve a defined shortage of primary care.

Yet nursing is not alone in this reversal or order. It has been pointed out that any number of now standard approaches in medicine to the treatment of various diseases or conditions grew not out of research at all but out of some other considerations. For example, radical mastectomy as treatment for breast cancer came to be simply because it was "so reasonable." Herniorrhaphy as the generally accepted treatment for patients with inguinal hernias is not supported by cost/benefit analysis nor any other appropriate statistics. Indeed, there is increased risk to the older patient undergoing elective hernia repair.

There is a new British study in which patients were randomly assigned to either home care or intensive care in hospitals after having suffered an MI. The study demonstrates conclusively that there was no improved survival among patients receiving intensive care. For older male patients, survival at home was significantly better. And there are obvious cost/benefit differences as well.

But it is simply a fact that neither medicine nor nursing can wait long enough to try to improve practice for all the scientific data to be in. Nursing is far too big a conceptual and empirical field to rest on the hope that there would ever be a day when we could claim that everything that we do is based upon tested hypotheses and valid evidence.

Thus, while nursing research is terrifically helpful in changing practice, it may not find its greatest value in inventing new practices, but rather in establishing the validity of those already in place. The research that supports Primary Nursing is testimony to this notion. While Primary Nursing may not have originally grown out of research, there is now a significant body of information which validates not only its effectiveness in direct patient care but the potential of significant cost savings as well as decreasing nursing turnover.

But one must continue to advocate research directed at building nursing's body of knowledge. We need more and more clinical epidemiological studies which help us identify clusters of patients at risk for either disease or differential response to treatment. We must have more and more studies which describe patterns of child development, maternal bonding, family relationships, and responses to care. We need further studies of how patients think about illness and disease, when they decide to seek treatment, and the extent to which different kinds of patients will differentially profit from health teaching or self-care. We need more studies of the efficacy of various nursing interventions from the interpersonal to the highly technical. And we need to worry less about intruding into the practice of medicine in looking at nursing's interventions or picking research problems than we need to worry about validating our practices. For example, a study of the effect of aspirin on clotting time seems to me perfectly justifiable as a nursing research study when one reason why nurses are not allowed to prescribe aspirin, at least for hospitalized patients, is its supposed effect on clotting time.

It becomes more and more clear in these days when nursing is discovering its inherent power that nursing research has potential quite outside traditional academic interests. That is to say, nursing research is a political coin.

We now have research in nursing which documents the cost savings of nurse-run rehabilitation programs for patients with coronary artery disease and patients with chronic illness. We have research which shows that nurse-midwifery services in a home-like birth setting save the consumer or third-party payers between $500 and $1500 per patient. We have a study in Georgia that documents that nurse-midwifery services to three defined counties compared with seven contiguous counties showed cost savings of over one million dollars in a one year period. We know that Primary Nursing in a renal transplant unit allowed patients to be discharged upwards of 3 weeks earlier thus saving 3 weeks of hospital costs. We know from Jean Johnson's very first study that preoperative preparation can decrease hospital stays for prepared patients. To the extent that contemporary economics dictates an obsession with the costs of everything, nursing research may help public policy decision makers reform health service delivery to control costs.

But nursing research also documents that cost effective services are not done at the expense of high quality. There is now overwhelming evidence that care delivered by nurse practitioners stacks up extremely well against traditional physician care in ambulatory settings. The collected research in nurse-midwifery shows that patients served by nurse-midwives are, for example, less often anemic at delivery, use less medication during labor and delivery, less frequently require forceps deliveries or cesarean sections, are more satisfied with care, and produce bigger babies with higher Apgar scores than comparison groups of patients served by traditional systems of care.

Knowing then, that nursing research does help establish the base for excellent practice, and knowing that nursing research can have political benefit, can we see some directions for nursing research in the '80s?

One direction for nursing research is best exemplified by the work of your speaker this morning, Linda Aiken. The kind of research she has done is incredibly powerful though it's the kind that is never covered in textbooks nor discussed as methodology. That is, the use of existing data, demographic or other information to shed light on an important phenomenon and point the way to public policy decision-making. Dr. Aiken's latest article on the nursing shortage, simultaneously published in the *American Journal of Nursing* and the *Annals of Internal Medicine* (a coup in itself) is a brilliant disquisition. I commend it to your attention as a superior example of a kind of research which needs badly to be done in nursing. Among the things most outstanding about this approach is Dr. Aiken's recognition of the effect of structural factors (number of hospital beds, salary structures, governance mechanisms, and so on) on the supply and distribution of nurses.

For a very long time in nursing research we tended to conduct studies which for methodological cleanliness reasons were conceptually limited to direct effects of nursing on patient variables. Such studies are still needed and in even larger numbers. However, it is now obvious that it will be impossible to understand nursing or its effects without reconceptualizing some nursing problems and possibilities as "systems of care." That is, it is clear that nursing does not operate in a vacuum, that structural variables condition both the independent variable—nursing—and the dependent variable—patient welfare—in ways we know too little about. We need to study structure of the practice site in order to understand better the effectiveness and efficacy of nurse practitioner practice. Studies of Primary Nursing are increasingly taking into account the structure of the delivery of care, particularly the decision-making options of that method of organizing nursing service delivery. We are realizing more and more that nurse-run programs can and should be tested for effect. But more importantly, we are learning that nursing care itself is a nurse-run program and needs to be understood as such. It was once easy simply to look at the effect of, say, nursing practice on patient outcomes. Yet we now know that nurse-midwifery practice itself is touched by structural variables of practice site, governance, standing orders or protocols, interprofessional relationships, space, and consumer input. We are just now beginning to redefine patient teaching, discharge planning, cardiac rehabilitation, school nursing, and primary care as systems of care in which the major actors and the major activity is nurses and nursing. Studies of systems of care are to be advocated, complicated though they may be.

Virginia Henderson has been right on many things for a very long time. She is right in the quotations I used earlier in drawing our attention to the need to depend upon clinical insight to decide what kinds of things need studying and in what way. It is the experience of clinicians that allows us to define nursing practices as systems of care. It is the experience of nurses in practice that makes us question nursing rituals. It is nursing knowledge that makes us look toward increased study of chronic illness and the effect of nursing on patients with long-term disability for as nurses we find ourselves dealing with such patients more and more often. It is clinical judgment which makes us question convenient methodological approaches to studies of nursing productivity or the effects of nursing in primary care for we know that what a nurse practitioner does in a visit is simply not the same as what a physician does.

On the other hand, I do not think it is clinical wisdom which makes some nurse researchers advocate seriously curtailing all experimental designs until we have conducted enough exploratory studies to understand what the phenomenon is with which we are experimenting. Such reasoning comes, I believe, out of academic naiveté about the nature of nursing knowledge, an arrogance of intellectual elitism that ignores the practice field. Not only can we not wait to find out the results of exploratory studies, but it is simply a fact that nursing knowledge is not built linearly from the exploratory to the experimental, the descriptive to the prescriptive. It is also a fact that the richness of professional argument about methodology makes such arbitrary dictates unreal, ephemeral, and slightly eccentric. Nurses know not only about practice but about what effects practice.

Two themes which might be highlighted for the future are money and power. We will need in nursing research to add to conventional research designs, wherever possible, costs and cost-benefit analyses for we know in our very souls that when money becomes tight, the first to be cut will be nursing, whether it's in the federal research budget or in a hospital's attempts to live within cost-cutting regulations. And we also know that the development of nursing over the last 25 years, certainly fostered in part by nursing research, has brought nursing to the point of direct economic competition for the health care dollar as well as for the consciousness of the consumer.

And we shall need to pay attention to two other themes which I believe area crucial to our continuing development as a learned discipline. First, we shall need to learn to value diversity, whether diversity comes in polemics about what kind of nursing research to do, in tedious arguments about methodology or statistics, in the setting of priorities for future study, or in the breadth of our own intellectual interests. We shall need to value our colleagues' work, even when it is not in our own area of particular interest or when it may be, in our idiosyncratic eyes, imperfect. For there is a great deal of fascinating thinking and research going on in nursing these days. Even when I, like you, think a particular approach is not exciting, we forget, too often, that the value of nursing research is not only in its findings, it is also in its ability to provoke new thoughts, whether those thoughts lead us to follow-up research, to criticism, or to new conceptualization.

And the other thing we simply must do is to learn to know the scope and variety of nursing research. At a recent professional meeting Claire Fagin, Dean of the School of Nursing at the University of Pennsylvania, presented a magnificent keynote address in which she tied together vast amounts of research in nursing and nursing practice. She was applauded for her paper by the entire group, but in the question and answer session on the next day, one individual characterized the importance of Dr. Fagin's literature review as having retrieved fugitive research. This is simply a misstatement. The research upon which Dr. Fagin's paper was based is widely available to those who wish seriously to look for it. It happens that some of the best research in nursing is published in the *Journal of Nurse-Midwifery,* a publication which, according to its editor, has a circulation of only 2000. Specialty journals in nursing now abound and it should be the assignment of any thoughtful nurse to dip into journals outside of her own area of interest every once in a while for there is wonderful work being done and we cannot allow our need to specialize, important though it is, to blind us to equally important work in another specialty. ...

For many years, those who wrote thoughtfully about nursing research advocated collaborative research between nurses and members of other disciplines, particularly the social sciences and of late, physicians. At one time, it was necessary that such collaborative strategies be pushed for nurses themselves were as yet naïve about research methods and study designs and needed the collaboration of members of older, more sophisticated disciplines. Now, I am more concerned that nurses collaborate with each other, for I believe that will be the sign of the arrival of the next generation in nursing. When we begin to know and love each other's work, we will truly have reached professional maturity. Perhaps you could think now of making that notion part of the theme for your 50th anniversary.

ENDNOTES

1. Gortner, S., & Nahm, H. (1977). An overview of nursing research in the United States. *Nursing Research, 26*(1), 10–33.

2. Henderson, V. (1977). We've come a long way—but what of the direction? *Nursing Research, 26*(3), 163–4.

3. Henderson *op cit.*

PRACTICING RESEARCH—RESEARCHING PRACTICE

I became Dean of the Yale School of Nursing in July 1972, and while I continued to teach research methods throughout the 12½ years I was Dean, my involvement changed as I became party to political and policy contexts in nursing and outside.

*These years—the 1970s and 80s—were the years in which advanced practice in nursing took off and in which nursing research entered the mainstream of federal and foundation funding. I was increasingly being asked to speak to nursing research groups as (I think now) something of a maverick. I did not have a doctorate, yet I was speaking about nursing **research,** the province of the doctorally prepared.*

I tried always to put nursing research in its proper relationship to nursing practice, and now I knew something about health services research which gave even more energy to my notion of nursing's contribution. I did not think much of what I considered the ponderous over-intellectualizations in nursing theory and nursing diagnosis that sprang up in this period. Wiser heads turned the nursing diagnosis movement into nursing interventions and outcomes and the grand nursing theory movement into "middle range" theory and we stopped wasting a lot of time and talent on fruitless chases of semantic illusions.

The timing of this speech is just about when nursing started to get uppity in the late 1980s. At least I was hoping I could help push the discipline that way. It seemed to me that nursing research was drifting off again, away from practice. One way to bring it back was to mine the clinical nursing research that existed and hope that would inspire more.

I left the Deanery in January 1985 and returned to the faculty to begin to develop curriculum in policy. I continued to advise student theses and teach research methods. A sabbatical after I left the deanery gave me the opportunity to begin working in health services research with the team that had "found" (in their words) Diagnosis Related Groups (DRGs) at Yale. That was an eye-opening experience as this paper shows.

This speech was the keynote address at West Penn Hospital in Pittsburgh for their Nursing Research Day, February 24, 1989. I gave it again to the Medical College of Ohio School of Nursing in May that year. As always, I used the research at Yale as a base.

Research is good for a lot of things, including providing occasions to have research conferences. Before talking about what research is good for, however, it might be a good idea to put it into perspective. Because there are some things research is *not* good for.

Research will not make nursing's political problems go away nor even make them very much more understandable. Research alone won't make the public pay attention to us or change nursing's image. Research won't increase the value of the profession when there are interprofessional battles to be fought. Research won't make you smart. Research won't make you famous. If you work in a university, doing research and publishing it may get you tenure. If you are a graduate student, research may help you get a degree. Research won't make you rich, though, and research won't erode the public's notion that we are all empty-headed, bubble-hairdoed, intern-admiring, unthinking creatures who couldn't possibly have chosen nursing over the mystical opportunity to become a physician.

Research isn't all that hard, though it may occasionally be tedious; while research does take some training to do it well, training alone does not make good research. Research is, however, more than mere data collection—the gathering of numbers. ...

At the bottom line, all research does is answer questions; it may answer them more or less well depending on how well one has posed the question, adhered to the rules of scientific convention, and respected clinical relevance. But to expect research to solve the political problems of nursing, create an autonomous body of knowledge, make one smart, change the public image, or otherwise have an impact on the non-clinical problems we encounter daily is expecting too much of a good thing.

Research may provide information upon which decisions can be based. And as a general rule, decisions based on good information are likely to be better decisions than decisions based on mere opinion, tradition, the authority of the decision-maker, or other people's agendas. Yet research by itself cannot tell us at all whether we *should* let nurses interpret EKGs, *should* change the TPN dressings once a day, *should* set productivity standards for nurses or nurse practitioners, *should* set our admission criteria for schools of nursing differently, or *should* change to problem-oriented records. Problems of "shouldness" are policy questions which can be addressed by thoughtful analysis. But it is a mistake to think that empirical encounters with the world through data gathering carry within them the answers to these kinds of questions.

I will suggest to you today that research has *two* roles to play in life, and that both are expanding, as are our practice roles.

The first role, of course, is in the improvement of practice. Now, none of us in this room are all that old. Yet within our lifetimes, we have seen clinical nursing research grow from an ideal as Virginia Henderson put it in 1956— the study of the work rather than the workers—to an entire discipline. Most commentators count as a landmark the publication, in 1963, of Dumas and Leonard's study of the effect of preoperative preparation on postoperative vomiting. ...

That wasn't all that long ago. Before Dumas and Leonard, preoperative preparation was a shave and an enema. Now, preparation for surgery, and for other noxious events, as Jean Johnson[1] has called them, is increasingly precisely tuned to patient condition, including social supports, and a whole body of theory has grown up to explain different interventions and their consequences.

Before Elms[2] and Mahaffey[3] and Wolfer and Visintainer[4] and Visintainer and Wolfer[5] among others, admission to the hospital was taking away an adult's or child's clothes, introducing the patient to the roommates, and that was about it. Now, whole programs of pre-hospital preparation for children and adults have grown up, with salutary effects.

Before Bocknak[6] and McBride[7] and McCaffery[8] and others, a patient's complaint of pain was a signal to check the prn medication orders, and if enough time had passed, give out the pill or the injection and hope it worked. Now, there are alternatives to medication, and there are ways to measure the effects.

Before Hasselmeyer[9] and Barnard[10] and Anderson,[11] premature babies were fed and changed and turned and occasionally held, but mostly they just lay there, growing silently. Now we know the effects of early infant stimulation on subsequent physical and psychological growth and early discharge as well.

And it is to be hoped that next year we can say that before Brooten,[12] it was not thought possible to let low birthweight babies go home until they had reached some magic weight in grams. Now we know differently, when nursing support can be provided for the parents at home, we know the enormous possibilities of saving scarce resources.

I take as evidence of the effects of nursing research in practice the fact that the *AJN* began last summer to run whole collections of brief reports of research which can change practice, in a regular series called "Working Smart."[13] The first installment told us that protective isolation may do more psychological harm than it does physical good, and that the outcomes of patients in protective isolation are no different than when a patient is treated regularly in a room with another patient, so long as caregivers follow hand-washing procedures. And it tells us that if we do the traditional shave prep the night before surgery, we bring the postop infection rate down to 2%. If we use a depilatory, we bring it down to 1.9%. And if we do nothing but have patients take antimicrobial showers the night before and the morning of surgery, we bring it down to 1%. And we know that stripping chest tubes can be detrimental and is indicated only when there is fresh blood in the tube and clots can be seen. In fact, stripping the whole length of the chest tube raises the negative pressure to more than ten times what it is normally set at. And withholding feeding in the early postnatal period in babies without respiratory difficulty may not only be baseless, it may be contraindicated, especially if the infant is hypoglycemic. Even ritualistically counting respirations has been questioned, and so has daily baths and weighing diapers of all babies, according to work cited in "Working Smart."

And we know that compliance is not nearly as simple as we once thought, nor could it happen the same way in patients who are internally controlled versus those who are externally controlled.[14] And we know that clinical judgment and patient satisfaction are increased when outpatient clinicians [nurse practitioners] pay attention to what the patient expects from the service and to what the present symptoms are attributed.[15]

One could go on and on and on. These kinds of studies are pushing forward the boundaries of our knowledge of practice and the effects of our work, and when converted into textbooks, lectures, supervised practice, and continuing education, they change the nature of nursing.

But there are other kinds of studies that have an effect on nursing as well, and those are the studies that are leading us to rediscover the nature of the work. I include in this category some of the work in nursing diagnosis, especially when it focuses, and it is increasingly, on clinical judgment. And I would add to that the work of Benner,[16] Tanner,[17] Pyle and Stern[18] on nursing expertness. These studies are helping us dig deep into the so-called intuition of nurses, to figure out how we do what we do and how it so often works, so invisibly. We are increasingly asking nurses in practice what bothers them, what insight they have into the work, what questions, observations, and knowledge informs them. And the work gets better and better.

There should be no area of patient experience that is out of bounds for nursing to investigate, since we are responsible for understanding how people experience illness, disease, disability, recovery, diagnosis, treatment, surgery, and discharge, as well as for how many resources are used in the episode of care. ...

We need to know about early newborn development as much as neonatologists or pediatricians do, perhaps more so, since we are in a position to help parents understand and adapt to the capacities of the newborn, thus promoting bonding, according to our literature. We need to know how social support works. We need to know how women experience infertility, violence, depression, and body image. We need to know how people make decisions about their health or about their children, including not only having them, but circumcising their boy babies. We even need to address holes in clinical knowledge you would think by now would be filled.

My favorite example is the length of a pregnancy. One would think by now we would know that, but it turns out, according to some nurse researchers, that we don't.[19] In fact, it turns out that there is a much wider range of "normal" than has been thought, and that is important when decisions are being made to induce labor because the woman is "overdue." We need to know how adolescents experience the pressures of growth, development, and choices. We need to know how people experience diagnostic labels, including mental illness. We need to know the capacities of the very old, the very young, and everybody in between, because our sister and brother nurses are in all the places where this information is important. ...

This kind of clinical nursing research relates to the first of nursing's two functions—the personal care, including prevention and health promotion—of people. But that is only one of nursing's roles and thus, one of nursing research's roles. We have another—the tending of the entire environment within which nursing takes place. ...

The relationship between nursing and technology has been written and spoken about endlessly as high-tech, high-touch. That dichotomy misses an important connection between nursing and the use of technology. It is becoming increasingly obvious that nursing is in a position to monitor, even dictate, the use of technology so that it is appropriate and cost-effective. ...

Just last year, an extraordinarily powerful study of intensive care was published by the George Washington University team, which includes a Senior Nurse Scientist, Betty Draper.[20] The team studied some 30 intensive care units throughout the country, looking at mortality rates, among other things, and controlling for patient condition with a measure they have developed called APACHE (Acute Physiological Assessment, Chronic Health Evaluation). They found, to their surprise, that there were wide variations in mortality rates, in spite of having patients who were just as compromised. They found that the variable that most explained the difference between the high and low mortality units was the authority of the nurses for participating in patient care decisions, and the authority of the head nurse to close beds if the load became too heavy. In the unit with the lowest mortality, primary nursing is practiced and there are clinical nurse specialists. One physician directs the medical care and the clinicians work together as a team. In the unit with the highest mortality, the researchers could not even get the physicians and nurses in the same room together for an interview.

There are other examples. Ultrasound is ordered during pregnancy for a number of purposes, including detection of intra-uterine growth retardation. One nurse studied the use of this procedure to determine its efficacy and found that in more than half the cases studied, the results were useless because the sonography was not ordered within the "window" of gestational age when it means something, and serial ultrasounds, required for definitive diagnosis, were not requested.[21] Surely nurses can participate in the decisions for testing, and surely nurse-midwives make them. ...

A recent article discussed the MUGA scan, a very high technology diagnostic procedure. The article usefully discusses the technique itself and what it shows. What is more interesting is that the nurse author explicitly says that it is a nursing responsibility to be sure that the pre-scan orders are correct and that the MUGA has been ordered for things it is likely to be able to accomplish.[22]

There is a whole body of research on tube feedings, done by nurse researchers, that can be drawn upon to make the technology work better for what it is intended for.[23] The research includes everything from exactly how to measure the portion of the tube to be inserted, to the effects, if any, of warming the feedings. And an article published only this week analyzes the practice of enteral feedings in one institution and shows the general imprecision of the technological use. Suggestions for changes in practice, both nursing and medical practice, emerge.[24]

Nurses are also in a position to invent or study alternatives to high technology. One nurse, for example, looked at the possibility of using certain EKG leads for early diagnosis of right ventricular wall infarction, for apparently, the treatment is quite different depending on where the infarction is, and that would be nice to know, early.[25] She found that it was possible to detect reliably the difference through one particular EKG lead, obviating the necessity for blood pool imaging studies (or whatever it is they do these days!).

Other nurses have studied nipple stimulation for contraction stress testing, as an alternative to oxytocin injection, which must be done in a delivery room, and which has the potential to bring on premature labor.[26] These studies have demonstrated that reliable and accurate non-stress tests can be achieved in a majority of women with this non-invasive procedure, which saves time, money, danger and stress.

Andrews has been studying the possibility of rotating the fetus from a posterior or transverse lie before the head engages in the pelvis.[27] She uses a combination of positioning exercises and the early results are promising.

And, of course, there is a whole body of literature in nurse-midwifery that effectively documents decreases in cesarean section rates and the use of forceps in nurse-midwifery practices.[28]

And finally, there is Jones' landmark study which documented the effect of Primary Nursing in decreasing the length of stay of kidney transplant patients.[29] Technology assessment is fundable too, with specific funding sources.

Technology is one way of talking about the environment within which practice happens. *The reason for the existence of the modern hospital (or nursing home or mental hospital or home care agency) is to deliver nursing care.* That suggests the nursing research directed at testing, evaluating and otherwise understanding the context for practice—what others have called health services research—is as much an agenda for nursing as patient care or clinical research.

Health Services Research has been defined as "organized, rigorous, inquiry concerned with the effectiveness of the delivery of health care to groups of people," and in general, it concerns itself with access to care, quality, quantity, and cost. And the relationships among them, known as efficiency and effectiveness.[30]

Health services research traces its roots to the sanitary revolution of the 1840s, when the concern was public health. The development of health services research was held back until there could be quantitative methods to measure not only mortality, but morbidity. And that depended upon the classification of cases. Disease classification, however, depended upon a workable theory of the causation, transmission, and natural history of disease, beyond the miasma theory so dear to the heart of Florence Nightingale. Disease classification eventually came to pass and morbidity could be studied; methodologies and statistical techniques still need to be evolved to deal with the problems of measuring effects.

Despite her wrongheaded and stubborn belief in the miasma theory (which actually worked, in India), Florence Nightingale deserves her reputation as the "passionate statistician." She was among the first to use mortality rates in comparing groups, as she compared deaths in Scutari with death of the military in England, when they weren't even fighting a war. And she argued forcefully for morbidity classifications, so that geographic regions, or hospitals, or wards within hospitals, could be compared. Indeed, her arguments form the basis for what we now know and love as DRGs (Diagnosis Related Groups).

While there is still important work to be done regarding disease classification, transmission, and so on, as the AIDS epidemic has taught us, health services research shifted after most infectious disease was understood and today the targets for such research increasingly include costs and the cost/quality equation.

Health services research can be classified simultaneously by the time frame of the study—prospective or retrospective—by its purpose and by its method. Since most health services research deals with large groups or large problems it is primarily retrospective, using existing data of various kinds.

For example, a graduate student in nurse-midwifery, who had been a public health nurse in Holyoke, Massachusetts, and who intended to return there after her degree, became concerned along with others that the infant death rate and prematurity rates for Holyoke were the highest in Massachusetts.[31] She also knew, from the nursing research literature, that prenatal care is the one variable found most to decrease low birth weight, which is the variable most associated with neonatal death. But it would not be enough merely to find out what the birth weights were for all of Holyoke (and it would have been difficult in any event), if one was interested in planning for services to be delivered there, as she was.

So she took all of the births in Holyoke for one year in one hospital, which represented the majority of the births, and examined the relationship between prenatal care and neonatal outcome. But knowing the town, from her public health nursing experience, she also included ethnicity and census tract of residence in her data collection.

She found the expected relationship between number of prenatal visits and neonatal outcome, but what she found that was even more valuable was a highly significant relationship between census track and ethnicity, and between those and outcome. Specifically, she found that for the census tracts with high proportions of Hispanic people, the neonatal outcome was considerably less good. That information can lead to more targeted planning for services to the particular population in the most need, and for Spanish-speaking personnel to deliver them.

We have examples of prospective studies as well, but they are fewer because they are so expensive to conduct. The classic study of Lewis and Resnick of a nurse clinic for chronically ill adults is one such instance.[32] And the experimental study of nurse-midwifery at the University of Mississippi Medical Center by Slome and others is another.[33] There, low-risk obstetric patients were randomly assigned to nurse-midwives or resident physicians and outcomes were examined. There were no significant differences except a higher rate of forceps delivery in the resident group and a longer second stage of labor, and a higher rate of appointment-keeping in the nurse-midwifery group.

Health services research can also be classified by its purpose: basic research, clinical research, and developmental or R and D studies.

The research that eventually developed DRGs is an example of basic, methodological research. And there is research going on in nursing today to develop patient classification systems for use in examining resource consumption. There are studies going on now to try to develop patient classes for long term care and for home care, classes which can be defined by relatively homogeneous needs for nursing. In long term care and home care, *nursing* is the resource consumed.

Some clinical nursing research is also health services research, when the service is conceived of as a "system of care." This kind of health services research is intended to provide solutions to particular problems; the only difference is that the outcome is measured in terms of groups and the service in general is more than a single nursing intervention.

The studies of nurse-midwifery effectiveness might fall into this category.[34] That body of literature generally conceives of the independent variable as nurse-midwifery itself, rather than as definably separate activities and outcomes from nurse-midwifery are compared, sometimes with outcomes from conventional obstetrical services. Similarly, the evaluation studies of nurse practitioners might be considered clinical health services research, especially when they deal with outcomes for patients served. And those studies have involved nurses both as subjects and as investigators.

Then, there are developmental or R and D projects. Here, previous research is used to propose production of useful materials, devices, or systems, and performance criteria are set in advance. The research on primary nursing might fall in this category, especially when length of stay is used as the criterion variable. A study in Georgia in which nurse-midwives were put into place to serve a rural population in three counties, which the four contiguous counties used as comparison is another example.[35] Here, the criterion variable also included costs and the results showed a cost saving of over $1 million in the nurse-midwifery counties.

And health services research can be classified by its design—experimental or non-experimental. The Lewis and Resnik Kansas study of nurse clinics was an experimental study, as were the so-called Burlington randomized clinical trials of the nurse practitioner.[36]

Descriptive or analytic non-experimental studies might include the School Health Project supported by the Robert Wood Johnson Foundation.[37] There, school-based health services were put in place in selected states and information on the kinds of problems seen and their outcomes was gathered. Again, the services provided were mostly provided by school nurse practitioners. A good deal of the early research about nurse practitioners was descriptive, reporting the scope of practices, number of people seen, and general acceptance of the new role.

Comparative studies which are not experimental are also not uncommon. Comparisons of primary nursing units with other units, of nursing services with other services, of nurse-midwives with physicians, for example. Or increasingly, studies of clinician caseloads. For example, Hays studied hospice patients to learn if those patients who had an inpatient hospice experience were different from those whose experience was entirely as a home-care client. She found differences which suggested that the present reimbursement formula which dictates that hospices deliver 80% of their services as home care may not be reasonable.[38]

Hamman studied the caseloads of nurse practitioners, faculty attending physicians, and resident physicians in the same setting. She found reliable differences between groups in both the process of care and the caseloads themselves. Nurse practitioner patients tended to have more diagnoses recorded and were more often members of ethnic minority groups. Resident patients were less sick than either of the comparison groups.[39]

There is an elegant comparative study which will appear in the nursing literature just as soon as I can get my student to get it out.[40] She looked at the effects of short staffing on patients, controlling for DRG. She compared two units in the same hospital, one which had a demonstrably short staff, by the hospital's own standards, for a 3 month period, and one which had adequate staff for the same period. Both units housed the same kinds of patients, and both units were budgeted for the number of staff considered adequate—this was not a case of staffing cuts. She found that there were more complications on the short-staffed unit, and the complications were generally preventable: aspiration pneumonitis, nosocomial infections, for instance. And she found that there were longer lengths of stay on the short-staffed unit and significantly more patient days beyond the geometric mean length of stay per DRG. Doing a quick and dirty financial analysis (this student is also getting her degree in management), she found that for the money it cost the hospital for the longer lengths of stay, four FTE nurses could have been hired.

Now, why make a point of all this?

The purpose of the modern health care system is to provide nursing care. Nursing does not occur in a vacuum, however, and the tending of the environment for nursing to occur is an important responsibility. If research is to help nursing advance, by making the practice better, then that part of the "practice" that tends the environment is an appropriate target for nursing research. Indeed, the funding priorities for the National Center for Health Services Research (NCHSR) [now the Agency for Health services Research and Quality, AHRQ] read like an agenda for nursing: health promotion, illness prevention, the organization and delivery of health services. Yet, in the 4 years that I sat on one of the research review committees for NCHSR, I don't think we saw more than about six proposals from nurse researchers. It is encouraging that the new National Center for Nursing Research has a branch within it to support studies of nursing systems.[41]

No nursing speech is complete without an exhortation to do more, better, so here is one.

The growing realization that the health care system is nursing might inspire us to efforts not only to build up the knowledge base from which our personal care practice springs, but also to build our base of knowledge and contribution about the contexts and environments for care.

One of those contexts is health policy. Policy-related research might well become a new subfield within nursing research, a field in which the clinical wisdom we have worked so hard to gather through our clinical work and research might inform and test health policy. The hospice study I alluded to earlier is one example. The possibilities of using nursing research in the service of improving the context for practice are legion.

There is a proposal now being considered to change the present requirement for RN staffing in dialysis units and eliminate RNs, substituting LPNs and dialysis technicians, as a cost-saving device, under Medicare. What needs to be studied is obvious, perhaps. Comparisons of units presently staffed with RNs with units who have substituted already (many of which are proprietary) would be in order. But such comparisons should deal not only with whatever measures of quality of care are possible (mortality, inpatient admissions, infections, length of stay on the caseload), but also we need caseload descriptions. Dialysis has been called "the first DRG," with prospectively set rates for reimbursement. But that was done in the days when dialysis was nearly exclusively for kidney disease. Now it is also used for everything from poisoning to diabetes to schizophrenia, and the casemix within dialysis units needs some work.

One of these days, the Health Care Financing Administration [now the Centers for Medicare/Medicaid Services] will get tired of the foot dragging of organized psychiatry about prospective payment and simply implement DRG-based rates in psychiatric services. Yet we already know that the psychiatric DRGs are not good predictors of length of stay. What is? My guess is that it is the behaviors to which psychiatric nurses pay attention, not the diagnosis at all, and it would behoove us to get some studies done and some data out upon which decisions for payment, as well as quality of care decisions, could be made.

And we need many more studies of costs of care. Right now, a target should be the cost-effectiveness of nurses in ambulatory care, since there is already a payment commission chartered by Congress to look into the possibility of changes in how Medicare Part B is administered. Now would be the time to get in on the ground floor of those policy decisions, with some data.

And we need data about what it really costs hospitals (if, actually, anything) for the education of student and graduate student nurses, as the Prospective Payment Commission winds up to eliminate the pass-through for medical education, which now includes nursing as well.

And we need studies of the effectiveness, casemix, and costs of nurse practitioners in HMOs, as we argue for substitutability. And we need more studies of the effects of prescriptive authority when it is granted to nurses. And we need studies of discharge planning, including assessment and placement of patients in long-term care and home care. And we need nurses to study the effects of the implicit policy of not attending to children in favor of the elderly, who can advocate for themselves. And we need to know a whole lot more about how the care of the chronically mentally ill can be organized and delivered.

There is a shortage of nurses upon us, and it is likely to get worse. That is both an occasion for research and an occasion within which to assert our truth: that nursing is two things—personal care and the tending of the entire environment. It is my hope (perhaps fantasy) that the policy attention that is being drawn to the nursing shortage will finally bring nursing publicly to where we have always privately known we were: the very core of the health care delivery system. When that happens, our research will be there, and I hope you will be too.

ENDNOTES

1. Johnson, J. (1984). Coping with elective surgery. *Annual Review of Nursing Research (Vol. 2)*. New York: Springer, pp. 107–132.

2. Elms, R. (1964). Effects of varied nursing approaches during hospital admission: an exploratory study. *Nursing Research, 13*(6), 266–268; Elms, R., & Leonard, R.C. (1966). Effects of nursing approaches during admission. *Nursing Research, 15*(1), 39–48.

3. Mahaffey, P.R. (1965). The effects of hospitalization on children admitted for tonsillectomy and adenoidectomy. *Nursing Research, 14*(1), 12–16.

4. Wolfer, J.A., & Visintainer, M. (1975). Pediatric surgical patients' and parents' stress responses and adjustment as a function of psychological preparation and stress point care. *Nursing Research, 24*(6), 244–256.

5. Visintainer, M., & Wolfer, J.A. (1975). Psychological preparation for surgical pediatric patients: effect on children's and parents' stress response and adjustment. *Pediatrics, 56*(2), 187–202.

6. Bocknak, M.A. (1962). Comparison of two types of nursing activity on the relief of pain. *Innovations in nurse patient relationships: Automatic or reasoned nursing actions.* New York: American Nurses Association, 5–11.

7. McBride, M.A.B. (1967). Nursing approach, pain and relief: an exploratory experiment. *Nursing Research, 16*(6), 337–340.

8. McCaffery, M., & Moss, F. (1967). Nursing intervention for bodily pain. *AJN, 67*(12), 1224–1226.

9. Hasselmeyer, E. (1967). *Behavior patterns of premature infants.* Bethesda, MD: USDHEW, PHS Publication #840.

10. Barnard, K. (1983). Nursing research related to infants and young children. *Annual Review of Nursing Research (Vol. 1)*, New York: Springer, pp. 3–26.

11. Anderson, G., & Raff, B. (Eds) (1979). *Newborn Behavioral Organization: Nursing Research and Implications.* New York: Alan R. Liss.

12. Brooten, D., Kumer, S., Brown, L.P., Butts, P., Finkler, S.A., Bakewell-Sachs, S., Gibbons, A., & Delivoria-Papadopoulos, M. (1986). A randomized clinical trial of early hospital discharge and home follow-up of very-low-birthweight infants. *New England Journal of Medicine, 315*(15), 934–938.

13. "Working Smart" (1986). *AJN, 86*(6), 679–684.

14. Lowery, B., & DuCette, J.P. (1976). Disease related learning and disease control in diabetics as a function of locus of control. *Nursing Research, 25*(5), 358–362.

15. Molde, S., & Baker, D.J. (1985). Explaining primary care visits. *Image, 17*(3), 72–76; Molde, S. (1986). Understanding patients' agendas. *Image, 18*(4), 145–147.

16. Benner, P. (1985). *From Novice to Expert.* Menlo Park, Ca: Addison Wesley.

17. Benner, P. & Tanner, C. (1987). How expert nurses use intuition. *AJN, 87*(1), 23–34.

18. Pyle, S.H., & Stern, P.N. (1983). The nursing gestalt in critical care nursing. *Image, 15*(2), 51–67.

19. Nichols, D.W. (1985). Clinical management of size/dates discrepancy. *Journal of Nurse Midwifery, 30*(1), 15–24; Nichols, C.W. (1985). Postdate pregnancy: Part I: Literature review. *Journal of Nurse Midwifery, 30*(4), 222–239.

20. Knaus, W.A., Draper, E.A., Wagner, D.P., & Zimmerman, J.E. (1986). An evaluation of outcome from intensive care in major medical centers. *Annals of Internal Medicine, 104*(2), 410–418.

21. Goodhart, L.J. (1976). The effect of modern technology on clinical practice: Ultrasound in obstetrics. Masters Thesis, Yale University School of Nursing, New Haven, CT.

22. Funk, M. (1983). Preparing the patient for a MUGA scan. *Critical Care Nurse, 3*(5), 57–61.

23. Moore, M.C., Guenter, P.A., & Bender, J.H. (1986). Nutrition-related nursing research. *Image, 18*(1), 18–21.

24. Flynn, K.T., Celantano-Norton, L., & Fisher, R. (1987). Enteral tube feeding: indications, practices and outcomes. *Image, 19*(1), 16–19.

25. Funk, M. (1986). Diagnosis of right ventricular infarction with right precordial EKG leads. *Heart and Lung, 15*(6), 562–572.

26. Summers, L. (1983). Nipple stimulation to induce uterine contractions for antepartum fetal heart rate testing. Masters Thesis, Yale University School of Nursing, New Haven, CT.

27. Andrews, C.M. (1981). Nursing intervention to change a malpositioned fetus. *Advances in Nursing Science, 3*(2), 53–66.

28. Diers, D. (1982). The future of nurse-midwives in American health care. In Aiken, L (Ed) *Nursing in the '80's*, pp. 159–180. Philadelphia: Lippincott.

29. Jones, K. (1975). Study documents effects of primary nursing on renal transplant patients. *Hospitals, 49*(24), 85–89.

30. Thompson, J.D. (1977). *Applied Health Services Research.* Lexington, MA: D.C. Heath (Lexington Books).

31. Frey, J.M. (1985). Factors influencing perinatal outcome in Holyoke, MA. Masters Thesis, Yale University School of Nursing, New Haven, CT.

32. Lewis, C., & Resnick, B. (1967). Nurse clinics and progressive ambulatory patient care. *New England Journal of Medicine, 277*(5), 1236–1241.

33. Slome, C., Wetherbee, H., Daly, M., Christensen, K., Mesley, M., & Thiede, H. (1976). Effectiveness of certified nurse midwives: a prospective evaluation study. *American Journal of Obstetrics and Gynecology, 124*(1), 177–182.

34. Diers, D., & Burst, H.V. (1983). Effectiveness of policy-related research: nurse-midwifery as case study. *Image, 15*(3), 68–74.

35. Reid, M.L., & Morris, J.F. (1979). Perinatal care and cost-effectiveness: changes in health expenditures and birth outcomes following the establishment of a nurse-midwife program. *Medical Care, 27*(3), 491–500.

36. Spitzer, W.O., Sackett, D.L., Sibley, J.C., et al. (1974). The Burlington randomized trial of the nurse practitioner. *New England Journal of Medicine, 290*(2), 251–256; Sackett, D., Spitzer, W., Gent, M., & Roberts, R. (1974). The Burlington randomized trial of the nurse practitioner: health outcomes of patients. *Annals of Internal Medicine, 80*(1), 137–142.

37. Meeker, R.J., DeAngelis, C., Berman, B., Freeman, H.E., & Oda, D. (1986). A comprehensive school health initiative. *Image, 18*(3), 86–91.

38. Hays, J. (1986). Hospice policy and patterns of care. *Image, 18*(3), 92–97.

39. Diers, D., Hamman, A., & Molde, S. (1986). Complexity of ambulatory care: nurse practitioner and physician caseloads. *Nursing Research, 35*(5), 310–314.

40. Flood, S.D. (1987). The effect of nurse staffing on patient outcome. Masters Thesis, Yale University School of Nursing, New Haven, CT.; Flood, S.D., & Diers, D. (1988). Nurse staffing and patient outcome. *Nursing Management, 19*(5), 34–53.

41. Merritt, D. (1986). The National Center for Nursing Research. *Image, 18*(3), 84–85.

RICHNESS IN PRACTICE,
DIVERSITY IN RESEARCH

This was an invited presentation as the Keynote Address to the ANA Council of Nurse Researchers' meeting in Chicago, September 28, 1989. It was a distinct honor to have been asked to address this group, especially as I still did not have a doctorate. By now, my opinions about nursing research were well known.

*In this speech, I was trying to beat the by-then well organized mainstream nursing research community over the head with my disappointment in the relative lack of nursing research commitment to actual studies of **nursing practice**, a horse I still will not consider dead. I suspect a replication of this little study I did would produce very similar findings in 2004, more is the pity. The studies about nursing practice outcomes are often being published outside the mainstream nursing research literature, in the health services, management, and information science literature as well as the "mainstream" medical journals. Those are the journals that influence policy. Point made.*

Well, no. The point is more complicated. Some of the complexity is hinted at here in terms of funding and other external pressures on nurses as researchers. I hope the humor and sarcasm in this piece come across as loving and understanding.

Occasions such as this are opportunities to celebrate progress and project the future. And we have much to celebrate as we note the creation of a Center for Nursing Research within the National Institutes of Health, as we count the growth of doctoral programs in nursing, as we see nurses involved in research review decisions in various of the federal agencies, as we monitor the flow of funds for research from foundations and corporations and national societies, and as we try to keep up with the number of professional publications, research conferences, newsletters, abstracts, think tanks, and study tours. Occasions such as this give us a chance to take a snapshot of things as they are today, to compare to past predictions and future choices.

Exactly 30 years ago, Leo Simmons and Virginia Henderson completed their review of 50 years of nursing research, published four years later.[1] At the end of their review project, Virginia embarked on the collection subsequently published as the *Nursing Studies Index,* a project that was to take 5 years. It actually took 12. Virginia worked at Yale with two primary assistants, Mrs. Laura McCarthy and Mrs. Elsie Mowe, and later, after Mrs. McCarthy retired, Mrs. Anne Bock. When I first came to the Yale School of Nursing, Virginia was deep in the project, working in one large office in the School, in the center of which were grey metal file tubs filled with handwritten IBM cards. Tea and cookies were served every afternoon, in china cups, and every Monday morning fresh flowers were delivered. At the completion of sections of the report, sherry appeared. It was a very English kind of atmosphere, with these three elder ladies working away quietly to record *all* of the literature about nurses and nursing. There were no computers, and all of the work of sorting and classifying the nursing literature since 1900 was done by hand without Medline, xerox, or Fax. The results of that project, besides the 20 pounds or so of four published volumes, was also to set us on a changed course, away from studies of the workers, to studies of the work.[2] Miss Henderson wrote that editorial the year I entered nursing school; she was 59 at the time and had already retired once. In November this year [1989] she will be 92. We won't discuss how old I am.

The point is only that within my professional lifetime, which doesn't seem all that long, research as a valued activity in nursing has grown beyond adolescence. It might still be a little too young for a mid-life crisis, which is probably inevitable. It's a good time to take stock. ...

Janice Gay and colleagues surveyed faculty of doctoral programs in nursing to identify the journals most often depended upon in teaching at the doctoral level.[3] With remarkable consistency, the same five journals were named: *Nursing Research, Advances in Nursing Science, Image, Research in Nursing and Health,* and the *Western Journal of Nursing Research.* Some 50 additional journals ranging from the *New England Journal of Medicine* to *Qualitative Sociology* were nominated. But the consensus on the five most frequently mentioned journals suggests that they are the "mainstream" of contemporary nursing's intellectual work and thus they formed the sample for the analysis reported here.

I reviewed the last 5 years of all five of the named journals—1984–1988. Letters to the editor, book reviews, comments on published articles, and editorials were eliminated.

The research questions had to do with describing this whole body of literature as well as with changes over time in the research. Articles were first classified as research or not, with several distinctions among the non-research articles. Then, the research articles were further analyzed by type of study, by whether the study dealt with patients or not, and then by categories of samples. Studies of nurses were further subdivided, as I will discuss later. The five journals are combined in the counts here. ...

TABLE 1 ARTICLES PUBLISHED 1984–1988 IN LEADING NURSING JOURNALS

Articles by category	Research 52.8%	Methods 18.9%	Concepts 8.9%	Prof Issues 4.7%	Reviews 4.6%	Theory 4.3%	Educ 2.9%	Hx 2.3%
Articles by study design		Descriptive/correl. 83.7%			Experimental 10.8%		Qualitative 5.6%	
Articles by population			Patients 55%				Not patients 45%	
Studies of nurses	Students 39.2%		Clin. Judgment 34.9%		Attitudes 20.5%		Faculty 5.4%	

There were 1055 articles entered into the analysis and in general, the number of published pieces increased from 182 in 1984 to 236 in 1988. The number of research articles also increased from slightly under half (47.2%) in 1984 to slightly over half (53.8%) in 1988. The majority of articles were research pieces; the second largest category was methodological articles, often instrument development or testing. The review articles more than doubled from just over 2% in 1984 to just under 6% in 1988. Included in this category were meta-analyses as well as review of a body of literature.

Conceptual/descriptive essays decreased over the period by two-thirds, from about 16% to about 6%. "Professional development" articles decreased as well from 6% to about 3%. These articles dealt primarily with computer applications and similar topics. Theoretical articles represented about 3.8% of all articles through 1987, with a hop to about 6% in 1988. The number of articles about education or curriculum decreased and most of them were about teaching research. There were 24 historical or biographical articles, or 2.3% of the total. Most of them appeared in the last 2 years studied. ...

Putting aside the non-research, history, and biographical articles, we can look at what kinds of research are going on. The first cut was to look at study design—qualitative or quantitative. For this and subsequent analysis of content, the sample is the 558 research articles.

I divided the quantitative articles into descriptive (including correlational and quasi-experimental) and experimental. The very large majority of studies were descriptive—83.2%. Qualitative studies reached their peak in 1987, when they accounted for 10.6% of all research in these journals in that year, falling back to 4.7% in 1988. The peak was primarily due to a special issue of *Advances* on qualitative research. The most remarkable trend line was the experimental studies. In 1984, they represented fully one-fourth (25.6%) of all studies, but dropped to only 5.3% in 1987.

Who was studied was a simple dichotomy: persons identified as patients—people entered in the health care system and its settings or not. Non-patients also includes samples who were not people—animals, or latex gloves, or IV solutions. Overall, just over half of the studies dealt with patient groups (56.5%). But there is an interesting trend over the time period. The number of studies dealing with patients has dropped and the number of studies of other entities has grown, and the greatest difference is in the first year studied when nearly two-thirds of the articles included patient subjects. By 1988, only slightly over half did.

Following Henderson's injunction, I looked at the category of non-patient studies to see how many were studies of the workers rather than the work. About one-third (29.6%) of total studies were about either nurses as students, as employed persons, or as faculty, which represents two-thirds of the non-patient studies. However, the category that most worried Henderson—studies of nurses' attitudes toward various things—is not the largest.

Of the 166 studies here, over one-third were about nurses as clinicians exercising professional judgment; slightly more were about student nurses. Only about one-fifth were attitude studies and they represent only 6.1% of all studies.

To examine the studies about patients, I built up a set of categories from a qualitative examination of the articles. First there were studies that dealt with persons theoretically "at risk," but not presently patients. A typical sample might be a study of variables predisposing to obesity, or a study of health behaviors of children defined as at risk for coronary disease. Many of the studies in this class could be considered health promotion studies. Then, the categories divided themselves into age groups, developmental stages, social roles, or illness categories. Thus, I classified studies according to their population: "at risk", newborns and infants with a separate category for low birth weight or preterm infants, children, adolescents (with an additional category for adolescent pregnancy), abortion, pregnancy, labor and delivery, mothering, fathering, caregiving, ill adults (acute or chronic and including studies of bereavement, survival from disaster and family coping), then the elderly, with a separate category for the confused elderly/Alzheimer's, and finally, a category for studies of mentally ill persons which included studies of depression in older persons or in new mothers.

In rank order, the samples most often included were acutely ill adults, followed by the "at risk" group, then chronically ill adults, then parents, mothers, fathers, caregivers, then pregnant women, then the elderly. No other group accounted for more than 10% of the studies. In the acute illness category, the most frequent conditions included were cardiovascular. In the chronic illness category, the most often studied were hypertension and oncological conditions. Of the studies of the elderly, the majority were of non-institutionalized, often healthy, old persons.

There were a few noticeable trends. Studies of the acutely ill decreased by half across the period while studies of low birth weight or preterm infants increased five-fold (although the numbers remain small). Studies of adolescents, which did not begin to appear until 1986, tripled. Studies of the elderly decreased by half, and studies of parenting and caregiving doubled.

As I was going through the journals, I kept a running count of studies which dealt with publicly or professionally perceived issues of importance. For example, in these 5 years, only two involved persons with AIDS. Only five reports singled out domestic violence. Slightly under 2% focused on the use of technology, including an interesting few which tested alternatives to technological intervention. Six explicitly cast the research problem in policy terms. Only four had anything at all to do with costs or money. Precisely one study dealt with DRGs.

This exercise ended with data from 1988 and only with the published literature in which there is a certain lag time. Therefore, I applied the same methodology to the abstracts of papers accepted for presentation at this conference. I was sent 77 accepted abstracts, and since this is a research conference, they all were either research studies or methodological pieces.

Of the research papers, 8.5% are qualitative, 3% higher than in the 5 year review. About 72% are descriptive/correlational, compared to over 83% in the literature reviewed, and about 20% are experimental, compared to half that in the published literature. More interestingly, almost two-thirds (62.7%) are studies of patients. Less than half (11 of 25) of the non-patient studies were about nurses, and they were almost equally divided between studies of professional performance and attitudes, with no studies of student nurses at all. Studies of acutely ill persons were the most numerous, followed, as in the literature reviewed, by studies of "at risk" groups, pregnant women, and the chronically ill (including a goodly number of studies of terminally ill persons). Newborns took fifth place instead of studies of parenting or caregiving. In this one set of papers, there are five dealing with AIDS, three on Alzheimers and related conditions, two on infanticide or sexual victimization. Four deal with applications or evaluations of technology, and two explicitly mention money.

Now, this is all simply descriptive. And obviously, there are many other journals which publish research.

If—and legitimate questions can be raised—if the literature contained in the journals most often read and assigned by doctoral faculty is any kind of definition of the mainstream of nursing research, what can we conclude about it?

The relative number of research articles and methodological articles has stayed about the same over the 5 year period. But the number of review and theory articles has increased, while the number of conceptual essays and educational articles has fallen. Perhaps this is a mark of the growing sophistication of the field, that it is now possible to summarize and synthesize research production into analytic reviews or evolving theories, particularly of the "middle range" type. Data-based comment has taken the place of arm-chair theorizing, surely a sign of intellectual progress.

The number of history or biography pieces is still quite small, but they only began to appear in the mainstream literature in the last 2 years of this survey. There is an encouraging move toward placing nursing and our history in social and policy contexts, and away from chronology. The more our history can be recovered, the less we will be forced to repeat it. Despite the growing interest in nursing history, as shown by the creation of two separate national organizations and a Center for the Study of Nursing History (to say nothing of several recent conferences), there are as yet few educational resources within nursing for serious scholarship in nursing history, and fewer financial supports. The study of history is at the bottom of ANA's research priority list. ...

If one can judge from the manuscripts that cross my desk, the biggest intellectual argument in nursing today is about the relative merits of qualitative or quantitative research, about knowledge arrived at by induction or deduction, and the related issues about "good science," phenomenology, critical theory, and epistemology. Perhaps what one senses as a growing acceptance of methods and approaches that are not traditional reductionist logical positivism is responsible for the marked decline in experimental studies and the slow rise of qualitative methods.

As a graduate student, I was part of the beginnings of appreciation for clinical experimentation in nursing. I was with Rhetaugh Dumas the day she got a call from Lucille Notter at *Nursing Research* saying her ground-breaking article with Robert Leonard had been accepted for publication.[4] That study, you will recall, was a classical experimental design with a randomly assigned experimental group who received special preoperative preparation, and a control group who did not, and the dependent variable was vomiting in the recovery room. While that article reads naïve these days, it has been credited with starting a movement toward studies of nursing practices as randomized clinical trials. (Rhetaugh was so excited she came to the office the next day with mismatched earrings.)

We forget how controversial the notion of experimentation was in those days. It was believed, mostly by people outside nursing, that it was not possible to control the clinical environment sufficiently to establish the validity of such studies. In fact, when Rhetaugh and Bob went around interviewing surgeons and anesthesiologists before designing the study, to get some sense of what the most vulnerable patient sample might be, there were barely concealed snickers. Surgeons believed that only the excellence of their operating technique had anything to do with how patients recovered; and anesthesiologists thought their gas-passing was the only thing that mattered. Only Rhetaugh and Bob thought nursing might make a difference, and when it was shown to do so, it was revolutionary. But the study was not popular in nursing and subsequent clinical experiments were slow to gain acceptance, as nursing worried about the ethics of withholding treatment from the control group.

In 2 or 3 years, Rhetaugh's study had been replicated several times, and nurse researchers were getting increasingly interested in teasing out the specific aspects of nursing that made a difference. The designs profited from the interdisciplinary contribution of sociologists like Leonard, psychologists, statisticians, and physicians. And the results made a difference to the patients served and to the image of nursing research in high federal places. For some—but clearly not all—research problems, the experimental design remains the most powerful and pleasing, as your recognition of Dorothy Brooten in this convention testifies.[5]

And yet, the overwhelming number of studies reviewed, while quantitative, were not experimental. True, the research problems chosen may not have lent themselves to manipulation [of the independent variable], and that may have been a deliberate choice of investigators. And one must acknowledge that experimental studies are time-consuming, difficult, and often expensive, and we still lack good choices of measures of outcome. That the percentage of experimental studies in this conference is nearly double that in the literature might be a sign that times are changing back. It may be that the present social and political context is making it more interesting and possible to examine the *effects* of nursing practice. Or perhaps the increased entry of experienced specialist practice nurses into doctoral programs and programs of research is providing us with new questions and thrusts for study. ...

Controversial as clinical experimentation was, it was not nearly as conspicuous as the entry of qualitative research into the lists. Jeanne Quint [Benoliel] and Barney Glaser and Anselm Strauss did us an enormous service by choosing to study death and dying, because the results of their inquiries were so immediately sensitizing that this new way of looking at complex human processes generated instant enthusiasm. Dickoff and James made "factor searching" credible in their framework of levels of inquiry[6] and as nurses have read in phenomenology, and as feminist theories of embeddedness and connectedness have been examined in nursing, it is becoming clear that some—but clearly not all—research problems profit from a qualitative approach. Yet qualitative studies are fiendishly difficult to design and describe in grant applications, and the mental work of data analysis is exhausting. The major reason qualitative studies are not accepted for publication in *Image* is that the data analysis is simply not completely cooked. Or else it's overdone, raised to such a level of conceptual complexity that it drifts away beyond Neptune's rings. A graduate student doing a qualitative study of nurse-physician co-therapy once staggered into my office after a long night of reading and rereading her field notes. She had come to the conclusion, she said, that if she played at it long enough, she could raise the level of conceptualization of the process to the point at which it would all be contained within the title of her thesis.

If one imagines the whole field of nursing's potential inquiry, it would be inarguable that some problems would profit from the kind of depth provided by qualitative methods and some would profit from clinical experimentation. What proportion of what kind of problem is impossible to guess. But one *might* guess that, of all the research problems out there, is it likely that 83% of them require a descriptive/correlational design.

While I did not keep track of it, my guess is that perhaps a quarter of the descriptive/correlational studies are really natural experiments, comparing groups of people who had naturally experienced something with groups who had not, or tracking people before and after the natural event occurred. Since it is not possible to manipulate the occurrence of disaster or trauma or cardiac surgery, these studies should perhaps be classes with clinical experiments, in terms of the increment of causal knowledge produced. However they are classified, they are still the minority of the majority of study designs, their number paling in comparison with the very high prevalence of correlational studies using demographic information to create natural groups to correlate and regress on the results of paper-and-pencil tests. Common sense would tell us that these kinds of studies might be conceptually difficult to design, and certainly data analysis and interpretation can be wearing. But they are easier to conduct. Or, as one colleague suggested, one reason why there appear to be so many such studies is that they are more fundable, depending as they do largely on validated measurements, reliable procedures and large samples. Without an in-depth critique, which I did not perform, it is not possible to determine the significance or importance of the topics chosen, the results obtained, or the usefulness of the information to clinicians. The question is only whether the distribution of designs in this small survey matches the distribution of potential research problems in nursing.

Nearly half (45%) of all studies were with populations who were not entered in the health care system at all, even as persons "at risk." Typical examples might include school children, healthy elderly persons at home, adolescents in gym classes, people in shopping centers, or nurses ourselves. Surely there is a part of nursing that legitimately deals with understanding the general human condition in the absence of illness or care, but when we know that about 65% of all employed nurses work in hospitals, a question might be raised about the extent to which the published research provides information needed by the majority of nurses.

In the April (1989) issue of *Research in Nursing and Health,* Margaret Williams editorialized on this phenomenon:

> Given that patient care issues in acute care settings are many
> and present exceptionally important questions...it is logical to
> assume that a large share of nurses' research would be con-
> cerned with these issues. Perusal of our research journals
> does not bear out such logic...[7]

Margaret suggests some factors that contribute to the difficulty of doing research in patient care practices—the whims of institutional review boards and their clearance procedures, the problems of trying to fit one's research around the patients' schedules for diagnostic procedures, treatments, family visits or supper, the necessity for physician approval and then the difficulty finding them to give it, the lack of interest on the part of the nursing staff, the shortened hospital stay. But, she suggests, many of these frustrations can be anticipated and dealt with and she gives six rules:

> First, it is easier to implement research as an insider than an outsider.
>
> Second, assume that service is *always* the priority no matter the stated commitment to research.
>
> Third, do not count on long-term support of studies at the unit level if administrative persons are not visibly supportive.
>
> Fourth, do not assume that IRBs will include nurse members or that they will meet frequently at preset schedules.
>
> Fifth, assume that physicians will, at best, be unenthusiastic about any studies that suggest less than optimal medical management.
>
> Finally, do not assume that unit personnel will gladly take on additional activities...out of pure interest in the study's outcomes.

And I might add a seventh principle: do not assume that the problem you have elected to study is interesting or important to the nurses who actually do the work of the place unless you have asked for their input into selecting the problems that matter.

Is it possible that this trend toward more and more studies of persons who are not patients, and more and more descriptive/correlational studies, is a product on the one hand of the fast track toward tenure many faculty nurses are on, and on the other, of the wish of doctoral students to rejoin the ranks of the employed and pay off their educational debts? And thus, research problems are selected more out of feasibility than significance? Or is the research tradition not well enough established in clinical institutions that important problems can be identified and the collaboration of researchers and clinicians fostered? Is this perhaps a temporary phenomenon of the race toward academic legitimacy that will disappear once that is achieved, allowing nurse researchers the time and energy to return to studies of patient care problems, assuming we remember how to do it?

While only about 17% of all articles surveyed dealt with people who were acutely ill (or recently the victims of disaster or family stress including death), nearly one-third of the studies which involved samples of patients were in the acute situation. Given the difficulties of this kind of research, perhaps we should be cheered by that number, and we should applaud our colleagues who managed to make it through the administrative and IRB systems.

The other high ranking categories of sample groups were non-institutionalized "at risk" persons, the chronically ill, the elderly, and women. One might make a paranoid observation about this distribution; that is, these are the people nobody else cares about and so it might be easier to have access to them. And of course, nursing has a distinguished reputation in moving into areas in which there was a vacuum...

Henderson said, studies of the work rather than the workers. On that criterion, there is encouraging progress, particularly in studies of nursing performance and clinical judgment. These studies are not the majority yet but they are creeping up on studies of student nurses. That pace may have been accelerated by the state-of-the-science conference sponsored by the National Center for Nursing Research.[8] In that conference, participants were hard pressed to identify knowledge ready for transfer into practice, and they outlined research agendas in nursing performance that will take us way into the next century.

Perhaps the relative paucity of studies of the work of nursing is an accident of sampling. I have worried in print that there seems to be a growing chasm in the nursing literature between those publications such as the ones surveyed and those which carry the bulk of nursing performance and economic analyses, and the studies of patient care practices.[9] It is of some minor interest that the circulation of *Nursing Management,* for example, is quite considerably more than the combined circulation of four of the five journals surveyed here.[10]

The nursing shortage and all its attendant publicity would make it seem as if issues in nursing resources and service delivery might soon be reflected in the mainstream nursing research literature. But do we mainstream nurse researchers consider those problems important? Are issues of patient acuity and nursing intensity, of working conditions and person-power supply, or organizational dynamics, turnover, job stress, and costs of care too operationally atheoretical to appeal to academic researchers or tenure committees?

I used this little exercise of examining the five journals both to stimulate my thinking for this paper and to see whether the vaguely recognized perceptions of the nursing literature I have been building up were grounded. For I also read the non-research literature and am constantly buoyed up by the immense richness of the issues nurses deal with. I'm not quite so entranced by the research literature. The very first article I ever wrote completely on my own was about this same feeling—that some, maybe even a majority, of the intellectual work in the nursing literature was not speaking to me as a nurse.[11]

It is only after there is some even half-conscious social consensus on policy direction that the important research questions can be stated and studied. Nursing achieved some kind of consensus perhaps with the publication of the ANA *Social Policy Statement* in 1980.[12] Among other things, the statement focused us on the definition and study of "the phenomena of interest" to nursing, especially in developing nursing diagnoses. I might suggest that this target has influenced the recent development of nursing research as well, as we seem to have turned our attention toward general human phenomena (of interest to nurses). A quick examination of the *Annual Review of Nursing Research* makes a case in point. Each volume has a section called "studies of nursing practice." But in every volume, the titles of those chapters are something like "pain," or "compliance," or "mother-child interaction," or "adult development." Phenomena of interest to nursing, surely, but not studies in, or of nursing practice. Is it simply silly to suggest that the largest phenomenon of interest to nursing ought to be *nursing?* We can break down interesting phenomena of human life and illness into more and more clearly defined bits, but to build that knowledge back up to equal the science of nursing requires a conceptual notion of the processes of practice.

At the risk of chomping down even further on the hand that is feeding me today, I would observe a certain troubling statement just issued by the Cabinet on Nursing Research, called "Education for participation in nursing research."[13] In it, the various degrees of participation are of nurses educated at the associate, baccalaureate, master's, and doctoral levels. The role of the nurse at the master's level, it is said, is to be the clinical expert collaborator with experienced investigators. This nurse is "particularly valuable" it is said, in "appraising the clinical relevance of research findings, especially of projects that focus on quality assurance of nursing care." Kind of a limited role in research since it does not at all address the crucial role of clinical experts in defining problems in the first place, but let's let it go.

When one gets to the section on doctoral education, the statement says the doctorally prepared nurse "contributes to nursing knowledge through conduct of research aimed at theory generation or theory testing" (note that what this theory is to be about is not specified). She or he is responsible also for acquiring funding and disseminating results. Nowhere in the description of doctoral education for research or the role of the doctorally prepared nurse in research is it hinted that she or he might also be prepared before or during the doctorate as a clinical expert, might know the important things to study, might even need or wish the collaboration of clinicians, or might have a role in reshaping nursing practice on the basis of the research.

In 1974, only 15 years ago, Carol Lindeman, then with WICHEN, conducted a Delphi survey of nursing research priorities. It was instructive to reread that work because it makes very clear how nursing research priorities are not immune from the social context.

In that study, the five highest priorities for which nursing should take the leadership were:

> Determine nursing interventions that promote adequate respiratory functioning in both medical and surgical patients.
>
> ...evaluate the effects of expanding the role of the nurse in patient care.
>
> Evaluate the nursing audit as a means of improving nursing care.
>
> Evaluate, in terms of patient outcomes, processes used to provide nursing care.
>
> Delimit and evaluate the functions and clinical parameters of the independent nurse practitioner.[14]

The mid-1970s, of course, were a time of intense interest in expanding nursing roles and functions, increasing the autonomy and control of practice, proving our worth. It would be interesting to examine the nursing literature since that study to see to what extent it was directive. I rather think the political agenda changed, partly because of the movement of nurses into all kinds of expanded roles, and the achievement of third-party reimbursement for nursing services. Now, the priorities for nursing research, as contained in the ANA's 1985 document include these top five:

> Promote health, well-being and ability to care for oneself among all age, social and cultural groups.
> Minimize or prevent behaviorally and environmentally induced health problems that compromise the quality of life and reduce productivity.
> Minimize the negative effects of new health technologies on the adaptive abilities of individuals and families...
> Ensure that care needs of particularly vulnerable groups...are met in effective and acceptable ways.
> Classify nursing practice phenomena.[15]

As an assignment in policy analysis, it is interesting to examine this shift over time. In 1974, the priorities were aggressive and were clearly focused on patient care. Today, they seem more passive and oddly, less respectful of nursing's contribution. For example, minimizing the negative effects of new health technologies assumes that those technologies are going to be put in place without our cooperation, and thus we deal with the human responses secondary—why is it always secondary?—to them. But the clinical expert nurses I have coffee with are involved every day not just in minimizing the effects of technology, but in designing alternatives and insisting on the right to decide when a technological imperative is in the patient's interest. And then they study the effects of the use of technology, a field called technology assessment, eminently fundable.

The political agenda behind the *Social Policy Statement* and subsequent elaboration on it was clearly to define an area that nursing could call its own and build a fence around it so nobody else could get in. That notion seems reflected in our modern research production and priorities, as they increasingly withdraw from the frustrations and complexities of modern health care and its systems. If we follow the guidelines for educating nurses for different research roles, will we create, or reinforce, the always present gap between those who do the work of nursing and those who study it?

Will we end up talking to ourselves?

In the 5 years surrounding the published literature considered here, cataclysmic change has occurred in health care. The USA went to spending nearly 12% of our Gross Domestic Product on health care, without making a dent in infant mortality, for example, which is nearly the worst in any developed country. Medical technology learned how to save very low birth weight infants, only to have them survive damaged, dependent on the health care system forever. Prospective payment based on DRGs was voted into place unanimously in the Senate. AIDS was identified, its transmission discovered, its epidemic proportions outlined, even as crack cocaine and its fallout proceeds to nearly wipe out a generation of young black men. Magnetic Resonance Imaging outpaced CAT scanning. Medicaid changed its rules to enroll more eligible mothers and infants. Oregon decided not to pay for organ transplants in its Medicaid program any more except for corneas and kidneys and explicit rationing as public policy was born. An imminent nursing shortage was identified, tracked, and used finally to break through the barriers of salary for nurses. The latest frightening statistic is that in New York City, 50% of newborns are HIV positive; 20% of all hospital beds in New York City—*all* hospitals, not just the city hospitals—are occupied by AIDS patients. Small area analysis has identified physician practice pattern differences which explain resource use. The JCAHO has embarked on an enormous project on the quality of hospital care, without, of course, nursing representation. Chorionic villus sampling started to be tested as an alternative to amniocentesis, with huge implications in ethics, counseling, and decision-making. Computers made information accessible instantly, including information on nursing resources and costs. Outpatient care has become the fastest growing sector of the health care delivery system, and relative value methods for paying for outpatient work are being tested even as we speak.

See, nursing is two things: the care of the sick (or the potentially sick) and the tending of the entire environment within which care happens. If one were to set a modern nursing research agenda, it might target those social mandates. The present research agenda for nursing speaks to the development of the profession. I am with Virginia Henderson who believes that nursing's lot in the world will improve when nursing's practice does:

> Whether or not nurses achieve full professional status is unimportant...unless this development results in, or is accompanied by, improvement in nursing care in all its physiological and psycho-social aspects.[16]

It will take all of us to do it.

ENDNOTES

1. Simmons, L., & Henderson, V. (1964). *Nursing Research—Survey and Assessment.* New York: Appleton-Century-Crofts.

2. Henderson, V. (1956). Research in nursing practice: when? *Nursing Research, 4*(3), 99.

3. Gay, J., Edgil, A.E., & Rozmus, C. (1989). Nursing journals read and assigned most often in doctoral programs. *Image, 21*(4), 246–250.

4. Dumas, R.G., & Leonard, R.C. (1963). The effects of nursing on post-operative vomiting. *Nursing Research, 12*(1), 12–15.

5. Brooten and her research team did very important studies of nursing programs of early discharge of low birth weight infants from hospitals, showing huge cost savings. See endnote 12, page 62.

6. Dickoff, W., & James, P. (1968). A theory of theories. *Nursing Research, 17*(3), 197–203.

7. Williams, M. (1989). Research and the acute care setting. *Research in Nursing and Health, 12*(2), iii–iv.

8. National Center for Nursing Research (1988). Nursing resources and the delivery of patient care: Report of the state-of-the-science conference. Washington, DC: USPHA, NIH Pub # 89-3008.

9. Diers, D. (1987). On research in nursing practice. *Image, 19*(3), 106.

10. Swanson, E., & McCloskey, J. (1988). Publishing opportunities for nurses. *Nursing Outlook, 34*(3), 227–236.

11. Diers, D. (1970). This I believe...about nursing research. *Nursing Outlook, 18*(11), 50–54.

12. American Nurses Association (1980). *Nursing: A social policy statement.* Kansas City: American Nurses Association.

13. American Nurses Association, Cabinet on Nursing Research (1989). Education for participation in research. Kansas City: American Nurses Association.

14. Lindeman, C. (1974). *Delphi survey of priorities in clinical nursing research.* Boulder, CO: WICHE.

15. American Nurses Association, Cabinet on Nursing Research (1985). Directions for nursing research. Kansas City: American Nurses Association.

16. Henderson, 1956, *ibid.*

CLINICAL SCHOLARSHIP

"Clinical scholarship" was the way I began to think about nursing that stood on narrative, carefully examined. I had been collecting dandy examples for some time out of personal reading and the required reading of manuscripts for the journal I edited. One snowy midnight, they came together and this paper practically wrote itself. Well, no, it's never that easy. (Published in the Journal of Professional Nursing, 11 (1), 24–30 *in 1995, used with permission.)*

Barbara Geach, cited here, became an Associate Editor for Nursing Outlook. *British (their education prepares much better than ours for writing and loving words), and daughter of two distinguished Professors, her own writing gifts as well as her vivid personality make a deep impression on all of us who know her. Her professional work is now reflective as major neurological damage from a brain tumor limits her movement and speech, but not her acerbic and witty correspondence that only occasionally includes observations on being a patient. Her personality is still wicked—in the best British Ron Weasley (of the Harry Potter books) sense of the word.*

The maturity of modern nursing practice makes it possible to talk about clinical scholarship. The increasing pressure on nurses for scholarly productivity makes it timely to talk about the variety of ways it can be expressed.

In her article on practice-based research, Roberts proposes a pyramid of kinds of activities that lead eventually to causal explanations, considered in traditional logical positivism the most valid (some would say important) form of explanation.[1] At the bottom of the pyramid is clinical observation and on that base is built surveys, description, cross-sectional, retrospective and prospective designs, and experiments.

In this article it is proposed that there is at least one other kind of intellectual activity that, although it also begins with clinical observation, does not fit the research model but might lead to increasingly sophisticated conceptualization. This activity is available to all practicing nurses and could form the basis for an additional way of defining, promoting, and rewarding nursing's intellectual work.

Clinical Work

Virginia Henderson is given deserved credit for calling attention to the proper focus for nursing research, i.e., the work rather than the workers. A decade of development of ideas about practice theory and practice-related methods followed. Over time, nursing research came to concentrate on the "workees," i.e., patients or potential patients, rather than the work or workers despite some spectacular examples of studies of the practice and effect of nursing.

Because as nurses we know what the term clinical means, we have no definition. For this article, the notion of clinical work is paraphrased from Berg's use of the term in describing a focus for research in social science. He uses the word clinical to mean direct involvement with and/or observation of human beings; commitment to a process of self-scrutiny by the scholar; willingness to change theory in response to the process itself; and descriptions that are dense and thick and favor depth over breadth.[2]

Thus, clinical scholarship might begin equally with observation of patients or practice, or with observation of one's own participation or reaction to patients or situations. Those situations occur in the practice of nursing, which is the care of patients.

Scholarship

The definitive reference on scholarship is Jeroslav Pelikan's monograph, *Scholarship and its Survival.*[3] Pelikan's notions stimulated later inquiry into the nature of higher education in the United States, and they lie under more recent reconsiderations of the nature of the university in light of changing demographics. Others have also written about scholarship in universities but their notions are more along the line of traditional research method.

Oddly, in Pelikan's lovely piece of work, there is no definition of scholarship. To scholars such as Pelikan (his field is history of the Christian church) scholarship simply *is*. He distinguishes between scholarship and science, by which he refers to the basic sciences, but resists defining either. However, he does propose attributes or characteristics of scholarship, the most important of which is the embeddedness of the scholar in the context:

> The difference between good scholarship and great scholarship is, as often as not, the general preparation of the scholar in fields other than the field of specialization. It is the general preparation that makes possible that extra leap of imagination and analogy by which scholarship moves ahead.[4]

We could read this as an argument for liberal arts education in nursing, but that is not the purpose here. Rather, it is argued that the use of the contexts of simply living in the world as well as practicing, known through education or experience, provide similar analogies that allow the creative leap. If the nurse also has a grasp of fields outside of nursing, or outside one's specialization, so much the better.

The first quality for scholars and scholarship, Pelikan says, is "the ability to use the mother tongue"[5], i.e., careful writing and critical editing. Because scholarship does not use data to speak for themselves, the words must speak with clarity, accuracy, and disciplined precision. The exquisite use of language is informed, Pelikan argues, by knowledge of other languages and other cultures, but again the argument here is not for a language requirement in nursing curricula. The very nature of nursing practice necessitates hearing and understanding the language of others, especially the language of meaning that patients assign to their experience. Scholarship requires making that understanding conscious.

The pursuit of truth has been the tradition of the scholar, whereas the scientist pursues proof or natural law. The pursuit of truth is paradoxically based on both trust and distrust—distrust of all prior assumptions, however cherished, that do not stand up in light of further inquiry and the trust that moral and intellectual integrity will characterize the work of colleagues and collaborators.[6]

According to Cardinal Newman,[7] the hallmarks of the scholar are a scientific formation of mind, an acquired faculty of judgment, of clearsightedness, of sagacity, of wisdom, or philosophical reach of mind, and of intellectual self-possession and repose acquired by discipline and habit. The enemies of scholarship would be fraud and deceit, superficiality and laziness, fuzziness of mind, lack of discipline, and lack of respect for the observed world or the work of others. ...

Scholarship, then, is certain habits of mind. Clinical scholarship modifies the noun only by focusing on observation in and of the work, including the perception of one's own participation in it. To these observations are applied disciplined habits of analysis (including careful attention to sources) and analogy that are carefully described and even more carefully edited so that, when written, the activity produces new understanding, new knowledge.

From Observation to Scholarship

It would be difficult to improve on Florence Nightingale's words about observation. "The trained power of attending to one's own impressions made by one's own sense, so that these should *tell* the nurse how a patient is, is the *sine qua non* of being a nurse at all".[8] Nightingale did not have technology interfering with data from the senses. But we would be wise to return to her admonition: "merely looking at the sick is not observing. To look is not always to see".[9]

To see is not always to notice, to recognize something observed (including felt by the emotional machinery) as different, signal, and worth reflection.

Barbara Geach's article on bedtime ceremonials provides a superb example.[10] As a psychiatric nurse working the evening shift, Geach observed more than one example of bedtime behavior that caught her attention. She describes one instance:

> Each night for the first three or four weeks of her hospital-ization for psychotic depression, she would undress very slowly, meticulously folding each garment as it was removed and placing it on a chair at the foot of the bed. A separate trip had to be made from the head to the foot of the bed with each garment. Then a nightgown would be put on, contact lenses removed, various objects rearranged on top of her bureau, and finally a very slow walk would be taken to the bathroom for her to wash her face and brush her teeth. The light was left on throughout all of this procedure, even though she shared a room with other patients.[11]

Note how the very language that Geach uses to describe this observation reinforces it: a trip *"had* to be made"; a walk *"would be* taken." The choice of these verbs is deliberate as is the choice of the adverbs, "very slowly," "meticulously." What is being observed and described is a process, and for what, verbs show the action.

Geach combines this case with two others. In one, the patient is disorga-nized, "screaming incoherently," "pacing continually".[12] In the other, the patient "at night kept wailing prayers to God not to have to burn her son...".[13] In all three of these cases, the behavior was repetitive and, Geach reasoned by analogy, ritualistic. Thus she turned to the literature on ritualistic behavior. That was helpful in distinguishing between rituals that are "successful" and those, such as seen in the case examples, which interfere with a function of living, i.e., going to bed and sleep, to the point at which the ritual itself becomes a source of anxiety.

"Bedtime is a time fraught with special meaning for all of us",[14] Geach writes, and the ways in which patients deal with the end of the day cannot only "be important indicators of illness; they may be profoundly meaningful to clients; and changes in their character may indicate and accompany over-all change for good or ill in the patient's condition".[15] Further, "participation [by the nurse] ... can provide a beginning for, and be an expression of, a nurse-patient relationship which gives the patient an emotionally corrective experience".[16]

For the first patient,

> A.B.'s behavior was as regular as any more appropriate bed-time ceremonial; it probably was an attempt to recreate a state of calm preparedness to go to sleep...One night, instead of simply giving A.B. medication, the nurse went with her to her room, helped her to straighten out her bedclothes, encouraged her to change into pajamas and get into bed, tucked her in, then, when A.B. again said, "I can't sleep,"

say to her: "Say your *Sh'mah*" (A.B. came from a strictly Orthodox Jewish family), A.B. smiled delightedly, said this short prayer with the nurse, and was asleep in less than a minute.[17]

When it became possible for the nurse to explore the meaning of this bedtime behavior with the patient, it turned out that "she had moved so slowly... because she was terribly afraid that...she was going 'insane'".[18] She needed to have control, but the behavior was an excessive form of control and was ineffective in calming her anxiety because she had to do everything perfectly. Further, "she was aware that 'sane' people did not have to check everything they said or did".[19]

Geach's purpose in this article was to mine the (literally) everyday behavior of bedtime for clues that might lead the evening nurse to more careful assessment and more clever intervention. Psychiatric illness often causes disruption in these kinds of activities of daily living and the degree of that disruption, and the pace at which the patient is able to resume previous performance levels is an index of illness in the first instance, and recovery in the second.

> The task is demanding, for clearly one had to follow the patient's lead to some degree and to employ ceremonials that fit reasonably well with the patient's culture and...religion. This will call for a delicate ability to fine-tune responses to the patient. The therapeutic effects of doing so, however, may extend beyond bedtime and into other aspects of the patient's life...If the result is only that a reasonable night's sleep has been assured, then this intervention will still have served a valuable purpose.[20]

The qualities of clinical scholarship shine in this article, i.e., the trained intelligence, the ability to turn to analogy, and particularly the context. The patients were linked by a similarity not in the behavior itself, but in the situation. The situation was put up against the normal context of bedtime, within which the behavior could then be seen not simply as ritualistic, but as truly ceremonial, opening the door to explanations different from recalcitrance or pathology.

Nightingale said observation may always be improved by training, will seldom be found without it, "Otherwise the nurse does not know what to look for".[21]

But what to look at and for is much more complicated. What nurses observe, look for, depends on our (sometimes inarticulate) theoretic perspective, or on what the relevancies are to the practice. Visintainer (1986) asserts that it is the purpose that determines what is considered relevant enough to be noticed, remembered, and acted on, and she supplies several examples.[22]

In one, a nurse admitted a young child for a tonsillectomy:

> The nurse...noticed that, although the boy was only seven, he seemed to "take charge." On the other hand, his mother

> seemed overwhelmed by the experience and sat quietly, often tearfully, by while her son answered questions and interacted with the staff...The child listened attentively to the preparation...by the primary nurse and was interested in learning all that was to happen the following morning. The next day he went off to the operating room reassuring his mother that he would be back soon.[23]

Again, note the words chosen: verbs for the child ("take charge," "went off"), adverbs for the mother ("tearfully") and the child ("attentively").

The boy came back from uneventful surgery but shortly afterward began to be "agitated" according to the aide. The primary nurse went back into the room to find the boy sitting up in bed, holding his throat, croaking, "something's wrong".[24] The nurse examined him, tried to reassure him, to no avail. She called the ENT resident who couldn't find anything either and prescribed Vistaril (Pfizer Labs, New York, NY). The nurse was uncomfortable about the order:

> She had known Bobby's response to the hospitalization... , his ability to understand what was happening and his management of anxiety and fear. In light of that information, his insistence that something was amiss convinced her that there was a problem, even in the absence of concrete signs.[25]

To the nurse, the interaction of mother and son, and Bobby's general coping ability were relevant; to the ENT resident, they were not. "For the nurse, that information was important *for the provision of care*"[26] (emphasis added), whereas for the resident, whose purpose was cure of the putative diagnosis of postanesthesia restlessness, the information was irrelevant. The nurse took the child back to the operating room where he made the correct diagnosis obvious by vomiting an emesis basin full of blood; he had been bleeding into the nasopharyngeal cavity, but it was hidden behind a clot too high to see.

In both Geach and Visintainer's examples, the nurses observed, acted, and did the right thing. That in itself is not clinical scholarship. In both cases the contribution is not just touching case stories, but rather is the product of intellectual work that raises the clinical instance to the level of theory.

This process is unreserved in Oliver Sacks' book, *Awakenings*[27] and made vivid in the film based on it. The book and the film portray the process of discovery. In the 1990 version of the book, Sacks provides a chapter[28] in which he describes Robert DeNiro, who played the patient Leonard, preparing himself for the role by locking himself in a hotel room, not moving for hours at a time. It is as clinical and evocative as his discussion of Parkinsonism. Sacks' character is astonished when a supposedly frozen Parkinsonian patient catches her glasses as he drops them into her lap. He watches the same patient shuffle across a checkerboard floor and freeze at its edge when clearly she was headed somewhere. In the film, the physician and the nurse paint the rest of the floor to continue the checkerboard and they watch (they awaken) as the patient walks slowly and purposefully to an open window, "borrowing" the regularity of the pattern on the floor to make her move. Sacks begins to wonder, both to marvel and to be curious, and his search for understanding leads to increasingly complex considerations of how it is "to be as one is"[29] which eventually draw on philosophy, linguistics, literature, and chaos theory as well as neurology. At the same time, Sacks was also doing traditional research on the effects of L-DOPA.

No theory could possibly describe, explain, or predict everything. Theory is a "working draft on an idea about the world."[30] As a working draft, theory is to be challenged and changed by encounters with the real world of clinical work. That process is explicit in theory-testing empirical research. It can be equally explicit in clinical scholarship. The clinical scholar must have a repertoire of possible explanations, "contexts" for Pelikan, "maps" for Visintainer, as well as the capacity to distill, to think of a name, and label for the present experience to enter into the mental Medline. One must have the capacity to envision what the present instance *is an instance of.*

In another article, Geach defines this process.[31] She was working with a schizophrenic patient who had missed a visit with his parents. As a faculty member, she was also supervising a student's experience with his patient, another schizophrenic with whom he was just beginning to terminate. Both Geach and White experienced intense, ego-alien emotions, despair in one instance, rage in the other, after disappointing sessions with the patients. Normally, such reactions are thought of as "countertransference," about which there is considerable literature, which they consulted. But the literature did not help. Their experiences did not fit the notion of countertransference as described. Geach and White defined an entirely new concept termed "empathic resonance" which describes the foreign, overwhelming, and paralyzing flood of unpleasant feelings and the acute sense of isolation and shame resulting in a reluctance to talk about it.[32]

Again, note the language: "despair," "rage," "paralyzing," "shame." In the article, the authors are describing not a process, but a "thing," a phenomenon, for which nouns and adjectives are the appropriate media. The two instances Geach and White report are linked not by the behavior, as in Sacks' work, nor by the situation, as in the bedtime stories, but by the internal observation, the feelings provoked, a datum as valid as watching a patient walk across a floor. The feeling is noticed, determined relevant to the work, tentatively labeled, put against available knowledge. When that knowledge fails to explain completely, the scholarship moves to develop a new concept and criteria that become part of the next nurse's repertoire.

Discussion

It is easier to discuss what clinical scholarship is not than what it is. It is not qualitative research, phenomenology, or hermaneutics. It is not mere journalistic reporting or even the traditional case study. Although clinical scholarship begins, as does clinical research, with observation, it builds differently.

Both research and clinical scholarship share a fundamental process—using comparison to advantage. In research, comparisons are between data before and after, or experimental and control, or last year and this year, or between different conditions of variables. Clinical scholarship compares between instances within the same context, or between what is observed (felt) and what is, could, or should be. Clinical research begins with a curiosity; clinical scholarship with the sense of wonder that we call "marvel." The satisfaction in clinical research comes with understanding what the data say; the satisfaction in scholarship comes in knowing.

Knowing, in post-feminist thought, raises intuition and other less-than-conscious ways of apprehending to consciousness.[33] It is suggested that there can be a rigor to that kind of knowing, called clinical scholarship. Simply feeling, intuiting, is not scholarship without informed, intelligent, and clinically grounded analysis.

In research, attention is paid to the numbers or concepts; in scholarship, care with the language is critical. In both cases, the activity is not complete until it is written down.

Excellent clinical research and scholarship share another potential similarity—they turn conventional ways of thinking upside down. The legend that storks bring babies is said to have started in Belgium when someone noticed that storks and babies tended to arrive at a house simultaneously. Actually, babies bring storks. When there is a new baby in the house, the fires are stoked and the increased rising heat attracts storks to nest.

Baranoski,[34] who is Visintainer, provides another example. She analyzes conventional reasoning about post-traumatic stress disorder (PTSD), especially in victims of disasters or war. She argues that the symptoms of PTSD are not abnormal and pathological so much as they are normal responses to an abnormal situation. Who ever thinks that their home will be swept away by flood or buried in ash? Who would think that experiencing war is just an everyday occurrence?

Clinical scholarship as discussed here is only one form nursing's intellectual activity can take. Other examples might be found in what Ganong calls "integrative reviews of nursing research"[35] to the extent that what integrates such reviews is informed and expert clinical knowledge. One such example is Maloni and Kasper's (1991) review on bedrest in pregnancy.[36] There, the literature about weightlessness in astronauts is melded with an exquisite understanding of obstetrical nursing to create a new amalgam of knowledge. Reviews of the literature are arguably scholarship; they are clinical scholarship when not only do they reflect the habits of mind described here, but they make visible the clinical intellect.

Clinical scholarship requires a maturity of practice that comes with experience, and especially specialist experience. Clinical scholarship is informed by reading, by thinking, by discussing with colleagues, by mentoring, by teaching, so as to generate a mental map kit of potential explanations. Berg suggests that who the investigator (scholar) is, in personal history and personality, must also feed both the scholarship and others' interpretations of it.

Just as the selection of a particular method of study in traditional nursing science depends on what the problem is, so clinical scholarship is particularly appropriate to particular kinds of problems. Perhaps it is no accident that the examples used here come primarily from psychiatric nursing and neurology. Psychiatric nursing depends on words and language to capture fully the patient and the patient's situation, as well as the processes of care. There are no lab tests, electrocardiograms (EKG), or heart sounds (except as metaphor). Perhaps, then, the exercise of clinical scholarship is best suited to those situations in which qualitative or quantitative measurement is either not possible, or not appropriate. Now that we know from Geach about bedtime ceremonials, it would be possible to do theoretical sampling and qualitative research, or even some forms of quantitative research, but those would lead us into incidence and prevalence, not into a deeper understanding of the phenomenon. Geach already gave us that.

Clinical scholarship as method is particularly suited to "concepts by intellection,"[37] those phenomena that have no easy empirical referents such as the kinds of clinical judgment portrayed here.

It is not possible to choose clinical scholarship as a method. Following the logic and sources cited here, clinical scholarship occurs to the nurse who knows it as an option. It is not a substitute for clinical research, nor is it a necessary precursor to traditional scientific method. It is, however, a responsible exercise of the special understanding that comes with continuous and deep immersion in the work.

ENDNOTES

1. Roberts, J. (1992). Practice-based research in maternity nursing: Issues and examples from studies of labor and birth. *Applied Nursing Research,* 5, 93–100.

2. Berg, D.N. (Ed), (1993). *Keeping the faith.* Woodbridge, CT: The Berg Group.

3. Pelikan, J. (1984). *Scholarship and its survival: Questions on the idea of graduate education.* New York: The Carnegie Foundation for the Advancement of Teaching.

4. *Ibid.,* p. 26.

5. *Ibid.,* p. 27.

6. *Ibid.*

7. Newman, Cardinal J.H. (1852/1976). In I.T. Ker (Ed) *The idea of a University.* Oxford, UK: Clarendon Press.

8. Nightingale, F. (1883). Nurses: Training of. In R. Quain (Ed) *Quain's Dictionary of Medicine (5th Ed)* (pp. 1038–1041). New York: Appleton. Emphasis in original.

9. *Ibid.,* p. 1038.

10. Geach, B. (1987). Bedtime ceremonials: A focus for nursing. *Archives of Psychiatric Nursing, 1*(4), 98–103.

11. *Ibid.,* p. 100.

12. *Ibid.,* p. 100.

13. *Ibid.,* p. 102.

14. *Ibid.,* p. 102.

15. *Ibid.,* p. 101.

16. *Ibid.,* p. 102.

17. *Ibid.,* p. 100.

18. *Ibid.,* p. 101.

19. *Ibid.,* p. 101.

20. *Ibid.,* p. 103.

21. Nightingale, 1883, *ibid.,* p. 1038.

22. Visintainer, M.A. (1986). The nature of knowledge and theory in nursing. *Image—Journal of Nursing Scholarship, 18*(1), 32–37.

23. *Ibid.,* p. 36.

24. *Ibid.,* p. 36.

25. *Ibid.,* p. 36.

26. *Ibid.,* p. 36.

27. Sacks, O. (1990). *Awakenings.* New York: HarperCollins.

28. *Ibid.,* pp. 369–386.

29. *Ibid.,* p. 225.

30. Visintainer, 1986, *ibid.,* p. 38.

31. Geach, B., & White, J.C. (1974). Empathic resonance: A countertransference phenomenon. *American Journal of Nursing, 74*(12), 1282–1285.

32. *Ibid.,* p. 1284.

33. Belenky, M., Clinchy, B., Godberger, N., & Tarule, J. (1986). *Women's ways of knowing: The development of self, voice and mind.* New York: Basic Books; Carper, B. (1978). Fundamental patterns of knowing in nursing. *Advances in Nursing Science, 1*(1), 13–23; Wolfer, J.A. (1993). Aspects of "reality" and ways of knowing in nursing: In search of an integrating paradigm. *Image—Journal of Nursing Scholarship, 25*(3), 141–146.

34. Baranoski, M.V. (in press, apparently never published). Post traumatic stress disorder: Normal reaction to abnormal events. *Psychological Bulletin.*

35. Ganong, L.H. (1987). Integrative reviews of nursing research. *Research in Nursing and Health, 10*(1), 1–12.

36. Maloni, J., & Kasper, C.E. (1991). Physical and psychosocial effects of antepartum hospital bedrest: A review of the literature. *Image—Journal of Nursing Scholarship, 23*(3), 187–192.

37. Northrup, F.S.C. (1947). *The logic of the sciences and humanities.* New York: Meridian (Macmillian), (p. 92).

EDITORIALS

In the early 1980s, Carol Lindeman, President of Sigma Theta Tau, Sr. Rosemary Donley, Editor of Image, *and Nell Watts, Executive Director of the society decided to Do Something about the Society's journal. They asked Linda Aiken and me and (forgive me, I can't remember who, it didn't work out) some other person to become Associate Editors and each take charge of one of the four issues per year. Every issue would have a theme. Mine would be "clinical scholarship"; Linda's would be policy; Sr. Rosemary's would be international nursing; the other person's would be nursing education.*

Clinical scholarship was to be the first theme. We announced the themes in an editorial and the manuscripts started to pour in. We got so many for the clinical scholarship theme that it took up two issues. This first editorial was the one that accompanied the first of the two issues (15 (1), 1983, p. 3, used with permission).

CLINICAL SCHOLARSHIP

When *Image* became *Image—The Journal of Nursing Scholarship,* it was decided to focus each issue on one kind of paper. Future issues will deal with public policy, nursing education, theory development, and other topics. This, the first issue under *Image's* new name, was planned to highlight "clinical scholarship" and there the fun began!

For what is clinical scholarship? Is it simply clinical research given another name? Or is it a particular kind of clinical research, such as case studies? Or is it the musings about nursing or some nursing concepts?

I thought I knew what clinical scholarship was when I wrote the call for papers and defined the focus for the issue. After having reviewed a fairly large number of manuscripts, and having corresponded with a fairly large number of people who wrote asking whether their papers would suit the new focus, I am instructed.

The original intention was to concentrate on the kind of writing that occurs so infrequently in nursing—the carefully analyzed clinical phenomenon or concept, the inductive reasoning from the empirical incident to the abstraction. So much for "clinical." "Scholarship" was intended to mean reference to already discovered theory or precept, logical analysis, penetrating search for coherence and clarity, digging to find new meaning or new relation to established knowledge. Re-examination of conventional wisdom, I thought, was one model; development of new understanding from existing experience or intelligence was the other big category. There would be a bit of creativity to clinical scholarship as well, whether the creativity came in inventing new ways to describe or explain nursing practice, or whether it became a linking together of previously unrelated theory or knowledge. At base, clinical scholarship would be firmly rooted in the practice arena, using the life experience of the nurse as professional and as human being to provoke insight.

The model I had in mind was Freud's work, delving as he did deeply into the human mind, then raising those findings and insights to the level of label and conceptual description. As the manuscripts rolled in, however, it came to me that there are other kinds of clinical scholarship beyond the case study.

There is, for example, secondary analysis of data that goes quite beyond the testing of particular hypotheses or the application of particular theories. There is an amassing of a variety of data to paint a new picture of a known entity. There are the essays of Lewis Thomas which touch on science and the practice of medicine in quite new ways, evoking in the reader a new grasp of what it is to think clinically.[1]

The major tool of clinical scholarship, I decided, is not conventional research method, but rather *thinking*. Analysis, synthesis, mental rather than empirical comparison of theory or idea, inductive reasoning or deductive, it doesn't matter. Along about here I finally turned to the dictionary which defines "scholarship" as "learning or knowledge acquired by study."

In this sense, then, scholarship is different from research, although research may well be "study." Scholarship implies brooding contemplation, the stretching of the mind for new insight that may characterize the problem formulation part of empirical research, or the data interpretation phase. Research method itself is not, in this definition, scholarship, but is the important following of convention or rule to provide valid and reliable data upon which to set the mind to work. Good research reporting may well fall into the definition of scholarship; mechanical reports which provide data but not insight do not.

The whole point of focusing on clinical scholarship at all, much less for an issue of the new *Image,* is to call attention to a way in which nursing can grow and change and become visible, in addition to clinical research, which is now well established. There is so much richness in nursing and in the thinking of nurses that we need to see and read. The most research in its most conventional sense can do is provide data upon which conclusions can be based, to answer questions. The work of the mind to raise those conclusions to the level of implication, interpretation, concept, or theory is the essence of scholarship, yet scholarship can occur outside of research as well. Scholarship may debunk myths, just as research may disprove previous theory or hypothesis. ...

We have little of this tradition of scholarship in nursing, at least as described here. Some of the journeys to develop nursing theory might also fall into this category, when they are linked to the clinical realities and when they result in theory as opposed to philosophy. ...

The attempt in this issue, then, is to display some examples of clinical scholarship. The hope is that publishing this kind of intellectual work in nursing may encourage and stimulate nurses to commit thoughts to paper, to begin to build a tradition of nursing scholarship that exposes nursing *thinking.*

ON CLINICAL SCHOLARSHIP (AGAIN)

*By the second editorial, I had been Editor of the journal for about 4 years and had begun to have fun with writing editorials to be catchy. The points to be made are the same. And they come with the same forlorn plea: **please, nurses, write it down!** (Image, 20 (1), 1987, p. 2, used with permission).*

Our fan club, all four strong, may think we are all too infatuated with clinical scholarship, this being the third editorial we have written about it. All right, this is one time the editorial "we" doesn't work; *I* wrote about clinical scholarship in the early days of *Image* as the *Journal of Nursing Scholarship.* (Before that, for the curious, it was just *Image.* Before that, by the way, was 1982. How time passes when you're having fun).

We know you're out there, you nurses observing, thinking, trying to get better at the work. Thinking about how you do what you do and why and when, the choices in decisions and the choices in where you put your energies.

There are tads and fancies in the way we define nursing. The latest is "caring." Now, that goes back a long way, to the distinction between nursing and medicine—a political difference, not a practice one. Medicine "cures;" nursing "cares." Since challenging the right to cure is treading on tender toes, nursing claimed "care" as exclusive territory.

Well, nonsense.

Caring is not all there is to nursing—nursing is a whole lot more. Any attempt to define the core of nursing—caring, diagnosing human responses— will be an incomplete definition.

That's where clinical scholarship conies in.

Clinical scholarship is the study of the nature and effect of nursing. It depends on the people who do that, who are engaged in the clinical work. It helps us know what nursing is and does.

Clinical scholars can be spotted in a half-hour's conversation, I wrote once. They talk about their exposure to people and events—the clinical work—with color, flavor, and texture. They describe patients or situations with acute observation, but always with what the observation produced as mental image or intellectual work. They weave the feelings produced by the work as transference throughout. But what clinical scholars add to the conversation are the ideas, theories, explanations, historical trends, data, or philosophy stimulated by the work. It is as if clinical scholars have heads full of data files, linked and cross-referenced, immediately accessed. A single case or event is not simply filed under the major heading—a patient with x condition in y situation. Clinical events are indexed as instances of larger phenomena, or are linked to like events and coded to other files. The computer analogy does not convey the creativity of the process one hears from clinical scholars, however, nor the gift for making unseen connections between things or ideas, mental leaps, intuitive lunges. The repertoire of clinical scholar is not just a collection of empirical observations, for what makes the process into scholarly work is the constant analysis that pits today's event against accumulated learning, and makes the learning available to help understand the event. And makes the scholar hunt for more explanations, more ideas, more theory, research or study to eat up the bytes of the storage disk. And finally, what makes clinical scholarship is a hunger for understanding as regular as the sensations that make one eat breakfast.

What distinguishes this process from simply superior clinical work is that the nurse writes it down.

We know you're out there. May we hear from you?

ENDNOTE

1. Thomas, L. (1974). *Lives of a Cell.* New York: Viking Press.

SECOND THOUGHTS

The majority of nursing research today is still less centered on the practices of the profession than on describing the actual or potential recipients of care. This is no longer an effect of the presence of social science or other outside academic influences but reflects the realities both of funding and time/space for data collection. Studies of nursing practice are not easy. They require access to complicated clinical institutions and their Human Subjects Research Review committees and a long time frame. At the same time, the increasingly complex work of clinical practice and management with decreasing resources does not leave much free intellectual space for practicing nurses to devise and conduct nursing research.

More to the point, studies of nursing practice require close connection between the researcher and the practice. The international movement of nursing into universities has its downside—educated nurses may feel as though they no longer need to get their hands dirty in nursing practice, since they are now dealing with high flying intellectual inventions or management challenges. The best of clinical nursing research continues to value, respect, and find new ways to include nursing practice.

The presentations and publications in this section leapt lightly over the pleas of others then to let research define nursing. Rather, we assumed that we knew what nursing was, thank you very much, and now we needed to uncover nursing's knowledge and build on it to make the practice even more solid, grounded, and effective. The effect of this stance is that nursing practice and our science come out of hiding to be judged by the same standards by which other science is judged. The discomfort occasioned by visibility is traded as a consequence of respect and public valuation. Through research, we have a language with which to talk about nursing outside the discipline where the politics and policy opportunities lie.

That I started to be a spokesperson for nursing research without a doctorate just happened. I didn't intend it that way, though I surely mined the maverick identity. And people asked me to speak, knowing that I would be off the left end of the curve.

When I read the contents here, a whole generation of human beings later, but many generations of nurses and nursing educators and nurse researchers later (a generation in graduate nursing education being maybe 2–7 years), the constancy surprised me. Or maybe it's only that I only ever had one good idea and I keep re-tooling it.

We are no closer to a partnership between education and service than we were 40 years ago. In fact, given the resource pressures both in clinical institutions and universities, the luxury of spending the time to develop collegial work has vanished. Where enlightened clinical institutions and universities may find common ground might be in what is now being called "outcomes research," which has both action-oriented implications and policy implications. Linda Aiken's recent work[1] on the relationship between nurses' perceptions of the work environment and patient outcomes, which underpins the Magnet Hospital movement internationally, is a shining beacon.

The model that is being developed in Australia in the Clinical Chair positions, especially at my third alma mater, the University of Technology–Sydney (UTS) could instruct us in the USA. UTS has a defined commitment to what they call "industry relationships" so they design their educational programs to speak to whatever the industry is. In nursing (UTS has no medical school, which means the faculty of nursing are the only credible health care voices), that has meant everything from clinical experiences of students to the Chair positions which put Professors on site in clinical settings, including the jail/prison system. It is a stunning model for the world.

Another way to build the connection between the academy and practice would be through health services research. There are few Schools of Nursing in the USA and even fewer internationally that have developed health services research capability, especially that capacity which allows the mining of clinical and operational data. At the same time, nursing informatics, which might have evolved to fill in this gap has instead evolved into software construction and implementation.

The "evidence-based practice" movement is surely helping to make research available to guide practice, using rigorous standards of evaluation, and some of that work is quite elegant. I just find it a bit remote from the daily grinding and uplifting practice. And so I continue to try to build bridges, now from the practice side to the academic. But that's another story... .

ENDNOTE

1. See, for example, Smith, A.P. (2002). Evidence of our instincts: An interview with Linda H. Aiken. *Nursing Economic, 20*(2), 58–61.

ADVANCED PRACTICE NURSING

ADVANCED PRACTICE NURSING

While advanced practice nursing such as nurse anesthesia and nurse-midwifery have been around for a very long time, and while critical care as advanced nursing practice is as early as post WWII, the role of the nurse practitioner, developed in the late 1960s and early 1970s, engaged the mainstream nursing profession in political and policy battles already achingly familiar to nurse anesthetists and nurse-midwives.[1] The history and development of the nurse practitioner "movement" has been described by many others whose names are now legendary in nursing: Loretta Ford, Barbara Resnick, Charles and Mary Ann Lewis.

The '60s and '70s in the USA were exciting times to grow up in nursing. Nothing was impossible. There was young energetic leadership in the Kennedy administration; the Civil Rights struggle opened all kinds of possibilities; then there was conflict and controversy in the Vietnam War era. The women's movement promised so much possibility. Social change was everywhere. But the disparities in access to health care among the poor, especially in rural areas, and among people of color could not be ignored. And in trying to address those disparities, other disparities were uncovered, including the uneven interprofessional power configurations (read: access to payment for services rendered). These same struggles play out in other countries; they aren't American inventions.

While I wrote about nurse-midwifery on occasion, and while I certainly worked on nurse-midwifery issues as a dean and a faculty member, this section is more about nurse practitioners. The nurse-midwives had their act together; what they needed from organized nursing, including mainstream nursing leaders like deans, was occasional support and still less occasional fire prevention or containment on the ground. Their political and policy agendas were clear.

Nurse practitioner issues were political and policy issues, in territory new to nurses: reimbursement, licensure/certification, prescribing authority, malpractice insurance. And mostly, the American Medical Association's well-funded and equally well-crafted resistance to anything that interferes with physician hegemony and income expectations.

On the ground, at least at first, nurse practitioners and physicians worked wonderfully together and, at least as I came to know it, the work was equally exciting to doctors and nurse practitioners. It was all this other stuff we had to deal with. There was, God knows, plenty of work to be done; NP's weren't taking the work away from anybody else. Especially in primary care in inner city community health centers and farm communities and Indian reservations and prisons and other unpopular places to serve. But those places and people lack political power, just as NP's do.

The papers in this section begin early in the nurse practitioner game. They were written for a variety of audiences. They are all overtly political, although that's not necessarily how I thought about them when I wrote them. Political writing is about what's "right" and depends on the writer's slant on beliefs and values. I confess: I am a left-leaning-liberal. In writing about nursing, though, what's "left" or "right"?

ENDNOTE

1. That mainstream nursing did not learn from the struggles of nurse anesthesia and nurse-midwifery is one of the sadder pieces of contemporary nursing history. And there is fault on both sides, as CRNA's and CNM's distanced themselves from organized nursing to achieve their remarkable successes. See Diers, D. (1991). Nurse-midwives and Nurse Anesthetists: The Cutting Edge in Specialist Practice. In L.H. Aiken and C.M. Fagin (Eds) *Charting Nursing's Future: Agenda for the '90's* (pp. 159–180). Philadelphia: J.B. Lippincott.

RESEARCH AND NURSE PRACTITIONERS: LESSONS FROM NURSING'S PAST

This is a speech given at the Rochester (NY) Conference on Ambulatory Care (read: Nurse Practitioners) on December 12, 1974. Loretta Ford was Dean of the School of Nursing at Rochester, and the late Barbara Bates, MD and Joan Lynaugh directed Rochester's sterling NP program. By this time, I was only 2 years into a deanery[1] and my thing was clinical nursing research. I didn't know from nurse practitioners but had inherited that agenda from the late Margaret Arnstein, who preceded me as Dean at Yale. Margaret's role in the NP movement has not been catalogued, and I surely do not know it all. I do know that her own history in public health nursing informed her as she saw primary care as a role for nursing. She was a friend of Charles Lewis, MD and his wife, Mary Ann, and Barbara Resnick, who started what we would now understand as the first NP clinic at the University of Kansas. Margaret also knew Lee Ford when she and Henry Silver developed an NP role in Colorado. She was Dean of the Yale School of Nursing from 1967–1972 and brought with her significant national and international standing.

*That was the history and at the time of this speech, I was early in understanding how to make what Margaret and Lee and others had gifted us with, work. I had zero, none, nada, **no** reservations about nurses moving into this primary care role. The breaking-through issues for nursing were too captivating to resist for a Type A nursing advocacy freak.*

In retrospect, this speech is awfully naïve for the audience. I was on a huge learning curve about NP's. I knew what I knew about research. I tried to put them together and it doesn't quite come off.

Odd how one remembers events. I remember them by what I wore. I had been criticized for wearing pants for public speaking (we're still in 1974). This time I wore a long blue and red patterned skirt over a very tight blue turtle neck thing that snapped in the crotch. It looked good but was neither comfortable nor functional.

It's a special pleasure to be with you tonight at this important conference. Like those of you who are visitors here to the Rochester programs, we at Yale have admired, envied, and cheered on the critical work that *started* here in developing the expanded role in nursing, and have watched with considerable excitement as the impact of Rochester's work has covered the nation.

This meeting is significant and special in other ways too. The attendance of such a large number of people in the dead of winter in the middle of a busy academic calendar shows the interest in thoughtfully considering future directions for the nurse practitioner movement and affords us the opportunity to begin to pull it all together. Critics of the nurse practitioner movement have worried that the emphasis on expanding the nursing role in the directions it is being expanded in ambulatory care will take us away from nursing. Some have gone so far as to suggest that nurse practitioners are wolves in sheep's clothing—physician's assistants under the skin. Yet the ideal in nurse practitioner preparation is to build on a solid base in nursing, then to expand the functions of the individual into areas of new scope and responsibility. Can we temper our excitement so we can learn from where we've been?

When we talk about the expanded role in nursing, we tend to confine it to a clinical expansion—the taking on of additional skills and knowledge so that the nurse may perform a wider scope of services to patients. I would like to speak with you tonight about another kind of expansion of the nursing role, for I see research in nursing as just that. Like other expansions in function, it too needs to be based in a solid understanding of its base—in this case, nursing research.

Research involving nurse practitioner work will not perhaps suffer from one of the psychological variables that nursing research has suffered from. In order to do research within any given area of work, one has to believe that that work is important. Otherwise there is no sense in studying it. It has seemed to me that all too frequently there is some doubt about whether nursing is important enough to investigate and that held us back for a very long time. Oddly enough there doesn't seem to be that feeling about nurse practitioner work. Oh, there are arguments about whether nurses really ought to expand their roles, and how that ought to be done if it's to be done, but there doesn't seem to be a great deal of doubt in those who are involved with nurse practitioner work about whether it's worth anything. Yet, research in nurse practitioner practice is so new as to be almost non-existent. While there have been a few studies of the practice of clinical specialists (who are, of course, in an expanded role in nursing), research on the practice of nurse practitioners by nurse practitioners has barely shown its head. The vast majority of studies in this area have been on patient acceptance and on comparisons of the practice of nurse practitioners with that of physicians. Rarely have there been studies of the outcomes, that is, the effects of different nurse practitioner practices on patients. Instead, we find numerous task analyses in the literature, a few cost comparison studies, and a few studies done by social scientists or physicians including the famous Burlington Trials study.

Taking seriously the epigram that those who ignore the past are forced to repeat it, I wish to submit to you some lessons from nursing we need to learn and profit from as we design a role for research in nurse practitioner work.

We are at something of a crossroads in our thinking and developing and teaching of the expanded role. We've come far enough to have the sense that this push is valuable and that it works, and we see now the healthy movement of nurse practitioner continuing education programs into degree granting curricula. So it is an appropriate time to reflect on where we've come and where we need to go. The first lesson, then, is that the proper focus of research in nurse practitioner practice *is* that practice. It took us nearly 100 years of nursing in the United States to learn this lesson in nursing research. Unless we know what in the practice of the profession works to serve patients better, we are hard put to design rationally educational programs to teach it, nursing or other services to administer it, or even granting mechanisms to fund it.

The purpose for research in the expanded role is the same as that for research in nursing more generally—to improve the care of patients. In fact, that's also the whole reason behind the invention of any kind of expanded role, from nurse-midwifery, perhaps the oldest of the expansions of nursing, to the more publicly recognized recent expansions of nursing in pediatric or family nurse practitioner programs. When the goals of nursing research and the goals of the nurse practitioner movement are so similar, one would think research and practice would become closer more naturally.

The most powerful studies that will evolve in nurse practitioner work will focus on problems in patient care, just as the studies which have begun to turn nursing research around have tested the effects of the practices of nursing on patients. Even when a particular problem may require descriptive or basic research before an adequate experimental design could be proposed, if one begins by seeing the solution of clinical problems as the god for research in nursing practice, one looks *at* research problems differently.

A problem for research is sensed as a feeling of irritation, a feeling that something is wrong, or at least not right, inadequate, or otherwise in need of change. A problem can be stated as a discrepancy, a difference between two states of affairs, what is now and what ought to be, what one knows now and what one needs to know, or between two sets of opposing facts. There are limitless differences around, though, so an additional criterion that makes a discrepancy a possible clinical research problem is that it has to be a difference *that matters*. And to matter, a difference has to meet the following test: if the discrepancy were removed, would patient care or patient welfare improve? There is too much to be done, too much demanded of nursing to fritter away our time on trivial problems. Forcing ourselves to state the potential significance of a given problem to the eventual improvement of patient care helps keep our eyes on the road, as it were, and our minds from wandering.

Lesson number two is this: Evaluation research has limited potential for advancing the cause of improvement in patient care of any other aspect of the expanded role movement. Evaluation is a component that must be written into all training grants, developmental projects, experimental curricula, and so on these days. I fear that most often that component is thrown in at the last minute with some stab made toward making it appear systematic and objective. It may even turn out to be systematic and objective, but we are deluding ourselves if we count as our contribution toward the systematic study of the nurse practitioner's work, simple evaluation.

We need evaluation of all our services in the expanded role and in the non-expanded one. But the kind of evaluation research that will take us farthest is not simply the multitude of task analyses, counts of success and failure in educational programs, superficial looks at costs of delivering care, or simple papers on patient and physician acceptance. The problem with most evaluation research is two-fold: first, it is often almost a theoretical. While one can evaluate the attainment of present objectives, few theories are stated or even implied, little attention is given to reconceptualizing the outcomes, events, or services, and thus there is comparatively little impact of the research—barefoot empiricism, as it were. It's just not enough. Secondly, the methods used in most evaluation studies make use of some of the tools of modern systematic investigation, but do not make use of the scholarship that characterizes real research. Studies may use research-derived techniques, including random assignment, systematic data collection, questionnaires, interviews, and other tested measurements, descriptive and inferential statistics, but these are often used more like a recipe for Duncan Hines double chocolate cake than complicated culinary creation based on thoughtful definition and combination of ingredients in abstract terms and highly refined means of evaluating the outcome.

If evaluation research is designed with the notion that out of it will come the necessity and the means for delving conceptually much more deeply into the nature of the practice and outcome of nurse practitioner work, it has the potential for serving to build up the body of knowledge on which future functions can depend. But unfortunately, most evaluation is neither designed so that it could be replicated, nor is it ever carried beyond the point of documenting the unique situation studied.

Such research was probably politically necessary in the early days of the nurse practitioner movement—say last February. But now we're more sophisticated and it has been documented endlessly and without major exception that nurse practitioners can be trained and that they are safe, accepted, and happy in their work. We need now much more than mere documentation.

An example. A group of nurse-midwives at a large eastern University-community medical center, were asked to develop prenatal services to a defined medically underserved area of the city, an area known to include a much higher proportion of mothers and babies at risk than the general population of the city, and an area known to account for three times its share of perinatal deaths. The nurse-midwives leapt at the chance but went in to the project loaded with more than just evaluation plans. From the beginning they defined their services explicitly, including the basic nursing scientific rationale and theory behind them. For example, a large component of their care includes nutrition counseling in the home situation as well as the clinic, and they buttressed their reasoning thoroughly with physiological and dietary theories. Another part of their conceptual framework (which is what is most often lacking in evaluation projects) included some notions of the relationship between psycho-social assets a mother or family might have and how well they cope with the changes of pregnancy on top of simply living in deprived circumstances. The services to be delivered, then, were proposed and defined in conceptual terms as well as simply empirical ones. From the beginning of the service, data retrieval systems were set up so that the service could build up a background of information used not only to document a service evaluation, but also to provide a gold mine of information for future studies.

The nurse midwives instituted their service almost exactly 1 year ago, in January 1974. To date they have seen some 30 women through their entire pregnancy, labor, delivery, postpartum, and family planning course with startling results. No baby from this population has weighed less than 7½ pounds at birth. Remember, this is a high-risk, economically deprived population. To the extent that birth weight is the greatest single predictor of potential for future child health, the effects of the expanded role of nurse-midwifery in this setting have already proved their point. But the year's worth of experience has also produced data and theory on which to expand further and become clearer about what it is in the service that works, and how that can be built in for the future.

One of the student nurse-midwives (for this is also a teaching setting–a contract stipulation when the service was started) is comparing the previous pregnancies of the women served with their current ones, and is finding that women who in previous pregnancies had all kinds of problems ranging from toxemia to schizophrenia, are sailing through the current pregnancy smoothly. Another student is tracking down the dietary histories of women with toxemia from a different population and her study may make a major contribution toward our understanding of the physiology of nutrition, diet, and toxemia of pregnancy. She got her research idea from the theoretical work that became background for the nutrition counseling parts of the expanded nurse-midwifery service role. A third student wants to try to incorporate an assessment of the mother's psychosocial assets—from family or other human support to internal psychological resources—into the initial add continuing assessment, to see if predictions can be made about the relationship of these variables to fetal and maternal outcome. If a relationship is found to hold, then the nurse-midwives have grounds on which to institute systematic psychosocial assessments and determine perhaps when, where, and how to provide additional services.

What makes this project both clinically and academically exciting is that it has the potential not only to demonstrate that the service works, but also to get a handle on *why* it works. It's the latter that evaluation projects often lack.

But the "why" is what is characteristic of academic research which has also invented the methodologies for studying cause and effect.

Constant evaluation of one's service to individual patients is supposedly built in as one step in the "nursing process." Evaluation research too often only extends this notion by adding more cases. But this kind of evaluation research has little potential for real improvement in patient care if all it contributes is numbers of patients cared for and superficial counts of outcomes. There's too much richness in the practice of the expanded role to be satisfied with these findings.

Lesson number three: Research on nurse practitioners themselves will not lead us very far.

There was a time, and indeed it may still be here, when multitudes of studies were reported in the nursing and other literature examining personality characteristics of nurses. Often the studies compared nurses in various specialty areas and found things like psychiatric nurses are intellectual, creative, and callous, while maternity nurses are warm, motherly, and dumb. The fact that such comparisons are odious to begin with is one problem, but the larger one is that it escapes me how such information will ever lead toward the improvement in patient care. It's even unclear what the implications of such findings are. We don't know whether the theory is that psychiatric nursing makes people callous or whether callous people choose it. What is more important is that we have no idea how these personality attributes or variables have anything to do with the delivery of health service.

Research on the workers themselves rather than the work has too long characterized a major focus of nursing research. I would hope that we could either put that focus aside as we begin to develop research in the expanded role or else learn seriously from our experience with nursing and redesign such studies to look at the relationship between personality attributes of nurse practitioners and the kind of care they give.

I would not wish to throw out all studies of the workers, but perhaps another lesson to be learned from our history of this kind of work in nursing research is that we may well have chosen the wrong variables. To measure personality factors which are by definition traits not amenable to major change (as the theory goes), except perhaps in psychotherapy, is a limited conception of the value of research on nurses. What we end up with are rather interesting psychological studies, but they don't move us very far ahead. We might seriously consider looking at other kinds of variables that might more appropriately characterize nurse practitioners and might have more relationship to the kind of care they give; for example, ability at self disclosure. One could hypothesize that such a personality state might well be correlated with capacity for intimacy and that capacity with the quality of patient care. Or how about problem-solving ability? How about internal-external control? For that matter, how about empathy?

This lesson to be learned from nursing research as we move into nurse practitioner research is quite clear. We haven't the time or the luxury to devote whatever attention and energy can be spared from the important clinical work to carry out studies which have little potential of improving the quality of patient care.

The fourth lesson is less methodological than it sounds: The most powerful research tactic for testing the effect of nursing is the experimental design.

Abdellah & Levine have credited Rhetaugh Dumas' study of the effect of nursing preoperatively or postoperative vomiting with breaking through the notion that clinical experiments were impossible or unethical. But there is still a preponderance of survey or descriptive study in nursing research and still some confusion about the proper place of clinical experimentation. Of course some situations are not amenable to random assignment and experimental manipulation. But it has been said that it may be more unethical to promote or continue unresearched practices than it is to systematically test them out, even if it means withholding a proposed practice from one group to compare with another.

What partly makes this time in the expansion of nursing practice exciting is that we are in a position to create the future of practice rather than have to spend our time trying to invent ways of explaining the rituals that have built up over centuries of unexamined activity. The rituals of practice in the expanded role aren't set yet in stone as some of them are in nursing practice, and because we come as nurse practitioner students prepared, hopefully, to question the bases of our teaching and learning, we won't fall into the trap of overly structuring our practice on no date base prematurely.

The classical experimental design allows the test of cause–effect relationships, and those tests lead further in the long run, into improvements in practice than do simply descriptive studies. They must begin to subject our cherished beliefs to empirical tests in classical experiments: do patients cared for by Nurse Practitioners *really* do better when the Nurse Practitioner includes a careful psychosocial history and assessment in her work-up? Does well-baby checking and parental counseling really have anything to do with anything in terms of patient welfare? Does prescribing a regimen of comfort and relaxation in addition to medical management of a disease process work? And, of course, does putting Nurse Practitioners in primary care situations really improve the access to and quality of care?

Taking the experimental design terminology a step further, we have lesson number five: Time spent in refining the definition of the independent variable—nurse practitioner practice—is time counted toward one's tenure in heaven.

The history of research in nursing tells us that early studies, even clinical experiments, on the effects of nursing on patients suffered from vague definitions of the nursing tested. These early studies often didn't replicate until the pieces of nursing practice began to be teased out. Some of that came in subsequent studies, some came in armchair thinking, reconceptualization of the nursing activities, and process. I would hope that we've come far enough in thinking about nurse practitioner practice that it would not be necessary to waste years dithering about what is nursing, when that question isn't even the right one. For research purposes, nursing or nurse practitioning is whatever one cares to define it as for the purposes of a study. I hope we've learned the distinction between a philosophy of nursing and a theory of it. All the philosophies there are, lovely in their gossamer goodness, are useless as definitions of the independent variable. There aren't all that many theories of nursing to choose from either, but there is the collective wisdom of nurse practitioners who together may come to some theoretical constructions of their practice that not only can be tested, but that can guide us in describing our work to others, and in further developing an understanding of so complex a thing as a combination of nursing and medicine. We can learn from the struggles of nurse theorists and from their successes how better to approach the definition and conceptualization of nurse practitioner practice.

Again, taking the experimental design terms, lesson six: Set a high priority on developing measures of the dependent variable—patient welfare—in nursing research in nurse practitioner research.

Most of the research that's been done on nurse practitioner care has included only the most superficial determination of the quality of care. What kinds of things could legitimately be affected by our care, in patients? Mortality rates, birth weights, compliance with recommendations, appropriateness of use of health services are only the tip of the iceberg of the possible things that might be tapped. An example from psychiatry intrigues me. Many new services were designed for the chronically ill patients when state hospitals began to discharge them in carload lots. What we're learning now is that while these patients may indeed stay out of the hospital, which is a *good* thing, they may also have such a minimal existence on the outside that it isn't much better than it was inside except for costing the state less. We need measures to tap the subtle nature of the quality of existence that could be affected by our services.

In reviewing some literature on social competence lately, and discussing it with some nurse practitioners, it occurred to me that if nurse practitioners are serious about what we usually call health education and helping the patient understand the reasons for our recommendations, then it is possible we are equipping patients with a set of skills, and perhaps even personality changes, that could well impact on other facets of their lives. For example, if the nurse practitioner helps the patient have access to the health care system (as was proposed as one of the reasons why nurse practitioners ought to be created) and if she helps him through it, does he then learn that systems aren't so impenetrable after all? And with that new knowledge, will he think better about his own ability to control his life, and will he then be more able to negotiate his way into a job, new living quarters, a school system?

There's another lesson in here we should learn from nursing research. A good deal of the early nursing research chose as measures of the effect of nursing some things that were not valid measures. The choice reflected our own ignorance of some physiological processes and our general naivete about what could legitimately be called a measure of the effect of nursing alone, uncomplicated by other things that happened to patients. Hopefully, the nurse practitioners advanced knowledge in human physiology, pharmacology, clinical medicine, and the like will help avoid these problems. But also because the scope of the nurse practitioners work is larger, she has a might wider variety of measures of outcome to chose from, and in some sense has a clearer notion of what he wants to accomplish.

We need to be brave and just the tiniest bit arrogant, too, in thinking of what nurse practitioner practice could affect. A television show a couple of weeks ago on children with learning disabilities sparked this thought: the program made the point that the tip-offs to a problem in learning are there but there are few eyes to see them. But a pediatric nurse practitioner or a school nurse practitioner, or a family nurse practitioner is in an enviable spot to have access to the behavioral and physical signs that indicate learning disabilities, and because of the nursing background, hopefully the nurse practitioner would be more alert to these subtle cues than teachers or other health professionals. The TV program went on to link untreated learning disability not only with failure in school, which is obvious, but also with delinquency, neurosis, even psychosis, to say nothing of limited potential for self actualization. A long term study of the nurse practitioner's ability to detect potential learning disability, and make the proper referral, and do the counseling and health teaching around this problem is almost a natural. And how wonderful to use as the dependent variables such large social phenomena as delinquency!

Another example: A pediatric nurse practitioner on our faculty works in the birth defects clinic where among other things she handles the continuity of care for children with spina bifida, myelomeningocele, and other such anomalies. As part of her care she routinely conducts Denver Developmental Screening Tests on the children and several times has picked up cues that a child's shunt was not working, had the child admitted, and prevented a long hospitalization and extensive surgery and trauma. Incidentally, her experience has an interesting methodological implication: the Denver may be much more sensitive than it is usually thought to be if it can pick up these kinds of clues, but is it also reliable in the measurement sense? Could other pediatric nurse practitioners administer the test and have the same findings?

Lesson number seven (and this is one nursing research should have learned from nursing practice): Not all patients are the same.

In nursing practice we are taught to individualize our patient care because different patients need different things. Yet in nursing research we often select samples and analyze data as if all patients were indeed the same, ignoring some important group differences. Of course, research would be impossible (except for case studies) if people couldn't be grouped together for analysis. But sometimes we've overlooked even the most obvious indications for stratifying samples. For example, studies of the effect of nursing on patients have often failed to analyze the data separately for male and female patients.

Dr. Alvan Feinstein's research provides an interesting model. He has tried to pull apart medical diagnoses—rheumatic heart disease originally, later breast cancer—in terms of extent of involvement, nature of symptoms and severity, in order to make more accurate predictions of the effect of treatment. In doing so, he's made some major contributions toward understanding the differential survival rates for degrees of illness, and convinced many that "a rose is not a rose is not a rose"—not every single case of rheumatic heart disease has the same characteristics and same outcome from treatment. His findings have made clinical medical practice more specific and his research has been instrumental in opening up a new field of inquiry for medicine—the practice of *their* profession.

A similar approach could be taken in nursing. We could try to separate out the characteristics of patients that have something to do with their experience of illness and treatment, and therefore could be effected by our practice.

The study I mentioned earlier where the nurse-midwife wanted to be able to incorporate some "diagnosis" of the patient's ability to cope with pregnancy, distilled from an understanding of her psychosocial assets, falls in this category. We still know far too little about which patients are likely to profit from which of our treatments or procedures and if we're going to improve the practice of nursing in the expanded role, such data is going to be crucial.

Lesson eight should be so obvious it doesn't, need saying, but it isn't, so it does: Replication is to be cheered and promoted.

The science that is the foundation for practice doesn't spring fully formed from the brow of Zeus but is accumulated over long years and repeated studies. The history of nursing research is filled with individual studies never repeated, robbing us of any claim to a solid base in nursing science. It's unclear whether the reason is that there's an implicit requirement for master's research and an explicit one for doctoral study that each study be unique and original, or whether it's that we've fallen into the old women's trap of not trusting each other and therefore not valuing our sisters' works. I fear that in the nurse practitioner game we may also trap ourselves by our own competitiveness and try to outdo each other in the wonderfulness of our research (as I sometimes think we've tried to do in our educational programs and in our practice) without considering the value to the profession of building up a bank of data from repeated studies.

Lesson nine is equally common sensical: Publish or perish.

I don't mean this at all in the orthodox academic sense. I do mean that we could get rid of some of our constant feeling of lonely struggling isolation if we shared our work with others, and also if they responded.

To subject one's work to the reasoned criticism of one's peers is so important a part of the scholarly professional life that it cannot be underestimated. There is so much good work going on in nursing, and all we see is the smallest fraction. We cannot begin to build a base of research on which to decide the future directions of nurse practitioner work until the research begins to creep into the literature. And we cannot wish to be respected by our academic peers or even the public until they know something of what we're capable of, and have data to see that it works.

Perhaps you've guessed where all this is leading—lesson ten: We must learn from the mistakes of the past and put service and research and the education for both back together.

The best kind of research will have to involve in significant ways as principal investigators the nurse practitioners themselves. This is not to say that collaborative research is to be outlawed or interdisciplinary efforts to be simply tolerated. But the nurse practitioner brings to the study of practice problems a point of view that no one else has, not other nurses, not physicians, no matter how closely they work together. For research to be useful to people in the expanded role, it has to have the credibility of a real understanding of what that practice is like. Further, the research must come from a real grasp of the problems in patient care faced by nurse practitioners as they perceive them. Research has to grow out of the real-life practice situation and no one has a better grasp of that than nurse practitioners themselves.

It took nursing in the United States exactly 100 years for the professional organization to make a commitment to the preparation of nurses in research in baccalaureate and masters programs. Please let us not wait that long to make a commitment to the preparation of nurse practitioners in research. Since the implication is here, I should say it out loud: I completely agree with Loretta Ford that nurse practitioner education must occur within the educational setting in degree granting programs and degree granting institutions. And it must be accompanied by research education. We have learned sadly in our history in nursing that we cannot advance the profession in diploma schools and through continuing education alone, and we have learned that one of the reasons that cannot happen is because such programs do not include an analytic scholarly emphasis. Yet here we are with legions of "certificate" nurse practitioner programs, and still very few in graduate or undergraduate schools. We simply must learn from our mistakes of the past, and not replicate them in the future. Quite literally, the survival of the expanded role in nursing may depend on our learning very quickly what we can from the history of nursing, and putting those lessons into our nurse practitioner programs immediately.

The expanded role gives us such an opportunity, working with our colleagues in medicine and other professions, to turn America's health system around. Not only so that people have access to the care they need but also so that the quality of that care is constantly improved. A nurse practitioner is only half trained if she learns the clinical techniques of the expanded role and does not also learn the tools and attitudes of systematic inquiry and scholarship. If she chooses to locate in rural Vermont in lovely autonomy or in a medical center constantly being abraded by the pressures of academic medical life is not so material. Our patients in Vermont, Rochester, or New Haven cannot afford to accept us simply because we're nice, available, friendly, female, and unusual in our new roles. We have a moral obligation to them, and to ourselves, to question constantly the dimensions of service and its effects, and to change where necessary, with planning and study of outcome. As a profession we also have the obligation to live up to the trust society places in us to act competently and we must be prepared to do so.

I propose to you that we are not living up to public trust so long as we continue to divorce research from clinical practice and provide the preparation for the former in doctoral programs in other disciplines, and the preparation for the latter in clinical continuing education.

Ladies and gentlemen, our challenge is this:

- to learn from our history and not make the mistakes of the past when there's a future out there with nothing but promise
- to recognize that we must overcome in nurse practitioner work what we've only begun to overcome in nursing—the sexist notion that women can do practical things but can't think, can take health histories and do physical assessments, but can't do the kind of abstraction research requires
- to think clearly about the practice of the profession as it fits with the world's realities and realize that we have the opportunity to teach others, including physicians and academicians, that research in professional practice is possible, that it improves services at the same time it serves the University's needs to develop new knowledge
- to question all that we take for granted about the ways things are and propose the way things ought to be because there's nothing stopping us. It's a revolution, no question about it, best stated in Bobby Seale's expression: "seize the time."

I leave you with another quote, this time from Mark Twain: "do what is right. It will please some people, and astonish the rest."

ENDNOTE

1. I was on the search committee that eventually made me Dean. I knew that I was not the first, second, or even third choice. Barbara Bates, MD was the leading candidate after two others—John Thompson and Rhetaugh Dumas—had taken themselves out. I was in favor of Barbara's appointment. Only she and I and the late Katherine Buckley Nuckolls, then Chair of our Pediatric Nursing Program and an obvious choice though she didn't put herself forward, knew about that apart from Yale's President and Provost. Barbara never told anyone either. She declined the offer of appointment, believing it was not appropriate for a physician to be Dean of a school of nursing. She was such an unusual physician that I still think it could have worked internally, but she was right. The symbolism would probably have killed nursing at Yale. There's a longer story that would have to deal with the then Provost's own impending career change to become a Jungian analyst, very into symbolism. The context is everything.

NURSES IN PRIMARY CARE: THE NEW GATEKEEPERS

As the Nurse Practitioner movement was seeded, so was the Physician Assistant (PA) role, and for the same reasons: the shortage of primary care providers in the context of expanding insurance coverage for primary care under Medicare and other mechanisms. There was an additional agenda behind the PA movement: the policy issue of what to do with very well-trained military corpsmen now being discharged as the military downsized in the 1970s. PA's were the children of physicians; NPs were the grown-ups of nursing. And I will stop this metaphor right here.

This article was originally a paper given at the Fifth Annual Symposium, Nurse Faculty Fellowships in Primary Care, sponsored by the Robert Wood Johnson Foundation and Vanderbilt University, Nashville, TN, April 30, 1982.

Let me take that apart. The Robert Wood Johnson Foundation was created out of whole cloth from the estate of Robert Wood Johnson in the early 1970s and became instantly the largest health care foundation in the country. From the beginning, the RWJF has taken a more activist role than foundations usually do, using the considerable power of their endowment to move their own agendas. Early on, they took on "primary care" as a special commitment. Most of their efforts were targeted to medical schools to change undergraduate medical education to emphasize primary care. The Foundation always puts together annual meetings of their programs that invite others in.

In this instance, I was not supposed to be the speaker. Ingeborg Mauskch, RN, PhD, important in my professional life as sponsor, was supposed to do this address. But she had a conflict—she was also on the committee that created the Holocaust Memorial Museum (she being a Holocaust survivor) and the dedication was the same day. She called me maybe 3 weeks before and asked if I could cover for her. I had been trying to break into the RWJ environment for years. Still, 3 weeks is awfully short to put together something like this.

Claire Fagin was in the audience and told me later the RWJ people in the front row were uncomfortable. I hope so (though I may have gone just a tad too far, as I reread this). This was a chance to say out loud what many of us were thinking behind the scenes. Claire got the AJN's interest to publish this (83 [5], 742–745, used with permission). My collaborator and informant and coauthor was Susan Molde, RN, MSN, then the Senior Nurse Practitioner at Yale-New Haven Hospital. Susan was the first NP trained under federal funding at Yale as an Adult Nurse Practitioner (the early work had been in pediatrics).

Primary care has been an exciting adventure for nursing, requiring great courage on the part of the pioneers. Now that we have established ourselves in primary care—in the role we know as nurse practitioner—it is time to look both back and ahead, to see where we have been and what we are becoming.

The first formal educational program for nurse practitioners started in 1965 at the University of Colorado.[1] It provoked unanticipated reactions. Although early studies of the new role consistently showed that we were accepted by our patients and our physician co-workers, the nurses and support staff exhibited resistance.[2]

Why? Some nurses felt that primary care was medicine, and that nurses who elected to practice primary care had defected, undermining nursing in the process. To others, the nurse practitioner was an interloper. The working relationships between nurses and physicians had always been modeled on traditional marital relationships—the physician was husband, the nurse was wife. In a sense, the nurse practitioner (or nurse-midwife) represented the proverbial "other woman," breaking up the "marriage." The "other woman" was independent, undeferential, free, and bitterly envied by the "wife."

Within nursing education, the primary care movement made nurse educators seriously question some of the profession's philosophical underpinnings. What *was* nursing anyway, and what did one need to know to do it? Nursing educators were quick to recognize the value of physical assessment and to add the subject to the undergraduate curriculum. That giant step expanded the basic nursing role. When nurses learned the language of assessment, communication between physicians and nurses improved. And skill with the tools of physical examination—the otoscope, ophthalmoscope, and stethoscope—brought nurses more knowledge, along with increased responsibility and accountability. A knowledgeable nurse is not likely to stand still when an intern (or anyone else) tries to tell her to do something she knows is incorrect or dangerous. Nurses who can make their own evaluations of patients are also less likely to call the doctor for small things. In effect, they control the physician's entree to the patient.

Nowhere was the conflict among nurses more obvious than in the ANA's first *Social Policy Statement,* which defined *nursing* as the diagnosis and treatment of *human responses* to health problems.[3] Furthermore, the *Statement* said that nurses diagnose and treat these *responses,* not the health problems themselves. Nurses in primary care fumed over that sentence, which they interpreted as saying that what they were doing was not nursing. The sentence was removed from the second printing of the *Statement*.

The extension of nursing into primary care also called into question the relationship of primary care nurses to traditional nursing service structures. Nurses in primary care may be caught between two competing hierarchies: On the one hand, there is an archaic reporting system that makes nurses accountable to other nurses who may not be prepared in primary care. On the other is a parallel physician-dominated structure in which all nurses are presumed to report to doctors.

Because the role of the nurse in primary care has been controversial, primary care nurses have had to be, like Caesar's wife, perfect in all things. As a result, primary care training promotes significant changes in nurses' attitudes—changes that make individual accountability essential and make the nurse even more impatient with mediocrity, rigidity, and chauvinism of any kind.

Accountability requires knowing that while the possibility of error is inherent in matters of judgment, considered decisions will most often be either right or reversible. Working in primary care also tends to make one aware of the *quality* of the data on which any decision is based. Whether it's a matter of care, curriculum, or policy, the nurse practitioner has learned to call for precision and logic.

Early on, nurse practitioners were obsessed with knowing everything about anything that could possibly go wrong with the body; their greatest fear was killing a patient. But, as experience grew, that fear dissipated. Concern for careful work-up and complete diagnostic evaluation has continued, but consumes less energy. Now, nurses recognize the limitations of medical science and are challenging traditional practices. They are becoming impatient with case conferences that emphasize obscure diagnoses. They have absorbed data from the social sciences and nursing research into their practices. Thus, their care is becoming truly holistic, the scope of practice is expanding, and studies are emerging to explain how nurses are able to do as well as—if not better than—physicians in the field of primary care.[4]

The original conceptions of primary care nursing held that nurses would care for patients who had routine or chronic health problems, thereby freeing physicians for complicated cases; and nurses in primary care would deal with, well, children and adults. It hasn't happened that way.

The first patients that nurse practitioners were allowed to add to their caseloads were the "undesirables"—the old, the poor, the alcoholic, the mentally ill, the noncompliant. Therefore, nurses quickly found themselves caring for the sickest patients, not the healthiest.

Patients who are difficult—because of their personalities, because they present management challenges, or because they are medically complicated—drift about within the health care system among attendings, residents, and interns unless they accidentally encounter someone who will spend the time to evaluate their complaints, look for effective treatment strategies, and assure follow-up. Such disadvantaged patients, with their multiple problems, require the kind of attention and follow-up that can be provided only by clinicians who remain on the scene. So they eventually end up in the nurse practitioner's caseload.

Another feature of medical center politics affects the nurse practitioners' caseload—when there is pressure on primary care physicians to capture patients for eventual referral to specialist colleagues, physicians may take on all of the new patients. Patients whose complaints are urgent, but not emergent, may then be assigned to nurse practitioners. When house staff are not scheduled for many hours of ambulatory practice, their patients may also be bounced to the nurse practitioners. Again, nurse practitioners end up seeing the *sick* patients—the ones who cannot wait for two weeks for their resident to come back to the clinic, or the ones who are being followed for a previously identified, major problem.

In health maintenance organizations (HMOs), a different phenomenon yields the same result. Because HMOs need to market themselves to potential enrollees, it is common practice to have new patients choose a primary physician and make an appointment with him or her for a physical examination. The physicians are then backed up for months doing routine physicals. Meanwhile, nurse practitioners, who usually do not perform admission physicals—the organization may fear that patients will be offended by seeing a nurse first—end up seeing the sick people.

Another turn of events is that in many primary care settings, nurse practitioners are now senior in clinical experience; and, in institutions where they have faculty appointments, they may have academic seniority as well. Nurses have taught generations of physicians how to practice in primary care, yet each new arrival believes himself "captain of the ship," entitled by training and social role to control the practice, including the work of nurses who may be senior in rank, experience, and expertise.

Nurse-midwives have long encountered this problem. Many of the settings in which experienced nurse-midwives practice use house staff as "back-up." Obstetrics residents have only 3 or 4 years' experience; interns but 1 year; medical students, 6 weeks. Imagine how a nurse-midwife with 25 years of experience feels when a green resident tells her what to do.

In retrospect, accepting the initial definition of the scope of practice for nurses in primary care—that of well-child, well-adult care—was expedient and probably strategically correct. Indeed, to have specified anything grander would have been so provocative as to ensure failure.

In 1974, the American Association of Medical Colleges sponsored a conference on primary care. At that conference, attended by some 500 people, mostly physicians, Rashi Fein, the Harvard economist, defined primary care as "...the development of systems of care emphasizing access to first contact, the treatment of basic (even if 'uninteresting') problems with emphasis on and concern for the total patient and his desires for support and care, and the opportunity to move from primary care to other parts of the care system in a smooth fashion."[5] At the same meeting, David Rogers of the Robert Wood Johnson Foundation said that any system of primary care ought to have certain basic capabilities. Among them:

- "It must have the ability to identify, from innocent-appearing situations, those few that are potentially serious, and provide properly for them."
- "It must provide appropriate science-based humanistic support for those it serves."
- "It must fit the way of life, the culture and the lifestyles of the people to be served."[6]

Add the definition of primary care published in 1971 by the Secretary's Committee to Study Expanded Roles in Nursing: "first contact care during an episode of illness, continuous care which is comprehensive and family-centered."[7]

What do we get when we add these definitions up?

Primary care is and always has been nursing. The statements above are not definitions of medical practice, which is defined by the laws of all states as diagnosis and treatment, prescribing for and operating upon disease. Of course, there are some functions of primary care that might fall into a definition of medicine, but the attitudes and values described in these statements are *nursing* values and attitudes, and they always have been.

Regardless of how or where nurses in primary care practice, the struggle for control of that field is the issue for the '80s. For primary care is the gate through which people enter the health care system, and she who controlleth the gate controlleth it all.

The issue of economic competition is rapidly surfacing. But until third-party reimbursement is available directly to nurses in primary care, we will not see economic competition as a full-blown problem.

In medical schools that are losing research grants, the pressure is on medical faculty to engage in direct practice and bill for it. Since medical faculty cost a lot of money, they must be extremely productive to be retained. To be productive, they have to do the kind of work that pays the most, which, in medical centers, is new patient visits, "executive physicals," and attending on the inpatient wards. Anyone who interferes with those sources of revenue will be challenged.

Maryland's nurses' superb and successful attempt to obtain direct third-party reimbursement is instructive.[8] Legislation passed in that state changed the *insurance* laws to specify that services for which others are reimbursed ought to be as reimbursable when delivered by nurses.

In Maryland, nurses were able to ride on the coattails of a history of defining reimbursable services as *skills*—an office visit is x dollars; psychotherapy is y dollars; physical examination is z dollars. What is so brilliant about the

Maryland strategy is that it glides right over the fruitless battles about who does what and how to define it?

The kind of competition predicted by the Graduate Medical Education Advisory Committee (GMENAC) report on excess medical manpower is not the biggest worry.[9] Although there have been federal enticements for medical schools to teach students about primary care, medicine is not changing its specialist focus. The number of general and family practice physicians has leveled off and is not growing. Primary care does not promise either the money or the status that specialization does.

Now that we know things have turned out differently than might have been predicted when primary care nursing started, we can begin to consider what primary care is and ought to be. We cannot escape the lessons of the past, but neither can we continue to survive in the present anomalous situation.

Primary care should be the door through which the patient enters the system, and primary care nursing has now developed that part of its role. In the next phase of development, primary care should move out of exclusive concentration on the first contact, urgent visit, triage, and screening functions, and into the arenas of comprehensive, family-oriented, continuous care.

The community mental health literature provides us with the concept of the "case manager."[10] In an ideal primary care system, every patient should have a case manager. It should make no difference whether the patient walks into the health care delivery system through the community mental health center, the nursing clinic, the emergency room, the office, or the neighborhood health center. The case manager is responsible for the first contact workup and should see to it that the patient's problems are completely identified. Then, the case manager should see to it that every other door in the health care system is open to the patient and that those who work behind the doors do what they are supposed to do and do it well. It may be that the case manager can provide for most of the patient's needs. Or, it may be that referral—not transfer—to other resources is needed. What is crucial to making this new primary care system work is that one person knows everything that is going on with the patient and can pull it all together.

This is a proper, indeed historical role for nursing, because only nursing is involved in all phases of the health care system.

Another feature of this new primary care system would be collaboration among nurses. If a patient required surgery, for example, the primary care nurse would help the patient select the surgeon, help the patient decide how to best use the surgical advice, arrange hospital admissions, make contact with the nurses who would be caring for the patient once admitted, and monitor the surgical outcome.

In this system, primary care nurses, including psychiatric nurses and nurse-midwives, are the first line of caregivers. The second line would, for the most part, also be nurses; the primary care clinician would see to it that the patient who is depressed gets a nurse-therapist, the depressed pregnant patient a nurse-midwife, and so on. On the third line would be pediatricians, internists, and so forth; on the fourth, physician specialists; and on the fifth, physician subspecialists. But the case manager could decide to jump from line one to line five if necessary.

Primary care and nursing have come a long way since 1965. We now know that putting nurses into primary care does not make them half-fledged physicians. Volumes of research show that primary care given by nurses is simply *different* from care provided by physicians. We no longer need worry about the validity of the role of the nurse in primary care, nor need we worry about malpractice or patient acceptance. If we *are* to worry, it might only be about how to reorganize the health care system so that the gains made are not eroded.

Clearly, if we can keep our wits about us there might come a day when primary care fulfills its promise. When that happens, we will have gone much further toward finally fulfilling *our* promise to the people we serve.

ENDNOTES

1. Ford, L. (1982). Nurse practitioners: history of a new idea and prediction for the future. In L.H. Aiken (Ed) *Nursing in the '80's: Crises, Opportunities and Challenges* (pp. 233–247). Philadelphia: J.B. Lippincott.

2. Storms, D.M. (1973). *Training of the Nurse Practitioner: A Clinical and Statistical Analysis* (Pub. 4). North Haven, CT: Connecticut Health Services Research.

3. American Nurses Association (1981). *Nursing: A Social Policy Statement* (Pub. No. NP-63) Kansas City, MO: The Association, p. 10.

4. Sullivan, J.A. (1982). Research on nurse practitioners: process behind the outcome? *American Journal of Public Health, 72*(1), 6–9.

5. Fein, R. (1974). Issues in primary care: the policy perspective. In *Proceedings, Institute on Primary Care.* Washington, DC: American Association of Medical Colleges, p. 25.

6. Rogers, D. Medical academe and the problems of primary care. In *Proceedings, Institute on Primary Care.* Washington, DC: American Association of Medical Colleges, p. 230.

7. US Health, Education and Welfare Department (1972). *Extending the Scope of Nursing Practice: A Report of the Secretary's Committee to Study Extended Roles in Nursing.* Washington, DC: US Government Printing Office.

8. Goldwater, M. (1982). From a legislator: views on third-party reimbursement for nurses. *American Journal of Nursing, 82*(3), 411–414.

9. US Health and Human Services Department (1980, Sept). Graduate Medical Education Advisory Committee. Non-Physician Health Care Provider Technical Panel *Report: Volume 6.* Washington, DC: The Department.

10. Krauss, J.B., & Slavinsky, A.T. (1982). *The Chronically Ill Psychiatric Patient and the Community.* Boston: Blackwell Scientific Publications.

Nurse Practitioners: Skirmishes, Strategies, Successes

This paper was never published. It was the keynote address to the NPACE (Nurse Practitioner Associates for Continuing Education) meeting in Albany, New York, September 27, 1984, 10 years after the first paper in this section. What struck me when I worked on it for this volume was how much I had been educated in political and policy issues of advanced practice in the interim.

I tried to catch the mood of nurse practitioners who were feeling put upon, caught up in complicated politics. Nearly exactly 20 years later in 2004, I could see myself giving an updated version of this speech as there are still silly legislative proposals, and increasing reimbursement obstacles to NP practice (the "incident to" provisions under Medicare being the most shining example). It's all about money. It's not about performance, competence, or quality.

The Nurse Practitioner role has rolled out internationally and other countries have dealt more creatively than the USA with some issues, especially prescribing. They may have learned from us. In New Zealand, for example, legislation was passed that granted prescribing authority to nurses, before NPs were even born there, under a governmental agenda to encourage competition in health service delivery. In Australia, especially in New South Wales, after a punishing lot of years, NP positions are being created by government, especially in the "outback" and in other underserved areas such as Corrections (jails/prisons). The individuals in Australia who have been important in pushing these positions through are nurses, and two of them are also trained in the law (Mary Chiarella, now Chief Nurse of New South Wales, and Amanda Adrian, then Commissioner of the Health Care Complaints Commission in New South Wales).

NPACE is still an important force, especially in the Northeast and I'm sure its conferences are as well attended as this one.

This paper is harder on Florence Nightingale than was probably appropriate. It was written before contemporary scholarship had mined Miss

Nightingale's life more contextually.[1] *Still, the notion that she was much more complicated than the self-sacrificing "lady with the lamp" was an important learning for me.*

The other context for this speech is that the political scientist, Paul Starr, who had just published his magnum opus The Social Transformation of American Medicine, *was the invited speaker. His book was thought by many of us to be more than ordinarily sympathetic to nursing. But his speech was arrogant and off-hand; clearly a nursing audience wasn't important other than whatever his honorarium bought.*

I was told the following story by the then Executive Director of the New York State Nurses Association, Catherine Welch. As hostess, she met Prof. Starr as he entered the airport terminal, introducing herself simply by name. He threw his trench coat (Burberry, of course) at her and said, "Carry this, sweetheart." I may have heard that story before I gave this speech which would account for why it had more passion and outrage in the delivery than even the words convey.

My mission this morning is quite simple: to tell you that nurse practitioners are just fine, we are not an endangered species, and anyone who thinks otherwise is simply deluded.

Now, lest you think *I* am the one who is deluded, let me develop this notion.

We forget sometimes that the notion of nurses doing primary care as nurse practitioners is not even 20 years old yet, if one starts the count from the first program in Colorado in 1965. If one starts the count from the early days of this century, when public health nursing began, nurses have been doing primary care for a long time and therefore there is nothing very unusual about it. When the immigrants got off the boat on Ellis Island in the early days, they were met by public health nurses, with stethescopes in their ears. When the early visiting nurse associations were started by Lillian Wald in New York City, for example, it was to provide primary care services to the poor, to mothers and children, and to people with tuberculosis.

Or, if one wants to go even earlier, when Florence Nightingale took her little band of 38 nurses to the Crimea, it was not to care for the wounded. There weren't very many wounded, in the first place. What there were, Miss Nightingale found, were 20 chamber pots and over 1000 men with dysentery. Her nurses were there to cure, not simply hold the hand or wipe the fevered brow. Cure meant baths, and good food, fresh air, and hygiene since there were no antibiotics and amputation was an iffy procedure.

Miss Nightingale went to the Crimea with her nurses in one of the greatest public relations coups we are ever likely to see. Her agenda was not altruism; it was to demonstrate to the Ministry of War that she could run things better than the Army surgeons and thus carve for herself a political place. Miss Nightingale believed she could take over the Army, first the surgeons, later the troops, and since the Army was the force for building the British Empire through colonization, eventually she could take over the world. Delusional? Perhaps, but we might remember this side of Miss Nightingale even more than we remember the legend of the lady with the lamp. She did carry a lamp, and she did drift silently through the wards at night, but she was not looking to comfort some handsome young man. She was looking for dirt in the corners, or sleeping on the job, to give her an excuse for firing the Army orderlies and substituting her nurses.

And when she wrote about it, she instructed her sister, Parthenope, to copy her letters and see to it that they got into the public press. She told her nurses to write about her, and she saw to it that letters she wrote home to families of soldiers who had died were printed in the papers.[2]

Miss Nightingale lived in the early days of the industrial revolution, which had improved social conditions to the point at which care of the sick, the elderly, the poor could be raised to public consciousness. She saw power in working with the sick, for who could deny that the work was important? And she saw the need to train women for this role, not simply depend upon their good impulses or charity. Her model of training was controlling and restrictive, for she was building a base of loyalty and discipline.

But most importantly, she kept records. She counted cases—mortality rates in Scutari, dollars, meals prepared, bandages rolled, and she wrote volumes of complicated letters which even today have not been completely catalogued.

I dwell on Miss Nightingale here to provide a framework for thinking about skirmishes, strategies, and successes, and I will return to the themes embedded in these anecdotes later.

To have a proposal that goes against prevailing wisdom or common practice is to provoke a skirmish. At the same time it is a strategy. Charles Lewis has written about some of the early reaction to the nurse practitioner clinic he and Barbara Resnick started at the University of Kansas in the mid-1960s. He reports that Mrs. Resnick was challenged by one physician to explain why she was looking through the charts. When her new role was described, the physician exclaimed, "My God, what won't they think of next?" One resident was overheard saying to another, "Look at this chart, this patient is going to a nurse clinic. Can you imagine, they're even letting nurses write in the charts now!" And this was January, 1966.[3]

But Lewis and Resnick prevailed, and their study of the effects of this nurse clinic on the chronically ill patients it served became a landmark article.[4]

Loretta Ford has written about the early days of the first pediatric nurse practitioner program at the University of Colorado. It was resisted primarily by pediatric nurses, including Ford's own colleagues at the School of Nursing. The federal government refused to fund it (in part because Lee Ford was a public health nurse, not a pediatric nurse, and because there was fear that pediatricians would gobble it up). The Children's Bureau, approached for training monies, refused to consider the project and instead designed its own substitute which relied heavily on physician control.

But Ford and Silver prevailed with help from private foundations and with careful attention to documenting the efforts of the nurse practitioners to both the lay and professional press. Perhaps you remember, as I do, a story in *Time* magazine about 1969, long before we really understood what nurse practitioners were, about a woman who had become the "general practitioner" in a small town in southern Colorado. I remember being stunned at the audacity of the idea and delighted to have nursing acknowledged in a mass circulation magazine.

There was an acknowledged doctor shortage in those days, you may recall, so the American Medical Association tried to propose that physicians take on the training of "physician extenders" so that physicians could be freed for the kind of work their lengthy training prepared them for. The American Nurses Association was not amused, but for the wrong reasons. There was also a nursing shortage, and the American Nurses Association did not think the solution to one manpower shortage was to raid another. The American Nurses Association also did not think physicians had any role in educating nurses for anything. It would have been nice in those days if the American Nurses Association had had the vision to be supportive, but that came much later.

The first nurse practitioner training monies appeared in the Division of Nursing budget in 1971. That's not even 15 years ago and within the lifetime of all of us, and the professional lifetime of many of us. It is useful to remember how recent this revolution is for it helps see over the hurdles of both the past and the present.

Of course, there have been fights along the way and there will be more. Arkansas tried to restrict the practice of nurse practitioners by demanding physician supervision, signed protocols, and a ratio of no more than two nurse practitioners to one supervising physician. That move failed.

In Tennessee, it took the nurse practitioners and physicians 5 years or so to finally agree on proper credentialling that shared the authority between the medical and nursing boards. North Carolina was the first state to have a nurse practitioner licensure law (and a registered nurse licensure law, for that matter). It provides limited prescriptive authority, with each nurse practitioner's formulary subject to approval of a joint medical/nursing board. The issue now in North Carolina is for nurse practitioners who work in non-traditional settings, for instance a state mental hospital, to have the authority to prescribe and monitor psychotropic drugs, which so far have been prohibited to nurse practitioners.

Prescriptive authority can be characterized as a political issue, and it will be that when negotiations to change state law to permit prescriptive authority to nurse practitioners are going on. But we must not forget, for the memory is our strength, that simply wanting to write prescriptions in one's own name is not the issue. The issue is that the people we must care for need not to have their care even more fragmented than it already is. Patients need to have medicines. Nurse practitioners know which ones they need. Nurse practitioners see the patients, take the histories, do the workup, read the previous record, and decide on treatment and management. Some of that is prescription. Why, then, should it not be possible for nurse practitioners to follow through and simply write a prescription (which is not a very big deal—four lines on a pad)?

In New Jersey, a nurse practitioner was sued for practicing medicine without a license. The suit was brought by the medical board, not by a patient. Her alleged offense was recommending a mammogram. With the support of the New Jersey nursing association, the case was thrown out when the medical board was declared to have no jurisdiction over nursing. What was really at issue here was not the performance of the nurse, it was the fact that she worked for a new HMO which had taken considerable business away from the local medical practitioners.

You all know the Missouri case. There, two family planning nurse practitioners were alleged to have practiced medicine without a license in examining women and then prescribing birth control and fitting diaphragms. It is not coincidence that the suit was instigated by, among others, the brother of the president of the state medical society. He lived and practiced as a family practitioner in the small town where the nurse practitioners had their satellite clinic. The nurses lost the suit at the trial court level, but the Supreme Court of the State of Missouri reversed in a magnificently argued opinion. The judges carefully traced the evolution of modern nursing, citing information from other states, the nursing literature, and the federal government to document that the activities of the nurses were, indeed, contemplated by an enlarged nurse practice act Missouri had passed in 1974.

That suit hit the public media and was covered on the MacNeil-Lehrer report. A prominent Missouri physician was interviewed and his major complaint was that the nurses had not paid their dues (gone through medical school, internship, and residency) and, therefore, despite the acknowledged quality of their practice, should not be allowed to do it. The president of the family practice physician national group was also interviewed. His major point was that it was okay if he trained "his girls" to help him with office procedures so long as he was in charge (and in control of their salaries, too), but it was not right for nurses to just be out there doing their thing.

It interested me to note that while the Missouri case was still being decided, a family planning nurse practitioner in Ohio was sued on the same basis. There, the story was even uglier, for that suit was brought by a physician who had sent his own secretary to see the nurse practitioner, to collect the evidence that she was practicing family planning. When the Missouri case was settled and the decision announced, the Ohio suit was dropped.

The Missouri case is significant on a number of grounds. One of them is the support the nurses got from the nurses' association, and from a number of national nursing groups including the ANA, NACOG, and the American College of Nurse-Midwives. Over 200 *amicus* briefs were submitted for this case, to the distress of the Supreme Court justices who complained that Missouri needed to change its procedures because this was not, after all, an election. The briefs came from medical school departments of obstetrics and gynecology, deans of schools of medicine, and so on. That should not surprise you. What might surprise you is that these people *supported* the notion that nurse practitioners could act on their own, with their own authority, and that modern health care simply demanded that nurse practitioner do activities thought formerly to be medicine.

Important as this case is, it is only part of an even more important phenomenon in health law. For a very long time, nurses were not even considered real enough under the law to be sued in our very own names for malpractice. Now, I do not wish to advocate that nurses do the kind of things that end up being malpractice suits, but the fact is that until very recently nurses could not even be named as defendants grated on one's psyche. We still have some of that to fix. Now, nurses can indeed be sued in our own names, but we cannot be named in institutional malpractice insurance policies. Only physicians can be "named insured." All of the rest of us are "and other employees." Part of that is because we are, by and large, employees. Part of it also is that malpractice insurance companies have not had a way to calculate experience-based premiums for nurse practitioners or nurse-midwives. There is not enough experience in settled malpractice suits against us to allow insurance companies to use their magic formulas for calculating premiums. The lesson here is that when nurse practitioners are questioned about whether we will raise malpractice rates for physicians who might hire us, or whom we might join in practice, the answer is no. There are no data—none at all—that suggest that nurse practitioners can or should raise employers' malpractice premiums, and do not let anybody tell you differently.

Until quite recently—the last 5 years or so—nurses could not act as expert witnesses in malpractice cases. Instead, physicians testified about nursing. That has now changed considerably and nurses are being called upon to advise lawyers on alleged incidents of malpractice, and to testify to the standards of care.

Yet another change in the way nurses are thought of under the law happened without even a peep of resistance about 5 years ago in Connecticut, and with very little more resistance in California in the same year. That is a change in the law that allows nurses to be part of "professional corporations," as doctors, lawyers, architects, engineers, and others can be. That means that nurses—nurse practitioners and nurse-midwives particularly—may buy a piece of the practice, and thus share in the profits and benefit from the tax provisions that the P.C. status covers. Thus, nurse practitioners do not have to simply live with the role of employee; we may now become partners in practice, sharing both the risks and the benefits.

While we're on legal things, a survey by *Nurse Practitioner* indicates that 18 states have legislation authorizing nurses to prescribe. According to the survey there is no law prohibiting prescription writing in many other states, and nurses are routinely recommending over-the-counter and prescriptive medications in 46 states.[5]

There are only six states remaining that prohibit diagnosis and treatment by nurses. There is legislation mandating third-party reimbursement for nursing services in government programs (Medicaid, Rural Health Clinics, CHAMPUS) and in privately sponsored insurance programs in 15 states.[6]

And all this in only 15 years or so.

There are, of course, forces of darkness who would wish this all to go away. Over the years, nurse practitioners have fought with organized medicine, organized nursing, organized pharmacists, organized P.A.'s, organized nursing education, state legislatures, Congress, and lawyers. And won and won and won.

It is inevitable as it was in the beginning, that nurse practitioners would encounter resistance. But what is important to understand is what the resistance really is, for it is easy for us to feel victimized by a random world. The resistance is not at all random. It may not be rational, but it is not random.

While we have been busy building up nurse practitioner practices and increasing our numbers and changing laws and whatever, other things have been going on that have now brought conflict. There is an alleged oversupply of physicians. The data for that statement comes from the GMENAC report, the Congressionally mandated study of physician manpower.[7] That study was stimulated when Representative Paul Rogers retired from the House. Rep. Rogers had been the one who initially declared in the early '70s that there was a deficit of medical manpower and that Congress had to fix it by increasing the supply of physicians by 50,000, immediately. Why 50,000? No good reason. When Rep. Rogers was asked what the target number should be, he turned to his health aide and asked for a number and that's what he got. The story also is that a friend of his had, the previous weekend, taken his child to an emergency room in D.C. for an earache or something and had had to wait 4 hours to be treated. The friend attributed the wait to not enough doctors, called his favorite friendly Congressman, and that's how we now have an oversupply of doctors. I do not joke; that's how policy is too often made.

Anyhow, how many of you have read the GMENAC report? It is actually very interesting and very useful to nurses and nurse practitioners. In the first place, it says there is an oversupply of physicians in certain very highly specialized areas—neurosurgery, for example. But it does not say there is an oversupply in primary care, or family practice, or general psychiatry. Nor does it actually advocate killing off nurse practitioners or training programs. What it does advocate (which is unenforceable) is keeping nurse practitioner training programs to the enrollment limits of about 1980. Since there were no enrollment limits in 1980 (only minimum enrollment rules for federal funding), that recommendation is empty.

There is an assumption that simply because there might be more physicians than we need, the competition between nurse practitioners or nurse-midwives and doctors would increase. That assumes that the work done by these groups of practitioners is the same, and thus we are striving for the same piece of a shrinking pie. Of course, there is overlap in function, but there is more than enough work to be done. But what is becoming clearer and clearer is that nurse practitioners own primary care; that nurse-midwives own normal obstetrics, and increasingly well-woman gynecology.

A nurse practitioner friend told me the following story. A primary care physician was trying to counsel her about her future in practice and, since he's a nice guy, was trying to warn her about the oversupply of physicians. He told her she ought to identify some small, specialized piece of the action for herself, and pursue that, as he had decided that cardiology was his piece rather than primary care. She said she had. "Primary care is mine," she said, and he grinned, scuffed his feet a bit and went away.

Medical education and medicine have become more and more specialized by organ system or cell unit. Physicians have even invented new specialties. Fetology, for example. Or human genetics as a practice discipline. Immunology—one can get board certified in that now. And that is just fine, for it leaves the science and practice of patient care—especially primary care—to us.

With increasing medical specialization has come increasing competition, because each specialty is smaller, and more dependent on the primary care specialists for initial diagnosis and referral. That means medical practice had gotten more competitive, and so what we hear about how we should worry about the oversupply of physicians is really physicians worrying about competition within their own highly specialized discipline.

More patients mean more dollars, not only to buy the Mercedes or send the kids to Harvard, but to pay off the office CAT scanner, or now the MRI. With increasing dependence on referral practice, the role of the gatekeeper— the one who greets the patient at the door and then opens all the other doors into the health care system—becomes crucial.[8]

Primary care is the gate into the health care system. Whoever gets to see the patient first determines all else that is going to happen. The first contact the patient has with the system largely defines whether he will return again, feeling satisfied with the initial visit, or whether he will shop around for something better. And where nurse practitioners have a range of referral resources, we can determine the income and practice size of others. Nurse practitioners, nurse-midwives control the gate and it is not even surprising that we absorb the political reactions of those who ambivalently want us to do the gate-keeping work (the initial history and physical and so on) but who do not want us to have the control that the gate-keeping work delivers.

The care of the worried well, of persons with minor acute illness or stabilized chronic conditions, which is what nurse practitioners were initially supposed to be good for, is the bread and butter practice. Well-woman gyne-cology is what supports an ob/gyn practice, not the time-consuming activities of labor and delivery, nor surgery. Well-child care, which is the equivalent situation in pediatrics, is the same. It is not surprising therefore that pediatricians who were the first medical specialty group to conceive the notion of nurses as partners in primary care are now trying to recover the ground that was lost when nurses did that. I love the notion, for instance, that pediatricians have rediscovered nutrition, or child development, or even adolescence.

When nurse practitioners began to be trained, there was an unexpected and unanticipated phenomenon which also has become a threat in clinical settings. When nurses came to know how to do physical examinations, diagnose, prescribe, and manage patients as well as physicians, and better than rotating interns or medical students, there was obvious reaction. When nurse practitioners began, there really wasn't anything equivalent in medical specialty practice to primary care. There still isn't, just as there isn't an equivalent to normal obstetrics, which nurse-midwives specially own. So a nurse practitioner who had done primary care for a year or 2 or 5 was the expert, unacknowledged, of course.

Now, through the Johnson Foundation and other sources, there is supposed to be something called primary care that is medical care. I find it hilarious (as well as fury-making) that nurse practitioners are now being hired in droves in medical schools to teach residents, interns, and medical students how to do the work we know how to do. My fury is not that nurse practitioners are selling out—they aren't. It is entirely reasonable that patients ought to get good primary care, and if training housestaff to do it is the local answer, fine. My fury is that the centrality of nurses, of nurse practitioners to the effort is unrecognized, and once again, nurse practitioners are hired hands.

That is not always the case. There is a fascinating report out of Jackson County Memorial Hospital in Miami.[9] The problem there was that the care of chronically ill patients who were very sick (and primarily diabetic) constituted a "service burden" to the residents that interfered with their learning opportunities. Therefore, a clinic staffed with nurse practitioners was set up. The residents then took on the care of the easily fixed simple cases that did not require follow-up and the nurse practitioners cared for the very sick. Not too surprisingly, hospitalization rates for the diabetics dropped and their ability to control their disease rose, thus improving cost effectiveness as well as quality of care. What the article does not say, because it is probably assumed we all know it, is that residents are really very powerful. Their feedback to the attending faculty is one variable in accreditation of housestaff training programs, and the competition for housestaff is fierce. They must be paid attention to. Not rational, but not random.

The incongruity of the contrast between hiring nurses to train or help doctors now and about 10 years ago is also funny. Ten or so years ago, nurse practitioners, the few there were, were actively prevented from having anything to do with housestaff, I am told, because the house staff were thought "too young," too tender and precious to withstand the force of a nurse practitioner making a diagnostic decision they missed. More important (but it took us years to learn it) is that medical education (not unlike nursing education, actually) is a very closed shop. Private, community physicians depend on residents for the 24-hour coverage of their hospitalized patients. They also depend on residents to call them for emergency room patients who arrive without a personal physician. Residents depend on faculty and private docs for references for their NIH traineeship, or their private practice referral system. Because nurse practitioners were entering this game uncontrolled (because they were not dependent on this kind of referral mentality) and uncontrollable (because they were nurses, working, by and large, as nurses in a nursing system) they were suspect. It is instructive even this late in the game to realize that what rolled down on the nurse practitioners in those days had nothing to do with clinical competence, putting in one's time, or anything else. It had only to do with the fact that nurse practitioners were not members of "the club" and the club would not trust their loyalty enough to accommodate them as equals, and the nurse practitioners didn't want to be members anyhow. Not rational, but not random.

Nurse practitioners brought to the practice arena the attitudes and values of nursing which include treating the patient as a whole person, supporting patient participation in decisions for treatment to test, patient teaching and advocacy, and lack of dependence on technology at the expense of clinical judgment. And people got nervous. In medical centers, physicians argue among themselves all the time about diagnosis or treatment, but they were not used to nurse practitioners entering the fray. In solo practices of long standing, physicians had developed their own ways of doing things and sometimes did not welcome suggestions from the new nurse practitioner kid on the block.

The largest and least rational of the sources of resistance is simply the fact that nurse practitioners are primarily women, and even when not, trained in a profession with deeply female roots and ways of viewing the world. Carol Gilligan studied moral decision making and the extent to which there are reliable gender differences in how men and women consider values, choices, and variables affecting decisions. Her data show convincingly that women place a real value on community, commonality, connectedness, and the context of things, while men (at least in her study) value logic and rationality, rules and social codes.[10] That finding has considerable import for explaining our frustration in nursing and primary care as nurse practitioners try not only to rationally diagnose, but contextually understand and treat. To know that the difference we might grope to verbalize about nursing and medicine in primary care is instead a gender difference takes a very large monkey off our backs. And makes it possible to sympathize with colleagues, men or women, brought up in a male-gendered profession.

It amuses me to note that some of the criticisms that were made of nurse practitioners, and perhaps still are today, were also initially made when nurses began to have formal training in hospital-based schools. One physician railed against nurses knowing the reasons behind all details of patient management. He said, "to attempt to give nurses instruction as to the reason why would be ... to inflict a heavy task upon them." That was in 1875. Another physician defined nursing as:

> an honorable calling, nothing further ... The great and princi-
> pal duty of a nurse is to make a patient comfortable in bed,
> something not always attained by the most bookish of nurses.
> Any intelligent, not necessarily educated, woman can, in a
> short time, acquire the skill to carry out with implicit obedi-
> ence the physician's directions.

That was in 1908.[11]

Or maybe 1928, or '58, or 1978, for the exact same argument was used when nursing education began to move into the university, and when nurse practitioner training moved into formal training programs and out of on-the-job delegation of scut work.

In the 12 years in which I have been involved and sometimes embroiled in clinical and educational issues about nurse practitioners, I have collected some of these same kinds of absurdities. There was a time, for example, when the chief of staff of a certain hospital seriously suggested that the hospital would have to insist that nurse practitioners get signed informed consent from patients to be sure that patients knew the nurse practitioners were not doctors. That went away.

There was a time when a new service chief declared that nurse practition-ers (by then, five of them in this clinic, all with longer tenures than his) could not see new patients anymore. That the doctor would have to see the patient first, sign him up and diagnose him, and then the nurse practitioner could take over management. That lasted about 2 months and quietly went away. Perhaps the physicians remembered the original reason they had recruited nurse practitioners: the docs didn't *want* to have to see all the patients themselves, especially those who were overweight or depressed, alcoholic or strange, or those who had "only" common chronic illnesses like hypertension, diabetes, or degenerative joint disease.

There was a time when a distinguished physician could write a positive letter to the *New England Journal of Medicine* about nurse practitioner effec-tiveness, but still worry in print that the experience of this country with nurse practitioners might parallel Britain's early experience with thalidomide and nobody complained.[12] He tried it again last summer, this time alleging that the inflated income expectations of nurse practitioner would kill us off and the journal was deluged with letters.[13] And this time they printed four of them, three from nurses.[14] All four said essentially that the author was misinformed, to be charitable about it.

There was a time when some nurse educators accused nurse practitioners of turning into mini-docs when they learned how to take a history and do a physical examination. Now, every single school of nursing teaches physical assessment and practically every nurse not only wears a stethescope around her neck but knows how to use it.

There was a time when it was thought that the way to fix the legal status of nurse practitioners was either separate licensure or alteration of the nurse practitioner act. For years and years, nurses organized annually to get their state practice act changed. Practically every state now has some kind of expanded legislation. Changing nurse practice acts was our own political agenda, and we did it with little public support. But now, it turns out that the public policy agenda—the "shoulds" and "oughts" that transcend party politics or national administration—might well be on our side. An organization called the People's Medical Society has taken its charge as enforcing and reinforcing the notion that the health care paying public (even when supported by public assistance) has the right to know what they are buying and to have choices. In that context, one of their early studies looked at the restrictive force of *medical* practice acts.[15]

The practice of medicine in Michigan, for example, is defined as follows:

> Practice of medicine means the diagnosis, treatment, prevention, cure or relieving of a human disease, ailment, defect, complaint, or other physical or mental condition by attendance, advice, device, diagnostic test, or other means, or offering, undertaking, attempting to do, or hold oneself out as able to do, any of these acts.

It has been pointed out that under this definition, a mother who gives chicken soup to a child with a fever is practicing medicine, and that is absurd.

The review of all the state medical practice acts, done on contract by a lawyer for the American Bar Foundation, concludes with several options including abolishing licensing of all health professionals. The option the study prefers is restricting the definition of the practice of medicine to only those activities that have inherent potential to cause serious bodily harm. Thus, advising, counseling, teaching, and other activities protected by the First Amendment guarantee of freedom of speech would not be included, nor would bandaging. The policy agenda for this study, remember, was not to restrain medicine, but to increase consumer choice of alternatives. And the study recommends that any future licensing laws require the licensed professional to give the rationale behind any test or treatment. Failing to do so would then constitute malpractice.

There was a time when it was thought that nurse practitioners would be unsafe as clinicians. A huge body of evaluation literature, now over 1000 articles, dispenses with that notion. Indeed, one review of the literature concluded that when nurse practitioners and physicians were compared, controlling for severity of patient condition, outcomes of nurse practitioner practice were superior.[16]

Then there was a time when the politics of interprofessional relationships made the AMA declare its opposition to funding of nurse practitioner programs, and its commitment to keeping nurses at the bedside. Those resolutions were not implemented.

Then there were accusations that good as nurse practitioners might be, they would only increase costs and in a society suddenly aware of the escalation in health care expenses, and maybe we had better cut back on nurse practitioners. But the data available showed quite the opposite—that nurse practitioners, when they could practice to the limits of their training and intellect, without artificial restriction—were cost-saving to institutions.

There was a time when there were worries that nurse practitioners would not stay in the work force, since it was thought that nurses did not stick with nursing. The data from Sultz's huge national follow-up study of nurse practitioners showed that over 90% were employed, that nearly all found their first position within 3 months after completing the program, that they did not leave the field for the greener pastures of more education or childbearing. Further, the data show that over half of nurse practitioners' caseloads were people in the lowest socio-economic group.[17]

And there was a time, which is still with us, when there were debates about whether nurse practitioners were "complementary" or "substitutable." Complementary to what, might have been the question, but it was not asked. And substitutable for what, might have been the other question, also not asked. It is simply a fact that nurse practitioners have moved into positions that used to belong to physicians, or sometimes social workers, or P.A.'s or psychologists, or administrators. To take a place to do important work, even when the place used to be some other discipline's, is not at all the same thing as substituting. Substitutes are temporary.

What has happened is that nurse practitioners have simply continued the nursing tradition that started even before Nightingale, of moving into gaps in the health care delivery system. Where physicians were not available (as in underserved areas, public mental health, Indian reservations), nobody has even worried about who gives the primary care.

It has been demonstrated in a large, well-controlled study in Salt Lake City that nurse practitioner services to nursing homes resulted in highly significant decreases in medications, especially psychotropics, significant increases in functional status of residents, and cost savings that more than covered the costs of the program. The authors (a study team from the Rand Corporation) point out that the feature of the nurse practitioner delivering primary patient care was not merely a substitution of a nurse for a physician, but an organized treatment program which particularly focused on assessment and management.[18]

The whole notion of complementarity is odd. It reminds me of early discussions of the nurse practitioner in which it was thought that she/he was somewhere between nothing and being a "full-fledged" physician. I always had a mental image of a bird with only half its feathers. That notion assumes that all there is to health care delivery is diagnosis and treatment of disease (which is really all physicians are licensed to do, despite different practice act language). To complement that would be to add some other services, which are unlikely to be reimbursable, and thus visible. To substitute would be to assume that *all* nurse practitioners do is the same stuff somebody else does, only cheaper.

It has become boring for nurse practitioners to try to define what it is we do, or what the dividing line is between medicine and nursing. It is not even an interesting cocktail party conversation any more. Nobody asks physicians what they do for a living, and if they were asked, they would stumble over the words just the way we do. Definition is not the point. Description might be, if we can get over being intimidated by the fact that whoever asks the question is unlikely to be impressed with the answer. We know what we do, and we do it just fine. When stuck for a definition, I often use Virginia Henderson's definition of the unique function of the nurse, because it says it so well:

> ...to assist the individual (sick or well) in the performance of those activities contributing to health or its recovery (or to peaceful death) that he would perform unaided if he had the necessary strength, will or knowledge. And to do this in such a way as to help him gain independence as rapidly as possible.[19]

Under this definition, if a patient could diagnose his own appendicitis and treat it, he would. If a patient could label his hypertension and prescribe medications for it, he would. The definition also implies preparing the person to negotiate the environment, whether it is the doctor's office, the family, or the acute care environment. (I have discussed this interpretation with Miss Henderson and she is not alarmed. After all, her first nursing position was with the Henry Street Settlement, under Lillian Wald's successor, Annie Goodrich.)

I hope not to make enemies by saying that I disagree profoundly with the notion that *all* nursing is (including expanded roles) is "diagnosing human responses to actual or potential health problems."[20] In the first place, it is not possible to diagnose a response to something that hasn't happened yet. In the second, and more importantly, this effort to define nursing has had the effect of turning a definition originally written for quite crucial political purposes (to get the word "diagnose" into the New York State Nurse Practice Act) into something never intended. Any definition of something as dynamic as nursing is incomplete, which is why no dictionary attempts a definition of the *profession,* only of the word. Further, while diagnosing human responses might well be a part of nursing, it is not all of it (how about care, for example, or counseling, patient teaching, advocacy, and so on). And surely, diagnosing human responses was never intended to be the *limit* on nursing practice.

Patients do not show up in primary care clinics with potential alteration in skin integrity. They show up with rashes, or pain, or wounds, or headaches, or whatever. In the course of dealing with the presenting complaints, the nurse practitioner ought to check into other things but she or he ought not to have to describe his or her practice with some kind of artificial semantic nonsense which does not match the reality of the work.

There are lots of skirmishes left, including some within the profession. We have heard and will, unfortunately, hear more about nurse practitioners being fired so that more family practice residents could be trained, nurse practitioners subjected to impossible working conditions under unnecessary supervision, restrictive practice acts, protocols, rules, or codes, peculiar administrative decisions which set nurse practitioner salaries too low and put a ceiling on earnings, productivity demands that make good care impossible. And those will continue.

But those are not organized effort; they are local and idiosyncratic.

When it comes to organized resistance or the skirmishes that involve legislation or law, we have *not lost* a single one. Obviously, we can organize together when we have to, and do a very credible job of political action. The fact that more and more nurses and nurse practitioners are getting professionally involved in both policy and politics ought to be encouraging. The lobbyist for the NLN, for example, is a pediatric nurse practitioner. There are nurses in many legislatures now, especially in the northeast. Some 20 nurses have been elected to membership in the Institute of Medicine of the National Academy of Sciences. A nurse is a special assistant in the White House. A nurse in the senior staff member to the Senate Finance Committee. And one in 44 women voters is a nurse.

But political action is neither hard to prescribe, nor very hard to do. The strategies that have brought about the changes and successes for nurse practitioners are not secret, Florence Nightingale knew them all.

Pick your target. If you want to take over the British Empire, start with the Army. If you want third-party reimbursement, start with the insurance law, because that is what governs it. If you want prescriptive authority, start with the pharmacy law which governs whose prescriptions may be filled. Don't mess with practice acts unless you absolutely have to—they are simply too hard to change and they are designed to be restrictive rather than enabling because they are part of a state's police powers.

Learn that you are not alone. Miss Nightingale had the Ministers of War and of Health in her back pocket. We have the attention of the Federal Trade Commission which is now pursuing vigorously several suits in Tennessee, which allege that physicians conspired to restrain the trade of nurse-midwives by refusing them practice privileges in Vanderbilt University Hospital, and withdrawing their physician backup's malpractice coverage when they joined private practice. A malpractice insurance company, which is owned and operated by physicians, has already signed a consent order to stop that practice.[21]

We also have allies in the consumer public. In Connecticut, the Commission on Hospitals and Health Care has just granted a certificate of need for an out-of-hospital birth center incorporated by a group of nurse-midwives and consumers. The certificate of need was granted despite a vote of the local Health Systems Agency against the proposal, and despite the negative testimony of the state obstetrical society and the two hospitals in New Haven. It was granted explicitly, according to the commissioners, because the consumers had demonstrated the need, and because data had been convincingly presented as to patient safety in such settings.

Which is another strategy. Use data, any chance you get. Any change argued from data is more impressive than change argued from bias or personal investment. That is partly why nursing has been so successful in fighting off the resistances of others whose best argument is they simply don't like the idea of nurses doing primary care. The phenomenal success of nurse-midwives in getting legal recognition in all 50 states, third-party reimbursement in Medicaid, and attention in the public press is a result of carefully accumulated data. In every nurse-midwifery service, from the beginnings of the Frontier Nursing Service in 1933, nurse-midwives have simply kept records of every patient seen, by demographic and obstetrical factors, and every single outcome. When it came time to argue or agitate for legislative change, the data were there.[22]

And data can be used for less grand but equally important agendas. One nurse practitioner I know keeps all of her encounter forms for the year and when it comes time for her annual evaluation, she counts the numbers of patients seen, the visit type—new patient, return, follow-up—and knowing what the institution charges for these visits, documents that she generates more than twice her salary.

Even records kept of who one's patients are, what problems they present, what medications they need, how often one consults with a colleague will turn out to be useful, and they are so easy to keep. Such statistics buried in your bottom desk drawer will just gather dust or mold. Descriptions of practice settings are publishable; a good deal of the basic nurse-midwifery literature consists of counts of how many of what kind of patient was seen over whatever time. Writing anything about one's practice—description, conceptualization, quandaries, political problems—is also a strategy. Florence Nightingale wrote incessantly and got it into the public press even without a peer review system. And it worked.

Another strategy: learn to read the political and policy agendas. In Connecticut, a third-party reimbursement bill for nursing passed on its first try. Part of the reason was that nursing knew the business community was concerned about the high costs of health care, and organized information about how nursing could lower costs of care. It is no accident that this year, after four futile years of trying, Congress has finally written new legislation to fund nursing at the federal level. The proposed funding levels are considerably above what has been available in the past. Why? It's an election year, with a party in power that needs the attention of women, and a woman vice-presidential candidate breathing down their necks.

A basic strategy is simply to know what has already happened somewhere else, and to consult the experts when change is desired. We are not alone. There are expert lawyers out there who can help get legislation passed, or can present our case to the Missouri Supreme Court. There are reporters who are sympathetic too, and often know more than one would think about nursing or nurse practitioners, because we make a good story. There is now a large body of literature available to buttress a case and if you don't have access to a medical library or the latest journals, call [or now, email] some school of nursing faculty member who does.

We have agendas in common with other nurses who are not nurse practitioners. Prescriptive authority, for instance, is as important to nurse-midwives and to med/surg clinical specialists who administer chemotherapy, T.P.N., or life-saving drugs in the ICU as it is to primary care types.

There are lots of folks on our side—from consumer groups like the People's Medical Society who share our values, to friendly physicians, to the courts and the Congress and the FTC. Nurse practitioners provide an alternative system of care, and the national mood is to seek high quality, lower cost alternatives. Take advantage of it.

Be a little pushy. If the *New England Journal* says something you don't like about nurse practitioners, write a letter. If there's a new senior physician whose attitudes about nurse practitioners are either unknown or negative, send him flowers on his first day and force him to find out who you are and what you do. And dig in your heels if you suspect you are being used. If you are asked for your c.v. or resume for some project somebody else is doing, don't give it unless you are sure it is in your interest. If you are told to take on new responsibility, make sure you get the credit for it too.

And get inside the system as much as possible. It is so much easier to make change from inside than from outside.

And seek visibility. Connect with a Future Nurse Club. Those people might never turn into nurse practitioners, but they have parents who are influential when you might need to call on them. Join a political party or the League of Women Voters. A lot of change strategy is taking advantage of reputation or connections made over time, and you will never know when the stranger you sat next to on an airplane might turn out to be a legislator, or other public figure.

While we might not want to be as deluded as Florence Nightingale was (she did actually have a vision and saw herself as Christ, complete with crown of thorns), we cannot ignore the fact that visibility and power are already with us. If you have been keeping score, you know that we have not ever lost a major battle, and the score on the skirmishes is about 94 to 3. It is hard to believe that when one is the lonely only nurse practitioner in East Overshoe, Nebraska or Littleville, Vermont, or when one feels alone even in a city where there are colleagues. That is why a meeting like this is not only for refreshment and education, but also for connecting.

It has been my pleasure to begin that connection this morning; now it's your turn.

ENDNOTES

1. Dossey, B.M. (1999). *Florence Nightingale: Mystic, Visionary, Healer.* Springhouse, PA: Springhouse Corporation.

2. Smith, F.B. (1982). *Florence Nightingale—Reputation and Power.* New York: St. Martin's Press.

3. Lewis, C. (1982). Nurse practitioners and the physican surplus. In Aiken, L. (Ed.). *Nursing in the '80's.* Philadelphia: Lippincott. (pp. 254–5).

4. Lewis, C., & Resnick, B. (1967). Nurse clinics and progressive ambulatory patient care. *New England Journal of Medicine, 277,* 1236–1241.

5. *Nurse Practitioner.* Survey Results (1983). *Nurse Practitioner, 8*(2), 41–42.

6. LaBar, C. (1983). *Third-Party Reimbursement for Services of Nurses.* Kansas City, Mo.: American Nurses Association.

7. Graduate Medical Education National Advisory Committee (1980). *Report to the Secretary,* DHHS. Washington, D.C.: U.S. Department of Health and Human Services (Pub. # HRA 81-656).

8. Diers, D., & Molde, S. (1983). Nurses in primary care: The new gatekeepers. *American Journal of Nursing, 83*(5), 742–745. Reprinted here just before this paper.

9. Becker, D.N., Fournier, A.M., & Gardner, L.B. (1982). A description of the means of improving ambulatory care in a large municipal teaching hospital: A new role for nurse practitioners. *Medical Care, 20,* 1046–1050.

10. Gilligan, C. (1982). *In A Different Voice.* Cambridge: Harvard Press.

11. Kalisch, P.A., & Kalisch, B.J. (1978). *The Advance of American Nursing.* Boston: Little Brown.

12. Spitzer, W.O. (1978). Pediatric nurse practitioners. Letter to the Editor. *New England Journal of Medicine, 198,* 163–164.

13. Spitzer, W.O. (1984). The nurse practitioner: Slow death of a good idea. *New England Journal of Medicine, 310,* 1049–1051.

14. *New England Journal of Medicine* (1984). *311*(8), 535–536. One of those letters was ours and it is reprinted after this paper.

15. Andrews, Lori B. (1984). *Deregulating Doctoring.* Emmaus, Pa.: People's Medical Society.

16. Prescott, P., & Driscoll, L. (1979). Nurse practitioner effectiveness: A review of physician-nurse comparison studies. *Evaluation in the Health Professions, 2,* 387–418.

17. Lewis, 1982, *ibid.*

18. Pepper, G.A., Kane, R., & Teteberg, B. (1976). Geriatric nurse practitioner in nursing homes. *American Journal of Nursing, 76*(1), 62–64.

19. Henderson, V. (1963). *The Nature of Nursing.* Philadelphia: Macmillan.

20. American Nurses Association (1980). *Nursing—A Social Policy Statement*. Kansas City: American Nurses Association.

21. Lerner, A.N. (1983, August 20). The impact of antitrust on the health professions. Remarks delivered at the 50th Annual Meeting of the American Association of Nurse Anesthetists. New Orleans, La.

22. Diers, D., & Burst, H.V. (1983). The effectiveness of policy related research: Nurse-midwifery as case study. *Image—The Journal of Nursing Scholarship, 15*(2), 35–41.

Nurse Practitioners: Letter to the Editor

This is the letter referred to in the previous paper. Dr. Spitzer's increasingly negative comments on NPs struck many of us as incongruous—this was the man who had done the very first methodologically credible studies of NPs in Canada. He was educated at Yale, after all. But he was now turning against what he has helped to create; Slow death of a good idea was the title of one of his articles. At the time, I don't know that I understood what was probably happening—he had gotten out too far ahead of organized medicine and had to back-pedal.

Over a lunch of very hot chili (I can see the table now), Susan Molde and I crafted what she has called a "temper tantrum." No more a temper tantrum than the balderdash upon which we were commenting. This was published as a Letter to the Editor in the New England Journal of Medicine *(311 (8), p. 585, 1984, used with permission).*

The writing here, apart from the fury that still crackles off the page, is in the style one must use. Cite the data. And, when you can, cite yourself, to establish your credentials. NEJM never publishes the positions or credentials of letter writers unless they are Senators or otherwise have a public agenda. So we are two lonely nurses here. The instructions for Letters at the time said they had to be confined to 40 lines, which we did, which is a good exercise for getting one's points done really fast and deadly.

It would be too much for us (and the other letter writers) to take credit for the fact that Dr. Spitzer has not been heard from on NPs since 1984.

To the Editor: For the second time in six years, Dr. Spitzer has issued a dismal prognosis for nurse practitioners (April 19 issue).[1]

In 1978, he acknowledged promising early research about the safety and effectiveness of nurse practitioner work but also called for continued surveillance, cautioning that the public's experience with nurse practitioners might parallel Britain's early experience with thalidomide.[2] Despite the outrageous analogy, his call for scientific testing of this innovation in health care was appropriate. We agreed.[3]

Now, he has recanted. Since he now accepts the data about the quality of nurse practitioner care, he is left with one naïve argument and one pernicious one on which to base a poor prognosis. What Spitzer reads as "internecine fighting" we take to be healthy debate. And although legitimate questions can be raised about whether any health care system can afford both nurse practitioners and physicians, the "unrealistic ambitions about income" of which Spitzer accuses nurse practitioners reflect not greed but comparable worth.

Spitzer's argument that nurse practitioners must be cheaper in order to survive is simply the latest in a series that proposed first clinical, then political, and now economic restraints.

The nearly 20 years of accumulated evidence tells us that we nurse practitioners can compete effectively on our own terms. We look forward to Dr. Spitzer's next retraction—due, we presume, in about 1990.

Susan Molde, RN, MSN
Donna Diers, RN, MSN
Yale University School of Nursing

ENDNOTES

1. Spitzer, W.O. (1984). The nurse practitioner revisited: slow death of a good idea. *New England Journal of Medicine* 310, 1049–51.

2. *Idem.* Pediatric nurse practitioners (1978). *New England Journal of Medicine* 298, 163–4.

3. Diers, D., & Molde, S. (1979). Some conceptual and methodological issues in nurse practitioner research. *Research in Nursing and Health*, 2(2), 73–84.

BETWEEN SCIENCE AND HUMANITY: NURSING RECLAIMS ITS ROLE

Writing for the general public is a different way of writing about nursing. To me, it requires putting nursing in terms that the audience is most likely to read and heed. That's not writing down, nor up. It's trying to get their attention and, having gotten it, shaping the message to be most catchy and palatable.

The following piece was published in the Yale Alumni Magazine *in 1982 (45 [5], 8–12, used with permission). This magazine went then free to the more or less 90,000 living Yale alumni, many of them in powerful positions in industry, government, and academia. I had written for this publication 10 years before, when I had just been appointed a University Dean.[1]*

And the feedback was wonderful. I heard from nurses who had been handed the magazine by patients they were caring for, saying, "maybe you'd be interested in this," and some of them became students at Yale. I heard locally from many of my University colleagues, often with surprise in their voices or notes that "a nurse could write so well." That gave me a standing as one of them that was important in what I needed to learn and do in that first year.

Ten years later, another opportunity surfaced. The Editor asked me to do a story on "modern nursing." This time I wrote it in the style I knew fit the magazine, including the "inside" references, the tiny academic conceit of a Latin phrase, and contemporary allusions to film. This time I negotiated for the pictures to accompany the article and several pages of follow-up interviews with nursing practitioner faculty and alumnae/i. We had a cover picture—a PNP faculty member doing a well-baby check on a really photogenic baby, who, as it happened, was the granddaughter of an important Yale Alumnus, something I had no way of knowing. But someone did and that information was printed with the photo credits.

It happened that there was also a big ad in this issue of the magazine for a company selling high-end imported carpets started by some Yale graduates. They got lots of copies and propped the magazine, cover up, in various

windows of bookstores and other retailers in New Haven, opened to their ad.
We got huge exposure, accidentally.
This is also, in my biased opinion, the best writing I ever did.[2]

The meticulous reader of the *Yale Weekly Bulletin and Calendar* of
November 2–9, 1981 might have noticed, in between announcements of col-
loquia on immunobiology, Sanskrit, and vector transformations, a lecture on
Florence Nightingale. The truly obsessive reader would have noticed something odd: the lecture was sponsored not only by the School of Nursing,
which might make sense, but also by the Department of History, the Section
of the History of Medicine, and the Department of Epidemiology and Public
Health. If the reader hungrily followed University politics, he might have
chuckled at the coincidence, for just the day before the lecture on
Nightingale, the Yale College faculty approved a major in women's studies.

It does not stretch the synapses too much to make these random observations fit. Florence Nightingale—founder of modern nursing, statistician, sanitarian, Victorian anomaly, brilliant and devious woman—is a figure in not only
the history of nursing and medicine, but the intellectual history of the nineteenth century, and lately she has been rediscovered as an important figure in
the study of women. As the attention of scholars and historians turns to Miss
Nightingale, so is public attention turning now to nurses as more than simply
an occupational group who dress quaintly. Nursing might even *(mirabile dictu)*
be the key to the reform of an obese and inhumane health-care system.

It is difficult to miss nursing in the public press these days, what with nurse
shortages in the headlines, nursing strikes enraging laymen and professionals
alike, and nurse-midwives confronting directly the medical obstetrics' stran-
glehold on women's health and normal childbearing. Nurses are refusing to
stay invisible, controllable, patronized, and underpaid. Nursing, like Florence
Nightingale, who started it all, not only is a metaphor for the struggles of
women for equality, visibility, and respect, but also is calling into question convenient societal assumptions about health-service delivery, health-care economics, and public policy. And like Florence Nightingale, modern nursing is
trouble.

In his essay "On the American Teacher," President Giamatti proposes that
among the reasons teaching as a profession has been called into question is
that teachers have not been able to define teaching so that it can be understood
and valued by others. Nursing is in precisely the same fix.

As with teachers, there is not a single person who has not had some contact
sometime, somewhere, with a nurse. It may have been the school nurse, spin-
sterish and cold, who measured your height and weight and was good for
excuses for getting you out of gym. It may have been the pert young thing who
brought your newborn baby to the waiting room and chirped, "It's a boy!" It
may have been, if you're old enough, a wan and tired woman in ill-fitting
fatigues who staunched the blood, eased the pain, and calmed the bone-deep

fear in Aachen, or Seoul, or Cam Ranh Bay, or marched with you to a prison camp on Bataan. If you're young enough, it may have been the nurse-midwife who was with you at the beginning of a new life, cheering, coaching, teaching, and participating with her humanity, not stealing yours.

It might have been the person with the pendulous bosom, the icy hands, and the icier voice who asked, "Shall we have our bath now?" as if you were not only filthy but infantile. Or it may have been the one who watched you all night in the ICU, or gave you your polio shot, or the one who held you when a loved one died. All of these were nurses, no matter what their training, degree, or credentials. Whether they were all good nurses is a more complicated question.

People think they know what nursing is, just as they think they know what teaching is. Mothers without 4 years of nursing school tend their sick children, and literally nurse the babies. Everyone at some time "nurses" a cold (and sometimes "doctors" it too). Similarly, everyone teaches. Yet professional nursing, like teaching, involves far more than either the title would indicate or the lay activity would suggest.

To understand what modern nursing is about, particularly those parts that attract the public eye, one must first understand what nursing means to those who do it. The nature of the work overwhelms all other factors: the interprofessional battles, the political wars, the intraprofessional confusions.

Nursing puts us in touch with being human. Nurses are invited into the inner spaces of other people's existence without even asking, for where there is suffering, loneliness, the tolerable pain of cure, or the solitary pain of permanent change, there is the need for the kind of human service we call nursing.

The intimacy that is the core of nursing gives us a peculiar aura, and just as some people feel awkward in the presence of a visibly pregnant woman—so clear is the fact of her intimacy—some people are embarrassed in the company of nurses. We are supposed to be dignified over vomitus, uncringing at the sight of blood, calm as we debride the decubitus, pack the wound, give out the bad news. Nurses must hear, but never tell, the secrets of the dark side of the soul, the hates and jealousies, the anger and violence, the cursings at fate, the bargains with God. The terrors of psychosis, the joy of a peaceful and happy birth, the erosions of poverty and discrimination that turn a body thin and sour-smelling are part of the nurse's world, all day, every day.

Because nurses have never had the prerogative of omnipotence, we find it comfortable and natural to be with the patients as human beings, without social distance. The tradition of nursing care is lodged in an explicit value: that it is our job to help others do what they would do for themselves if they had the skill, energy, or will. And, when recovery is impossible, to assist others in the ultimate act of dying, dignifying the individual with all his personal history, idiosyncrasies, needs, values, and desires.

Some of what nurses do looks so easy to the untrained eye. How could putting a bedpan under someone take 4 years of college? How could feeding a helpless, aged woman take a degree? How could mixing a formula, taking a temperature, asking about a health history merit a curriculum? By itself, any task is more or less simple; but nurses must do all of these, and many more complicated ones, and do them with grace, the reassuring illusion of speed, and some purpose and plan in mind.

When done either superbly well or dreadfully badly, nursing seems so simple, for what is invisible in any human service is the thinking behind the act. The questions we ask the family of a patient in the emergency room are not at all random; we are diagnosing, determining the problem, defining the things to worry about. The options a nurse-practitioner presents to the patient—this test is effective but costs $60, and there are other ways of getting the same information, although they may be less specific and may take longer—are carefully thought out. Intensive-care nurses develop an occupational ear with which to listen for the subtle wheeze, the ominous groan, the restless rolling that might predict dangerous change. Nursing requires the use of all the visual, aural, tactile, and psychological senses, for they detect the data upon which one acts. The intellect sorts and classifies, questions and predicts, for it is imperative to the practice of nursing that the nurse understand enough of how the human body responds to illness and treatment that she may distinguish what is okay from what is trouble, what requires her skills and what requires the talent or training of others, what is normal and what is anomalous. A good deal of what is now social work, respiratory therapy, occupational therapy, physical therapy, psychiatry, and medicine began as nursing. The cure for typhoid fever, for instance, before immunizations and antibiotics, used to be entirely nursing care—alcohol baths to lower the temperature, fluids to treat the dehydration. It used to be true that nurses' work concentrated on helping the patient recover from the interventions of surgery. The surgeon amputated, and the nurse controlled the bleeding, prevented infection, and prepared the stump for rehabilitation.

The mid-twentieth century was a time when nursing stood still while advances in medical science, pharmacology, surgery, diagnosis, technology, and administration moved so far and so fast that the turf nursing once called its own was invaded. Nursing's struggles of the past few decades have been to catch up to the changes in modern health service delivery and begin to reclaim the central role it once had.

The activities of nursing that directly connect the nurse and the patient are crucial, but what is less often understood is the extent of nursing's entirely separate but equally compelling responsibility: no less than managing the whole experience—the entire environment—of the health care practices of all other professional groups. The nurse is in charge of all of the health care system and must make it work in the service of those who need and want it. It is the nurse who must see that the room is warm and the ice is cold, the dinner is served properly and on time, the doctor is called and informed, the family is comforted, the lab gets its results back on time, X-ray pays attention, the floors are swept, and the costs—ah yes, always the costs—are kept down.

The deepening realization that this is the way it is for nurses is what is making us so uppity these days. It is not only the pressure of eight or twelve or sixteen hours a day of trying to care well for sick people when we can't get the laundry to send the sheets, or the nursing administration to provide enough staff, or the doctor to listen, show up, or cooperate, or that we can't prevent pain, death, and disfigurement. It is not just being on one's feet and running, trying always to catch up—our work is endlessly unfinished. It is not just the 5 minutes snatched for lunch or the coffee going cold in the lounge, nor the mounds of paperwork that must somehow get done and recorded and filed.

Nurses are burnt out, not only because the work is grueling, but because it goes unrewarded. "Burn-out" is a phenomenon now so pervasive that research is being done on it by everyone from circadian rhythm biologists to endocrinologists to psychologists and stress-management experts. Studies done in the last 2 years show that what nurses want as top priority is not salary (though that would help), not better working conditions (though that would help, too); rather, we want respect, and we want the freedom to practice to the limits of our knowledge and talent without institutional or interprofessional interference.

There are about 1.4 million nurses in the United States; about 75% of them employed at any given time. Nursing is the largest group in health service delivery and the largest primarily female profession. Despite general economic gains in the field, nurse salaries are on the average about the same as those of secretaries or, as cited in the case of *Lemon v. City of Denver* (a federal suit alleging sex discrimination), tree trimmers. Nurses' salaries average about 75% of the salaries of teachers. Perhaps what grates on us most is that whereas in 1945 the dollar difference between the median nurse salary and the median physician income was about $7,500, in 1980 the dollar difference was *$66,500.* You might ascribe our ingratitude over this discrepancy to green-eyed envy, but what makes the inequity intolerable is how little the patient understands the role of the nurse and how much the public believes the fantasy that the doctor, no matter how good, bad, or indifferent, is the captain of the ship and the shaper of all things medical.

When a patient receives a hospital bill, he has no way of knowing what proportion of it is accounted for by the nursing care he received. While most hospital bills now itemize laboratory fees, prescriptions, special procedures, and tests, nursing costs are buried along with brooms, breakfast, and the building mortgage. Until it is possible to isolate the costs of nursing, it will be impossible for nurses to argue that they deserve more of the respect called salary and for hospitals to justify their salary schedules. Because nursing is economically invisible, it is possible for both nurses and administrators to discount nursing, to lump us into an amorphous, faceless mass. Nurses have been thought to be interchangeable, and until very recently there were plenty of nurses to go around, so there was no incentive for an institution to do anything about working conditions, salary, fringe benefits, or lunch breaks. Nurses were expendable; a questioning, unhappy, or uppity nurse could always be replaced with another newer and cheaper warm body.

There is a nursing shortage, and it is desperate, but public policymakers are now reluctant to see it because to acknowledge that there is a shortage is to have to admit to nursing's importance and to face up to the inequities in the business that is health care.

For a very long time, nurses who wished to escape the daily grind, the rotating shifts, the evenings and weekends and nights and double duty left clinical work for teaching and administration. That pattern began to shift in the late 1950s, and the pendulum has indeed swung so far that there is a recognized and undebated shortage of nurse faculty and nursing service administrators. Those nurses who wish to practice to the limits of their training and brains have increasingly moved into positions of clinical specialization, and a whole set of new hyphenated nursing categories has grown up: nurse-midwives, nurse-practitioners, clinical-nurse-specialists, nurse-clinicians, nurse-researchers. Like their sisters in institutional practice, they confront the same issues of visibility and control of their own work and autonomy, but there is an additional twist to the problems of these new professional categories: economic competition.

There has been a good bit in the press in recent months about competition in the health care industry, as various administrations have tried to attack the problems of uncontrollable health care expenditures. Competition policy has been pinned to the "free market," which in this context means that the consumer must choose which brand of health insurance to buy and assumes that only those brands offering better benefits and services will survive.

It would be a mistake for public policymakers to restrict attention only to competition in the health *insurance* game, for it is increasingly clear that competition between nurses and others, primarily physicians, is the issue for the eighties. Nurse-midwives, one of the oldest of the specialist practice roles for nurses, have hit the competition problem earlier than other groups, but the issue affects other specialists as well.

Nurse-midwives do not pass themselves off as obstetricians and do not pretend to do the range of things obstetricians do. Nurse-midwives are specialists in the care of the essentially normal patient (85% of all pregnant women), and are determined to involve the patient in all possible decisions regarding her care and her participation. National certifying examinations provide the public evidence of the safety and competence of nurse-midwifery practice, and a complex system of accreditation of educational programs buttresses the quality of the teaching and, therefore, the practice of nurse-midwifery students and faculty.

Where patients are eligible, informed and given a choice, more and more are now choosing the style of practice nurse-midwives deliver. While the number of nurse-midwives and their patients is still small, it is conspicuous enough to provoke resistance. This is often couched in terms of patient safety, or of quality of care, the assumption being that physician care is *ipso facto* "first class," and anything else is not. Even Congressional committees have now recognized that patient safety is not a cause to be concerned about nurse-midwives (in more than 55 years of nurse-midwifery practice in the United States there has never been a settled malpractice case against a nurse-midwife, for example). Given a declining birth rate, a surplus of obstetricians, and a national mood of consumer choice, it is hardly surprising that there is inter-professional rivalry, for the issue is not quality of care; it is money.

Nurse-practitioners—nurses with advanced preparation in primary care—are now encountering the same level of resistance, for they have built a better mousetrap. Data now show convincingly that well prepared nurse-practitioners can deal quite safely with 70% to 90% of the patient problems that occur in the office or ambulatory visit, while simultaneously delivering the traditional nursing services of counseling, teaching, and patient advocacy. Primary care—the first visit to a health-care system during an episode of illness, and the continuing care during that illness, including coordination of the care by others—is the gate through which patients enter. Who controlleth the gate controlleth it all.

Specialist practitioners make the most dramatic case for competition as an issue. But broadly conceived, if there is to be a finite number of dollars for health care, and if there is to be an "unavoidable" excess of physicians by 1990, and if nurses of any stripe demand their share of the pie, competition is the inevitable outcome.

In the 60 years of the Yale School of Nursing, it has always been in the forefront of the field, as any professional school in a distinguished university should be. Today, as we prepare college graduates and nurses for advanced practice as nurse-practitioners, nurse-midwives, and clinical-nurse-specialists, we run directly into the established boundaries of territory and power. We have taken as our agenda the reform of the health care system, through the education of our students, the research of the faculty, and where possible, collaboration with others. The role of reformer is neither easy nor comfortable, for the reformer or the reformee. Our nursing programs are calling into question everything from the nature of nursing education (where we fight our professional organizations) to the scope and limits of professional practice, from the ways human services have been constructed and rewarded to the intellectual questions that can and must be raised about the kind of understanding—scholarship—that can be brought to bear on what are finally issues that are fundamental to the serious study of the relationship between science, service, and social policy.

It is difficult for nurses to fight off the tendency to be bitter. Like the character in *Network,* many of us are "mad as hell, and we're not going to take it anymore!"

Florence Nightingale was powerful in part because of how she managed herself and her time. She decided deliberately, in 1857, to make others cower by adopting a regal mode of presenting herself—appointments were made with one person at a time, with Miss Nightingale reclining in an invalid's posture on a couch, meanwhile writing volumes of complicated correspondence, couched in Victorian eyelash-batting. We don't have that option today (nor would we want it).

The people who are coming into nursing at Yale these days are all college graduates (including Yale College graduates). They are smart, aggressive, idealistic, impatient, and deeply committed to human service. They tolerate mediocrity, including chauvinism, badly. They ache to give of themselves in a special way called nursing. Nurses will no longer contain what we have learned the hard way about health, health care, sickness, suffering, mutilation, shame, brutality, ignorance, discrimination, hope, and human dignity.

A school of nursing exists in a place like Yale to link the University's academic values to the public interest, just as nursing applies the abstractions and discoveries of science to the problems of people. The first dean of the Yale School of Nursing, Annie W. Goodrich, understood how and why a great university should house a nursing school. She wrote that to be a nurse requires that one speak "the tongue of science and that of the people." When she wrote that in 1923, it was literary and visionary. In 1982, it is our mission.

ENDNOTES

1. Diers, D. (1972). It's a good time for nursing. *Yale Alumni Magazine 36*(3), 8–13.

2. I had great editorial advice from Andy Ward, a novelist and columnist, husband of Deborah Ward, RN, Ph.D. (YSN '77), now Professor, School of Nursing, University of Washington who was one of my NP colleagues at Yale. Andy took time out of his own writing to shape mine.

SECOND THOUGHTS

The papers in this section move from fairly conventional academic ways of speaking about nursing to pointed prose to overtly political writing to writing for an educated lay public in a style tailored to that audience.

The progression both in content and style were forged by experience and by opportunities to take what I was learning and doing and make it visible, or at least audible. And then taking the feedback from speaking to re-form, reinvent and otherwise revise ideas and ways of expressing them for the next audience.

It is difficult now to capture for those who did not live through it, how tough the times were for nurse practitioners in the early days. The tough stuff was in the politics and policy, not so much in the daily clinical practice. And the tough stuff wasn't really about practice, it was about power and control and money, not venues in which nursing was comfortable. We had to learn fast.

I took the high ground (a war metaphor, but that's what it felt like) to encourage nurses and NPs to do what they knew how to do and do it right, believing if they did, the data would show it. And the data did, of course.

The problem with doing something controversial, such as implementing advanced practice, isn't that the idea isn't the right one, the implementation pretty good, the data convincing. The problem is with defining what the problems, the barriers, are. In advanced practice the issues were entirely political and I spent a lot of energy trying to help beleaguered NPs and nurse-midwives and nurse anesthetists redefine their toxic experiences. What advanced practice nursing was doing wasn't wrong, it wasn't even unpopular, and it surely wasn't unsafe. It was simply confronting established social policy and order and money and power. When the rhetoric on the other side got extreme, we knew we were doing it right.

The trick, then, is to back off from the confrontational rhetoric which was important at the time, and turn to some other forms of expression that celebrate the nature of the work. Of course, the political posturing doesn't ever stop but it can get less draining as we learn that's what it is: posturing. And we learn how to posture our very own selves. And we learn when to associate nursing's agenda with others'.

I made trouble with the speeches in this section, deliberately, consciously, with purpose aforethought. The courage of the pioneer NPs and clinical nurse specialists was in front of and behind me. I felt the obligation to speak for and about them and their work; the privilege of the position I held gave me the platform. I tried to give NPs words and ways of talking about their work that might sand off the rough edges of local politics.

The adrenaline of public speaking and the responses of those who liked what one said is a very high high. Whether all that air consumed in speaking makes any difference is impossible to calculate.

NURSING, POLICY, AND LEADERSHIP

NURSING, POLICY, AND LEADERSHIP

Data and research lead to an understanding of nursing's work. The contexts for practice, which include organizational decisions, government programs, ethics, and party political strategy are also "data." Often these contexts are hidden.

I have observed that nurses feel victimized by a random world. The world is not random; it may not be rational, but it is not random. There are real reasons why things happen. The works in this section were aimed at providing new explanations for nurses about policy perspectives, or at providing new understanding to the public, including policymakers, about nursing.

The policy-making process is generally outlined as getting on the agenda or agenda setting, policy formulation, policy implementation, policy evaluation, and modification. If nurses wish to move beyond our parochial interests, it will be necessary to know what the policy process is, as well as how to use the tools of research and narrative to influence policy.

Until the policy agenda is understood, it is difficult to associate one's own disciplinary interest or research to it. When it is possible to associate nursing's interest to existing policy thrusts, it is a win-win.

By virtue of position and thus a platform, a place to stand, any Dean of a School of Nursing is supposed to be a "leader" in the profession. I was and am not very interested in nursing education issues such as entry into practice, credentialing, and so forth. I was and am very interested in helping nursing position itself to do what we know so well how to do as both basic and advanced practice, and then to *claim credit* for that work.

A long time ago when the possibility of being a Dean first surfaced, I had to think through what I would do as Dean. Since I didn't know how to dean, I would have to fall back on what I did know—my own values about nursing. I swore a great oath: "never badmouth nursing in public." Looking back, that was probably influenced by the growing consciousness fomented by the women's movement, and the recognition that oppressed groups will take it out on each other. I refused to act as oppressed or to speak of nursing as oppressed. Rather, I wanted to celebrate nursing whenever I had the chance.

Speaking about leadership is essentially inspirational. One cannot lead without being positive about the work and cheery about the possibilities.

TO PROFESS—TO BE A PROFESSIONAL

This was a speech originally given to District 4 of the New York State Nurses Association and published in the Journal of the New York State Nurses Association *(1984,15,[4], 21–29, used with permission) without any changes. It has been reprinted several times in other journals and collections of readings.*

At this time, I was on parallel speaking tracks: advanced nursing practice and nursing practice/leadership. In my head, they were the same, only the audience differed and thus the examples or narratives. This speech would have been given about a year earlier than the "Skirmishes" speech in the previous section, but both of them were in New York.

It is a great pleasure to talk about professionalism and about nursing as a profession. I will take the posture that we are no longer searching for our profession; we already have it.

I begin this paper by turning to the dictionary, for much as I think I know what the words "profess" and "professional" mean, it is always good to be grounded by Webster. Among the meanings of the infinitive, "to profess," is "to lay claim to some belief insincerely." That may be what we are accused of doing in nursing—simply claiming we are a profession when others may think not. We may feel forced to be ambivalent about nursing, about being a nurse, and we may feel defensive in explaining nursing to others, or embattled as others attack. We have been thought to be mere pretenders to professionhood.

I would propose that the problem with nursing in today's world is really quite simple, and like everything else in nursing, quite complicated. The bottom line is this: the problems with nursing, as I've heard them, are *not nursing's problems.* That is, there is nothing seriously wrong with nurses or nursing. What is seriously wrong is that we—nurses and nursing—have changed a lot over the years and the world has yet to catch up with us.

Thus, the trouble nursing seems to be in or that nurses feel so badly about is good trouble and is not our problem. The world simply has an outdated view of nursing and our task is not so much to defend our thoughts or our work, but simply to yawn and patiently teach people what nursing is today. Seeing the task that way makes it a whole lot easier, for the pressure is then not on nurses to interpret so that others can understand us and our issues; it is on others to understand for they are so pitifully unknowing.

All of us get dumb questions from time to time. We are asked, for example, what is the difference between medicine and nursing? Sometimes that throws us into a fit because it is so hard to define for the unknowing what nursing is. But if one simply considers that question dumb, or at least uninformed, then it can have a snappy answer: doctors are authorized by the states to practice medicine, which is to diagnose, treat, prescribe, and operate—on disease—not people. Everything else is nursing.

A colleague of ours, a distinguished nurse dean, was recently put on the spot at an interdisciplinary national meeting by the dumb question, "Is there really a body of knowledge universally accepted as nursing? What is nursing research anyhow?" She replied, correctly I believe, that she found the question insulting. Had the questioner read any of the nursing literature? Of course not. Well, had he read any physics lately, or economics, or cell biology? There is hardly universal agreement in those fields either, so why should he expect a higher standard for nursing?

A male student in my school was asked by friends, when he announced his intention to go to nursing school, "Why do you want to be a male nurse?" His reply, which I cherish, was, "I already know how to be a man. What I want to be is a nurse."

A colleague and I have collected the responses one gets when one is introduced as a nurse at a social gathering, or when one introduces oneself as a nurse to the stranger in the next airplane seat. The responses fall into four categories: 1) "Oh, really, how nice. Excuse me, I need another drink;" 2) a rambling story about the other person's experience with hospitals, surgery, birthing, or an aged parent; 3) a random pass, as if one were automatically an available, experienced sexual partner; 4) "Oh, I could never do that, all those bedpans and blood and all."[1]

These kinds of visceral responses make the nurse feel strange, to stand there in one's best basic black and try to make polite chatter. Indeed, it can make one feel as if one doesn't belong in this social situation, as if one has egg on one's blouse, a tattooed Nightingale lamp on one's forehead, or a red "RN" on one's chest. It takes a while to realize that the reactions one gets in polite social conversation are not the problems of nursing. They are the problems of laymen who simply do not know how to deal with nurses outside the institutional setting where we can be set apart by uniform or role or function.

Nursing is metaphor, meaning that the nurse is not real, in these kinds of social settings. The nurse is merely symbolic and reacted to as a symbol.

Nursing is a metaphor for the class struggle, for example, and in more recent times, for the struggle of women for equality. True or not, nurses are thought to be maids or domestics. While domestic service is a perfectly honorable way to earn a living, one does not ordinarily run into servants as guests at cocktail parties.

Nursing is also a metaphor for motherhood. Nurses are the archtypical mothers and it makes some people nervous to have awakened in a social scene the regressive feelings of being a child.

Nursing is also a metaphor for the kind of power the Amazons used, or Lysistrata. Thus, nurses evoke in others an atavistic fear of women, based in the remembered or fantasied experience of lying in bed with a woman in white towering over us, helping to do the kinds of intimate and personal things that if we were well, would be done in the privacy of our houses behind a closed door.

Nurses are thought, and quite correctly, to know the kinds of secrets that scare the layman. Nurses have confronted death, have heard the late night secrets, have been present at birth, and have seen mutilation, pain, terror, agony, and hope. Those who have seen such things are untouchable for their knowledge is frightening and makes others feel weak, timid, or naive.

But at the same time, nurses are thought to be mindless, even in the choice of profession. Bright nurses are thought to have simply "settled" for being a nurse, either out of lack of ambition to be a physician, or lack of money for the training. It is rarely thought that nurses might *choose* nursing over the mystical opportunity to be a doctor, a lawyer, or whatever the other upscale choices are.

The cocktail party is a stereotype of the social setting in which nurses encounter the middle-class lay public. We are there pinned by conflicting images, all of which we are supposed to embody. We are simultaneously weak, strong, motherly, castrating, dumb, smart, powerful, warm, cold, and any other contrasts you wish to add. And when we feel mutely confused with this kind of attack, we tend to think it is our fault, there is something inherent either in the profession or in our inarticulateness that does us in. But it is impossible to be graceful, smooth, and clever when metaphors about nursing contradict each other and do not match the reality. It isn't that we profess insincerely; we need to be reminded every now and then what nursing is and does and where it is going.

There is no point to nursing unless it is to serve. Indeed, there is no point to nursing education unless it prepares for service and no point to nursing research unless it guides, documents, reinforces, informs practice.

It is of interest to me that within the last 2 years, several university-based professions have realized what nursing long ago discovered: that practice professions are not like the humanities and liberal arts in which knowledge is sought for its own sake. An engineer who knows the theories of stress will build bridges that fall unless that knowledge is built also in the vicissitudes of practice where winds do not always behave and human error is an eternal possibility, and short cuts make a joke of architectural drawings or specifications. A lawyer who learns the practice of law only through a cram course before taking the bar examination may be a legal scholar, but is unlikely to be helpful to a client with a mundane but important personal problem. A minister who knows the history and theories of sacred theology will not inspire a congregation to higher moral or ethical behavior unless he is also trained in applied psychology and human behavior, for the ministry too is a practice profession. And knowing—having the knowledge—to practice is a very complicated thing, more so in nursing than in any other profession because the sheer scope of our social mandate is so huge.

Nursing is primary care, secondary care, and tertiary care, no matter how those are defined. Nursing is health care and sickness care, prevention, health promotion, and rehabilitation. Nursing is community care, home care, institutional care, mental health care, and increasingly, self care. Nursing is there at the beginning of life and the end. Nursing treats individuals, families, groups, communities, and where it is practiced as administration, institutions. Nurses observe, listen, test, assess, diagnose, monitor, manage, treat, and cure. But above all, nursing is caring.

As a profession, we have any number of divisions among us, divisions of training, gender, education, philosophy, state, organization, setting, and regulation. But the one thing upon which nurses agree is that the essence of the practice, and thus the knowing, is caring.

In the first place, it is not easy to care for people—any people—any time, anywhere. It is especially difficult when there are no ties of blood or common interest that bind the nurse and the patient. In nursing, caring requires authentic altruism that must be titrated precisely so as not to overwhelm on the one hand, nor be lost on the other. Caring takes enormous energy, even when genuine liking is present, for it is impossible to care equally for or about everyone. Yet that is precisely nursing's assignment.

Caring cannot be forced. It may be built through the luck of a happy childhood, fostered through friends, family, teachers, nurtured by direct learning, and crafted, finally, through application. One's quantum of caring is diluted and then replenished but must always be there. The nurse must find it in herself if it has drained away in the pressures of an unrewarding position, in a corrupting institution, in a bleak and confusing world. When the spark of caring is gone, the nurse is truly burned-out.[2]

Nursing done right is physically, emotionally, and intellectually fulfilling. Many people think nursing is simple—just take nice people and turn them loose. But to be caring, to deliver tender loving care, is exquisitely difficult. If being tender and loving were merely inborn characteristics, there would be no need for psychology, sociology, or the humanities. Sensitivity trainers, psychiatrists, and social workers (to say nothing of police) would be out of a job. Nursing, practically alone among the human service professions, deliberately tries to train its young in empathy, sensitivity, and compassion. Nursing goes far beyond that because those attributes alone aren't enough either.

Nursing provides its students with ways to tool, hone, sharpen, deepen, and direct the tenderness and love with which most people are equipped. Indeed, nursing realizes that care which is simply technical or merely procedural and not tender and loving is not quality care. Similarly, care which is simply tender and loving but not thoughtful and planned is not good care.

Caring for and about people cannot be dismissed as merely intuitive. But intuition has been defined as "unconscious intelligence." Nursing is not just comfort, care, coordination, collaboration, or just applied psychology, physiology, sociology, anthropology, or diluted medical science. Nursing is all of these things and more. It requires an effort of considerable intellectual acuity—which looks to an outsider like intuition—to thread one's way through all the knowledge, technique, and tenderness one has and to come out with the right action to serve the patient's particular need.

Caring is not restricted to the situation in which one nurse is alone in a room with one patient. It is also an exercise of caring to manipulate a budget so as to provide enough staff to handle the patient load. It is the application of the concern for caring that makes a curriculum change to include more carefully analyzed clinical work, buttressed by selected readings, self-study, and validation by examination. It is caring to help a community organize to mount an immunization program, or provide school lunches, or construct a rape crisis center, or promote an alcohol counseling program. And it is caring that fires nursing up to change legislation to make needed resources available not only to the people, but to nurses themselves.

Nursing has chosen to try to professionalize the field through higher and higher education, as if requiring doctoral preparation would make the field more professional. But professionalization will come only when *practice* is professional, improved over what it is today by intelligent caring, not through simply credentialing individuals. Having one's occupational claims of expertise acknowledged is the first step in the pursuit of professionalism. The significant flaw in the decision to raise educational standards lies not in advanced education per se, but in the absence of a monopoly over the work that will be performed once the training and education are completed.

I suggest there are two ways in which the professionalization of nursing will happen. The first is determining what kinds of knowledge will best serve the development of a monopoly over the work. The second is realizing that the long-desired monopoly is just about to fall into our hands and we should be ready for it.

There might be three kinds of knowing to be prescribed for nursing as a profession of practitioners. First, there is the kind of knowing that prepares one for civilized life—the content and experience that allow one to participate in the life of one's times, with an appreciation for history, ideas, the studies and sciences, the explorations, and the frontiers of thinking. Because nursing's social mandate is so large and the need for nursing's contribution to the reform of health service delivery so apparent, an argument can be made that this kind of knowing is basic.

Yet, this kind of knowing may also suggest that the students be more experienced in life than nursing's new students generally are. This kind of knowing has been called the liberal arts, but liberal education has become so pre-professionalized that it is not the civilizing influence it once was. Perhaps, this kind of knowing is something that should come later in one's nursing education rather than earlier, for I doubt that late teenagers just coming out of their own personal developmental crises are able to truly appreciate the great ideas, the philosophies, the grand schemes of the past or future. Perhaps such material is useful after, rather than before, one has learned and experienced the world of work—when one feels more of a need to be able to place professional identity and gifts in a larger framework of society, when one knows enough to be able to find a place in political science, economics, sociology, and when one has seen enough human behavior under stress to want to know history, psychology, or group process.

Also, the notion that liberal education is confined to the undergraduate years or the first 2 years of a BSN program does not give enough credit to the liberalizing effect of graduate education. We might think of how to make more of that point.

The second kind of knowing is most conveniently labeled science. There is a growing realization that nursing education, in its efforts to carve off a piece of turf and call it exclusively nursing, may have gone too far and neglects to provide students with knowledge of the human body and how it works.

The advances in human science over the past quarter century suggest that now it may be easier, rather than harder, to teach all of the science students need. We know so many more of the principles of physiology, cell biology, or biochemistry that it is no longer necessary to force students to learn by rote and memorize things that now have conceptual explanations. The sciences of human behavior have developed to the point at which it is no longer even interesting to sit nursing students in a survey course on psychology, when social psychology has whole bodies of knowledge directly pertinent to the phenomena of nursing. Psychiatry has moved from the analytic to the biologic and a psychiatric nurse who does not have a grasp of the dopamine theory or who does not understand the relationship between the limbic system and behavior is simply not prepared for practice. A pediatric nurse who is not fully grounded in clinical child development will be unable to practice to the potential limits of patient or parent need. A nurse in a cancer setting will be unprepared if she does not have enough of a grip on cell biology to interpret particular chemotherapeutic regimens when the patient asks.

The content of science, however, is now too huge to be encompassed by any single human mind. What now needs to be learned and known are the processes of human body and mind, so that new content discoveries can be linked to past learning.

We are still conceptually young in nursing. Where nursing education has not been closely tied to practice, some intellectual excesses have produced education which fits people for no kind of practice at all. Some so-called integrated curricula do not well prepare a student to deal with patients who are not integrated. I would argue also that some attempts at nursing theory, when they come out of the armchair rather than the practice field, do not help us advance. Self-care theory, for example, useful as it may be in some situations, does not seem to work when the patient is the high-risk newborn, the comatose individual or, perhaps, the floridly psychotic. And when we use an intellectual process—taxonomy—as if it were a political process, and believe if we can just find new names for nursing phenomena we will have a profession and be recognized, we are dreaming. There seems to me to be no particular advantage in calling pain "alteration in comfort," potential or actual, if we do it just to prove we are not doing medicine or using medicine's words.

There is, then, a third kind of knowledge or knowing and it is called nursing. I mean the process of patient care, the diagnostic process, the application of all kinds of knowledge to the immediate situation, the discovery and assessment of patient condition, and the uses of information for decision making. I also mean the kinds of knowing we used to call nursing process, the therapeutic use of the self, the nurse-patient relationship. I also mean the techniques and talents of physical care which, along with many other things, have washed out of some nursing curricula. The kind of knowing called nursing is learned in its exercise though it may be planned and analyzed in the conference, tutorial, or classroom.

The three kinds of knowing will be basic to the future practice of nursing in ways that have not been required of nurses in the past. It will be essential that nurses know the methods and processes of scientific explanation of the human body. It is necessary now, in some situations, such as intensive care, or the trauma center, once the patient has been treated for the fractures and shock and he is transferred to the hands of the primary nurse. She adds or subtracts oxygen as she repeats blood gas levels; she adds or deletes intravenous medications; she preserves skin integrity and prevents infection which in these compromised patients would be fatal. The nurse in this situation must know a great deal about cells and fluid balance and electrolytes and pressures of blood and spinal fluid, about neurons and permeable membranes and synapses and the neurophysiology of consciousness. The technology of monitoring the body is already with us and the possibility of preventing complications in any patient with impaired physiological processes is already here.

The job of nursing now and increasingly in the future will be to know the range of ways in which the human body and its workings can be controlled by machinery and medication. Even now, nursing is in the position of making decisions about when and how to use the results of technology and chemistry. We are especially in the position of limiting the use of devices, capsules, pills, and machines when their use is questionable or when the patient has been subject to so many specialists' orders and prescriptions that the care becomes uncoordinated because no one is in charge.

Nurses of the future will be.

Things are about to change for us, not so much in the work itself, but in the responsibility and authority over it. Without even asking, the health care system is being forced to confront nursing as central, powerful, and reimbursable. There already have been changes in institutional reimbursement under Medicare. Hospitals will now be paid for their services under a prospective, rather than retrospective, reimbursement system. When health economists or public policy-niks discuss these phenomena, as Paul Starr has done in his book, *The Social Transformation of American Medicine,* and in a speech he gave at a conference I attended recently, it is amazing how little account is taken of nursing. Starr and others simply assume that nursing will fall into sync with the decisions being made by others. While he was at some pains to point out some of the consequences of new reimbursement patterns on nursing, such as cutting hospital nursing staffs, he has not grasped the point. The point is that the new system of hospital reimbursement transfers the power of decision making—economic decision making—into the hands of nursing. The only reason for the existence of the modern hospital is to provide nursing care. That is why hospitals were created and why they are the social institutions they are today. Thus, the service provided by hospitals and billed to Medicare or other third parties is essentially nursing service. Now, the Health Care Financing Administration has said that hospitals are costing too much and so they have proposed to fix it through a system of charges with nationally referenced standards.

The Diagnosis Related Group (DRG) formulas for pricing hospital costs were invented to control the behavior of institutions and physicians, not nurses. Yet, we already hear that nursing will have to suffer, staff will be cut, and we should realize what this issue is.

For way too long, nursing has been buried in the hospital bill along with brooms, breakfast, and building mortgage. It has not been in the interest of institutions to treat nursing as a revenue center and so nursing has been economically invisible. Under the new system of reimbursement, that will stop. That may well be painful for nursing, but we will have little choice. Since hospitals were designed to deliver nursing service, it will be in their interests to figure out just what that service is and how much it costs. DRGs in their present form are used to pay hospitals on the basis of case-mix by diagnosis. Yet nurses have long known that it is not the diagnosis alone that determines what kind of nursing service is needed, and that is especially not true in cancer nursing. Therefore, it will become an institutional interest to have nursing define the care given, and thus, why it costs whatever it does.

In an economic climate in which institutions will be forced to justify expenses and in institutions in which a large chunk of the expenses are called nursing, we will finally be brought out from under the bushel to say what we do and spend our time on. And that will force us, usefully I think, to make our care more directed and precise, while not eliminating the social conversation and easy dialogue that makes patients feel cared for and secure that somebody knows what they are doing.

There is an inexorable chain of logic here. If institutions will be pressed, as they already are, to justify their costs, and if the largest chunk of the non-capital costs in hospitals is nursing, then the eyes will be upon us.

At first, the eyes will turn to us because it is inconvenient or uncomfortable or politically unwise to look elsewhere—at ancillary services, or other contributions to the hospital bill. But eventually, if not immediately, it will become clear to hospital economists and financial managers that they will need to depend on nursing to help the institution survive economically. If we are clever about it, we will be standing there poised to be helpful. Already, we know how important nursing has become to decisions about hospital discharge. Since length of stay is the unit of analysis on which prospective rates are set, we are in the policy mainstream right now. Nobody but nursing has the data that will be desperately needed for institutions to plan their prices and reflect not only minimal care, but *quality* of care.

The next step in the logic, at least as we might shape it, will be to separate nursing costs from other direct and indirect costs. The instant that happens, nursing will suddenly be in a position of authority we have longed for. If we are going to be responsible for the costs of care, we must also have the authority to determine how these costs will be defined, controlled, monitored, and accounted.

The reimbursement tinkering to date has concentrated on what had to happen first—a way to define quantity of care as a factor in hospital costs. Whether the DRG system survives or some other comes in is not very relevant; something like it will be with us for a long time simply because it makes so much sense. The greater quantity of care given (so long as it is appropriate), the more it costs, and thus, the higher the price to the third-party insurers.

The next step will be, however, to add to the measures of quantity some measures of quality. For it is simply logical that if care is better, it ought to be priced higher. That's the American capitalist way and there is no reason to think the health care industry will work any differently from any other.

No one but nursing can define and decide upon measures of quality of institutional health care, for nobody else is there all the time.

What we are in then, is not a health care crisis but a revolution, and one of the things it is already accomplishing, whether we like it or not, is returning nursing to the central role it had in the old days. In this revolutionized health-care system, nurses will not only be seen as essential and central, but will have to be rewarded for that centrality as well, whether the rewards come through money or through increased ability to participate in public policy.

With these new kinds of professional responsibilities, nursing will have the authority we have been saying for years that we wanted. We will also have a visibility that we have never had before and that in itself will get us over the hump to being considered one of the "learned professions." The future is already with us and we cannot hold it back.

As a new high holy days prayer book, put together a couple of years ago by the Reform branch of Judaism, says: There was that law of life, so cruel and so just, which demanded that one must grow or else pay more for remaining the same.

ENDNOTES

1. Fagin, C., & Diers, D. (1983). Nursing as metaphor. *New England Journal of Medicine, 309*(2), 116–117, simultaneously published in *American Journal of Nursing, 83*(9), 1362.

2. Diers, D., & Evans, D.L. (1980). Excellence in nursing. *Image, 12*(2), 67–71.

LESSONS ON LEADERSHIP

The more I grew up as a "leader," the more frustrated I became with all that was being written and spoken in nursing about how awful it was to be a leader. I didn't think so. Or, I thought, if it was so awful, get out. Sure, it was complicated in thousands of ways, but it was exhilarating too because nursing was growing and changing and gaining public attention and federal money.

This was originally a speech for the annual induction ceremony of Alpha Zeta Chapter, Sigma Theta Tau, at Columbia University, on February 28, 1979. It was later published, slightly revised (I cleaned up some grammar) in Image *(1979,11 [3], 67–71, used with permission). I remember the event as being very high up in some kind of NYC tower, overlooking the west side of Manhattan. Speaking to New York nurses is always a challenge; they add another degree of complexity. They are quick and tough. To connect with them, I used humor more than I had done before. Someone at the publisher wrote a great header: "Leadership in nursing deserves attention, but the topic is not all that grim. In this article, the lessons for prospective leaders are given, with a light touch." Now that I read this, I think I probably wrote it; I recognize the prose style.*

A non-systematic scanning of the nursing literature shows that there is considerable confusion about what leadership is, and who the leaders are. One might gather that nursing leaders are, in no particular order, unmarried, arrogant, retired, educators rather than clinicians, short people, mostly from New York City, mouthy, haughty, cutting, powerful, unattractive, or dead.

A leader in nursing is frequently defined as head bureaucrat.[1] Leadership and management are often equated as if the only thing a leader does is manage an on-going organization. Or, nurse leaders are defined simply as those who are famous. A recent book and an even more recent doctoral dissertation requested nurses across the country to name the nursing leaders. These individuals were then questionnaired or interviewed for the study's purposes.[2]

The lists of people produced are, indeed, famous; whether or not they are also the leaders is a much more subtle question.

Claus and Bailey's model of power and influence in health care gives some needed clarity to notions of leadership.[3] They define leadership as a set of actions that influence members of a group to move toward goal setting and goal attainment. Inherent in the actions are situational variables, personal, organizational and social power bases, formal and functional bases of authority, and accountability. Other elements in the spectrum of leadership actions are sound managerial and human relations behaviors and the use of influence strategies that will promote a willingness to follow. Thus, leadership is viewed as multidimensional, encompassing the wise use of power, managerial functions, and human relations processes.

In this model, the leader is one who exercises certain activities drawing on her own strength, and the power derived from position, from personal sources, and from the delegation of which the authors define as the **right** to take action, and uses as processes for accomplishing goals, managerial activities, and interpersonal or human relations process. The outcomes of activity are accountability, defined as liability for one's own actions, goal attainment, and human outputs in the form of motivation, performance, satisfaction, and growth.

What is not included in the model (but discussed somewhat in its elaboration) are the softer aspects of *leadership,* those things that do not fall conveniently into boxes in a diagram such as vision, political processes, creativity, charisma, and certain important kinds of knowledge of other people's motivations and pressures, and the ability to read the dynamics of a situation.

From the literature and experience, it is possible to deduce certain common themes in nursing leadership. For convenience and for fun, they are labeled here "axioms" for potential leaders.

AXIOM NUMBER 1: THE UNIVERSE IS NOT RANDOM, NOR ARBITRARY.

It may be at times irrational, but there are real reasons why things happen the way they do.

This is stated as the first axiom because, all too often, nurses feel victimized by a random world, subject to the arbitrariness of personnel policies, administrative decisions, or physicians' personalities.

The non-randomness of the universe is illustrated by the following example. In a certain hospital a crisis in nurse staffing is about to happen. There are a number of open positions and a memorandum from the president of the hospital has just announced that in budget planning for next year, no new positions will be created, and any staffing deficits will have to be filled using existing financial resources. Head nurses are working double shifts on some units and positions are frozen.

A staff nurse in this institution becomes more and more frustrated and feels more and more victimized by an unfeeling, inattentive administration, or so she reads the situation. Complaints to her supervisor seem not to accomplish anything, and, indeed, complaints of the supervisors to the administration seem fruitless. The nurses are convinced that the situation is the result of random and arbitrary decisions in which they did not participate, and of which they are ignorant.

One who is to be a leader in this situation, following axiom number one, might begin to ask some penetrating questions. She might inquire about what the financial aspects of the problem are. She would find that the hospital has a budgetary problem with its regulatory agency and with its current yearly budget. "Why?" she asks. Because the census is down under what was budgeted. "Why is the census down?" she inquires. Because fewer patients are being admitted, and those who are admitted aren't staying as long as they used to. "How come fewer patients are coming in?" she pursues. Because there is a new hospital in town with a brand new building, trying to build up its clientele, doing massive public relations efforts with physicians, promising surgeons early operating times and free parking. Further, there is a new chief of surgery in her hospital, who has decreed that first priority on operating room time will go to the full-time faculty of the school of medicine, and the community physicians have removed themselves (or been removed) from the schedule of coverage of emergency room patients who do not have a private physician, so the bulk of admissions from that source are going to the resident house staff. The community doctors are annoyed, and are taking their patients to another hospital.

Pressing further, she would discover that in her community there have recently been several strikes of workers in industrial plants. Unemployment is seriously up. So a significant number of people who might need hospital care are not seeking it because they can't afford it.

Finally, pressing to the limit, she finds that some physicians feel the nursing care in her hospital is so bad (because of short nursing staff in part), that they do not want their patients admitted there, thus, simply increasing the problem.

The leader in this situation, whether she is in the defined position of leadership or not, has discovered that the problem confronting the nurses is not simply victimization, nor is it a random event. It may not be rational, but it isn't random. Once a situation is defined not to be random, and, thus, not unsolvable, something can be done about it.

AXIOM NUMBER 2: MONEY MAKES THE WORLD GO 'ROUND.

Understanding this axiom leads to different ways of analyzing problems that confront nurses daily. Knowing that money makes things happen and prevents things from happening can make some negotiations of leaders more understandable, and more effective.

For example, a common problem in ambulatory-services nursing in medical centers is that there is often a move on the part of physicians to run their services without professional nurses, or with as few of them as possible. The move is interpreted as physicians' lack of concern for patients, or their not believing that nursing has anything to offer people and nurses simply become inflamed or demoralized.

But a little prodding will reveal that this issue isn't interprofessional politics, it's money. Many hospitals and medical schools are decentralizing budgetary authority and individual physician department chairmen or section chiefs are being told that their operations must break even. It simply costs more to hire professional people, and when the physician-director is paying the bills, that's how the decisions will be made. All the arguing that patients need nursing care even in ambulatory settings, or that nursing has a professional body of knowledge to bring to bear on patient problems will fall on deaf ears because it's not the issue.

The issue is money and to effectively solve this problem, money has to be found, or made, or otherwise appear if nurses are going to continue to have a role in these settings. How can money be manufactured? Nursing can be marketed, just as medical services can. It is not inconceivable that more patients might come to a service in which they not only get good medical or surgical care, but they get attended to as human beings, are taught about their conditions, and are provided with humane interest and follow-up. More patients mean more money.

There is considerable flap just now in some circles about nurse-midwives. Outright attempts to close down a birthing center in New Jersey have hit the national press. Any institution with a nurse-midwifery training program, or any one that wishes to base its obstetrical services on nurse-midwives, encounters resistance from physicians and administrators. It is too easy to interpret this situation as simply physician patronization or general doctor nastiness. Defining this problem as a financial one opens up other possibilities for retaining one's mental health as a nurse-midwife, as well as ways to counter the attacks.

Obstetricians have learned from their women patients that nurse-midwives are a direct economic threat. That threat must be fought off, and since the threat can't be publicly defined in financial terms because the physicians would look foolish complaining about the potential decrease in their inflated incomes, it must be fought off by other, less rational means. And that's what's happening.

AXIOM NUMBER 3: EFFECTIVE GOSSIPING IS A SECRET LEADERSHIP STRATEGY.

Information access and control is power. Gossip, in the sense of inside information, usually about people or relationships, can be used in the service of nursing goals. But we are not used to thinking that way—it seems so female and unprofessional.

In a recent instance it was necessary for the nurses in a particular hospital to contact members of the hospital board to stop something they believed inimical to good patient care. The list of members of the board was public, and the nurses began to use it. An informal information-passing system evolved in which the nurses polled their colleagues and pooled their data to figure out which board members might be touched by which arguments and which ones had the most clout. One nurse knew the husband of a board member and called him up. Another knew that getting to one lawyer on the board would reach all of the lawyer members because they were old friends. One board member was known to be being groomed as the next president of the board; he was called repeatedly. Still another was known to be the unannounced head of an important board project; he was swamped with calls.

Since nursing is at the center of health care, and everything else revolves around nursing, nurses are very often in possession of important information just from being there and hearing others talk. Such information can be power when carefully, discriminately, and discretely used, and used in the right place at the right time. Politicians work on the basis of "it's not what you know, it's who you know," and since nurses are often at the bottom of the power heap, we know fully who is above and who is making waves.

Management decision making doesn't happen entirely in the defined committees and task forces and subgroups. A lot of it happens in the parking lot, or the cafeteria, or the cocktail party. Such occasions for contact and communication are to be sought, not avoided, and are perfectly legitimate occasions to make an impact. Far too often we believe the table of organization really works the way it's drawn and neglect the possibility of affecting decisions through far less formal routes.

AXIOM NUMBER 4: IF YOU'RE GOING TO HAVE THE RESPONSIBILITY, TAKE THE AUTHORITY TOO; OR, IF YOU DON'T HAVE THE AUTHORITY, DON'T TAKE THE RESPONSIBILITY.

Nurses have been good at feeling responsible and being responsible in patient care.[4] We have collectively worked long hours for low pay because the patients' needs come first. We have also been sucked into taking responsibility for things over which we have not had authority, and the examples are legion.

For example, on one nursing unit which had converted to primary nursing, there was a particularly obstreperous and arrogant physician. He was forever screaming at the nurses for things they did or didn't do, including things they weren't even supposed to do. When primary nursing came to pass, he was significantly annoyed because he couldn't figure out who to talk with about his patients, and he had to go to several nurses to get his information or deliver his orders since they had individually accepted responsibility for small panels of patients.

One day he came steaming onto the unit to see his patients and found that some lab slips had not yet been returned. He threw a tantrum and screamed at the head nurse to do something about the lab. She said to him very quietly, "When I have the authority for the clinical laboratory department, I will take the responsibility to see that they do their work on time. Then you can scream at me, but not until then." And she pointed him toward the telephone and gave him the number of the lab.

It's a useless and draining exercise for nursing to try to clean up the errors, faults, sloth, or mistakes of others over whom we have no authority. It is also doomed to eternal failure. It is very hard, however, for nurses to relinquish the traditional notion that everything that happens to a patient, or everything that happens in the institutional environment, is nursing's responsibility. When the health care system is structured that way, we can come back to exercising that responsibility. But until that happens, nurses have to learn the leadership tactic of knowing, and saying out loud, "That's not my problem."

On the other side of the coin, there are times when nursing, having the responsibility, has to seize the authority as well. Where nursing has the responsibility for delivering high quality patient care, and where either the staff are not qualified, or there are too few, or there are too many patients, some nurses have simply stopped the admissions process until the patient load became normal again. Such an action is the purest kind of leadership, and very difficult to bring off without considerable support. Which leads to:

AXIOM NUMBER 5: POWER AND INFLUENCE ARE A LOT OF HARD WORK.

Leadership takes a good deal of mental and physical energy that has to come from some place. For some, the sheer energy of ideas is enough to fuel the fires. Others develop more systematic sources of support in colleagues, friends, and family. Responsibility itself can be a source of energy as well as a source of support. Nursing's adoption of sometimes too-encompassing responsibility in patient care is only in part something that was foisted on us. There is something quite energizing as well as seductive about having all those people leaning on you, depending on you.

There are informal sources of support which leaders need to cultivate or at least make conscious. One is the support that comes from having defined for oneself a set of principles in sufficiently abstract terms that can guide one through the morasses of decision making. The support of doing something that's right, that follows from an important principle is not to be doubted. Such principles may be ethical or moral, or of social consciousness, or even of sheer practicality. They become commitments, a personal set of standards to judge events and behaviors by, as well as a kind of map to outline at least the boundaries of the territory within which one will operate.

One such commitment or principle might be that people have the right to feel in control of their lives, and accountable for their own actions. That principle might then be the base from which decisions about innovations will be made, especially when, as is inevitable in any innovation, mistakes will be made. If one is committed to personal accountability, then systems or structures which permit people to make mistakes, live with them, and learn from them will follow, rather than hierarchical structures that attempt to minimize mistakes.

Closely allied to the support that comes from a personal set of commitments is the support that comes from believing in something. For some, this may be religious or existential belief; for others, it may be more pragmatic. For instance, simply learning to believe that nursing is important is an enormous source of strength in nursing leadership.

Which leads nicely to:

AXIOM NUMBER 6: PARANOIA GIVES ONE AS CLEAR AND TRUE A VISION OF THE WORLD AS POLITICS OR RELIGION.

Sometimes, it is realistic to be suspicious and to interpret some situations as "they're out to get us." Sometimes they are. These days this feeling comes more often than it used to, and for quite good reason. What we are experiencing as nurses right now is backlash—an effect of the increasingly significant moves nursing is making both politically and in the delivery of services, and a reflection on the increasing power of women.

The informal nursing literature is full of horror stories about this kind of retribution and backlash. Nurse practitioner clinics are closed when local physicians realize their economic impact. Schools of nursing are threatened when they state their right to practice without the control of others. A President vetoes our one piece of legislation thinking that nobody will respond and he won't get any fallout from the decisions.

It is too easy to have one's nursing confidence undermined by backlash. But the other side of paranoia is to realize that we must be doing something right to be so important as to evoke these kinds of irrational responses. Backlash is a symptom of something else, and an implicit recognition that one's efforts have paid off. Thinking about it this way makes it easier to take sometimes, and provides more confidence for the next battles to be fought.

AXIOM NUMBER 7 is a related one: ONE WHO STICKS ONE'S HEAD ABOVE THE CROWD WILL SOMETIMES BE A TARGET.

Leadership goes hand in hand with visibility. Those who are defined as leaders are more visible; having visibility makes one tend to be defined as a leader. The visible ones will attract attention and not all of it will have the wonderful feeling of fame.

One of the most difficult things nurses have to learn is the impossibility of being universally loved and adored. Some may shy away from opportunities for leadership knowing that the wish to be loved is more important than the opportunity to lead.

It is all too easy to take personally the slings and arrows that are attracted by one's leadership position. Leaving aside for the moment the personal qualities that might invite attack, it is simply a fact that a position of authority will call out in others sometimes irrational reactions among the led. Here, the group dynamics theories of the Tavistock people, especially Rioch and Bion, are helpful.[5] These theories point out that people will go to enormous lengths to avoid dealing directly with the ambiguity of leadership. They will fight, flee, pair, undermine, and otherwise react and the leader must realize that all of that will happen outside of her or his control, all of it is totally predictable, and most of it isn't personal at all.

AXIOM NUMBER 8 is a different kind of axiom: VISION DOESN'T NECESSARILY MAKE A LEADER, BUT A LEADER WITHOUT A VISION ISN'T.

Any formal leadership position is a means to an end. There's not much excitement in simply managing the thing and seeing to it that it functions efficiently and that the papers get moved around in some kind of order. What is exciting about leadership is the way it forces one to have a vision quite beyond the exigencies of the daily grind. Without a vision the work is meaningless.

The kind of vision that's important is the long-range, idealistic sense of vision that looks down the road 20 or 50 or 100 years to see what should happen, then uses today to help make it happen. Without a vision, a dream, it isn't possible to set priorities or plan beyond a year or so, or decide what might be sacrificed in activity today in the service of something that will bring the vision closer.

Vision is not simply goal setting, which is much shorter range and much less fun. The grand illusions, the big thoughts, the arrogance of trying to reform the entire health care system are the visions of leaders. Such visions have to be clear enough to give direction, but fuzzy enough to be ultimately unreachable. They must have the gossamer quality of a dream or a mirage in the desert, and that same quality of unreality and unreachableness. One has to have a sense of humor about one's vision, else its unreachableness becomes too frustrating. But one has to have one, in part to make sense of the aching hard work of the day, in part to provide some inspiration outside even the long range plans. A vision serves as an energy source, a star to guide us, a hook on which to hang dreams of glory. Goals, on the other hand, are achievable end points, termini to measure progress. Accomplishing one set of goals just leads to having another set, like an endless staircase to be climbed. A vision, a dream, keeps enticing one onwards, to see it more clearly, to bring it closer to hand. And a good vision will outlive any leader; it gives one a legacy.

AXIOM NUMBER 9 is more empirical: LEADERSHIP IN NURSING CAN'T BE CONFINED TO NURSING ISSUES.

Rozella Schlotfeldt, Ada Jacox, and Virginia Cleland, among others, brought a class action suit against TIAA (a tax shelter annuity plan for university faculty) because of discriminatory policies unfavorable to women in their retirement annuity policies.[6] Dr. Schlotfeldt has written about her involvement in this suit:

> I think such action makes an important social contribution; I thought that was right. I told ... the President of the University that inasmuch as he had gone on record as saying that he wanted to eliminate all discrimination within the university, I was going to help him. I told him that it was necessary to name the University in the TIAA suit and I made the assumption that he would encourage me to be actively involved in the action. His response was that he would encourage faculty to do anything that they thought was right in order to right a wrong ... Leaders surely must take positions on important issues. They must also, I believe, contemplate the future and determine wherein change is needed; and the help to bring it about ...[7]

The kind of social responsibility exercised by Dr. Schlotfeldt and others is a further mission of leadership in nursing. She writes that this activity brought considerable criticism within her own setting. What it did not bring, oddly, was any publicity in the feminist press. It should occur naturally to the feminist movement that the issues of women's retirement benefits might deserve some thinking, and some applause to these courageous nurses who brought the suit, and who had to name their own employers as defendants. Yet, one suspects that because they are nurses, their action, which benefits all women in universities covered by TIAA, is invisible.

The opportunity for nursing to exert leadership quite outside its own sphere has vastly increased with the H.S.A. (Health Systems Agencies) legislation (PL 93-641). In H.S.A.s nurses have the opportunity to influence the shape of decisions on any number of issues in health planning, manpower planning, cost containment, and reimbursement for services. Indeed, H.S.A.s need nurses, for our more complete perspective on the delivery of health care is essential to make health planning a more rational process.[8] If we seize the opportunity for participation now, we will have the luxury some years down the line of not having to gripe at decisions that affect us and our practice since we will have helped other decisions emerge. If we don't participate now, then we will have no excuse.

Finally, **AXIOM NUMBER 10: ALL WEAKNESS CORRUPTS AND IMPOTENCE CORRUPTS ABSOLUTELY.**

Not to reach for power is to limit one's potential for awareness and development of self esteem, limit one's consciousness, one's ability to use sources of energy and power, and to obtain the abundant life.

To the extent that leadership offers the chance for the abundant life, and the challenge of the careful exercise of power and influence, it is to be sought, not avoided, applauded, not derided.

ENDNOTES

1. Slavinsky, A.T. (1972). Leadership: problems and possibilities in nursing. *American Journal of Nursing, 72*(8), 1448–1449.

2. Safier, G. (1977). *Contemporary American Leaders in Nursing—An Oral History.* New York: McGraw-Hill; Vance, C. (1978). *A Study of Influentials in Nursing.* Unpublished doctoral dissertation, Columbia University, New York.

3. Claus, K., & Bailey, J.T. (1977). *Power and Influence in Health Care— A new approach to leadership.* St. Louis, Mosby.

4. Miller, J.B. (1976). *Toward a New Psychology of Women.* Boston: Beacon Press.

5. Rioch, M.J. (1971). All we like sheep (Isiaha 534:6). Followers and leaders. *Psychiatry, 34*, 258–273; Bion, W.R. (1959). *Experiences in Groups.* New York: Basic Books.

6. Jacox, A. (1979, August 11). How much is a nurse worth? *American Nurse, 11*(7), 4–5.

7. Safier, 1977, *ibid.,* p. 38.

8. Novello, D.J. (1976). The National Health Planning and Resource Development Act: What it is and how it works. *Nursing Outlook, 24*(6), 357–360.

The Emperor Has No Clothes

At the time this speech was given, in Boston at Beth Israel Hospital, BI was the jewel in nursing's crown. Primary nursing was implemented, advanced practice nurses were going strong, Joyce Clifford, the Director of Nursing and Mitch Rabkin, MD, the head of the hospital, had a lovely partnership. Nursing was valued and valuable. BI is a teaching hospital with all of the baggage. But it was working spectacularly.[1]

My former student, the late Eileen Hodgman, had a position at BI to assist in developing professional practice. Her values were at the core of BI's and she worked to make the culture change. "E," as her friends called her, asked me to do this speech, which was preaching to the converted, but I was trying to raise the thinking about nursing leadership.

Beth Israel and the wonderfulness of the nursing service was sacrificed (my opinion) on the altar of mergers and acquisitions[2] in the craziness of the 1990s.

In this speech can be seen the threads that eventually found public view in a piece Claire Fagin and I wrote, published simultaneously in the New England Journal of Medicine *and the* American Journal of Nursing, *a coup noted by absolutely nobody. "Nursing as Metaphor" has been reprinted many times so it is not contained here.[3]*

As I put this section together, I was astonished that the seeds for another speech were here as well—the notion of nursing as craft. That plays out in the next section, in the "Adventure of Thought and the Adventure of Action."

The fairy tale from which I stole the title for this paper goes like this: long, long ago, in a small middle European country, a young man succeeded to the Emperor's throne. But he was a strange young man who believed that he was always beautifully dressed though in fact he wore no clothes of any kind. But he was the Emperor so his followers indulged his fantasy and even complimented him daily on the color of his non-existent cloak, or the length of the invisible plume on his invisible hat. The Emperor walked throughout the land, for he was a popular man despite his peculiarity, and the peasants and merchants gathered round to rave about his beautiful apparel. The country folk and the court all knew, of course, that he was naked, but fearing retribution if they said so, great efforts went into teaching little children how to act when they saw the Emperor, and warning newcomers to the country not to comment upon his nudity.

One day the Emperor was in a parade in a small town fair and in the crowd was a father and his small child, come new to the country to trade. The child was quick and lively, excited at the chance to see a real live Emperor for the first time. As the parade came even with the father and child in the crowd, the father held the child up on his shoulder to get a better look. The child, who knew no other way to view the world, cried in great astonishment, "But the Emperor has no clothes!" whereupon the crowd, hearing the truth for the first time, fell upon the Emperor and deposed him.

This little allegory means something to me about leadership which is why I chose it. It *doesn't* mean, as I've heard it guessed when some people saw the theme for this paper, that the doctor is automatically the Emperor, though one could have some fun with that thought. Nor should it be implied that the deluded Emperor in the story is a characterization of leadership which I plan to enlarge upon, though that could be fun, too.

In nursing there is a prevailing myth, recounted in our professional literature, and even stated in public forums that there is a lack of leadership in the profession. I'm never sure what that allegation is supposed to mean but I suspect it means a certain invisibility of nurses in high and public places, a certain undercount of nurses among the activists or defined power figures in clinical institutions, universities, congressional hearings, federal bureaucracies, and the public press. Such a view of nursing leadership is so narrow as to be almost meaningless. Today, I would like to address some aspects of leadership in nursing from the point of view of the child watching the naked Emperor, to point out some realities both of nursing leadership and of the context within which it happens.

If there is any truth to the rumor that there is a lack of leadership in nursing it may be that we, as nurses, feel more often led than leading, more often compromised and manipulated, put upon or put down, unvalued or undervalued, powerless and handicapped rather than powerful and authoritative. These feelings are real, not imagined. But the great secret is, *it isn't our fault*! There are real reasons why we feel this way, and why we sometimes even act powerless.

There is lots written about power, authority, and control in the nursing and organizational behavior literature, and you can read that as well as I can. Today I want to talk about some other aspects of leadership in nursing as a way to reveal some truths which may point the way to new activities or new thoughts about the issues in the practice of the profession and in its boundary negotiations. This is not a paper on leadership strategies either, for those are also remarkably well developed in the nursing and social psychological literature. Interpersonal communication, conflict resolution, assertiveness tactics, group dynamics, even charismatic qualities are exhaustively discussed in whole libraries of books and journal articles. I want to discuss some lessons on leadership that aren't written down anywhere and don't fit nicely into available concepts or strategies.

In the great tradition of Murphy (whose first law is, "If something can go wrong, it will,") and Parkinson (whose first law is, "Work expands to fill the time available,") here are some Laws for Leadership:

LAW 1: IDENTITY AND IDENTIFICATION ARE NOT THE SAME THING.

Identity is said to be the most powerful element in establishing the territory of any individual or group. Identity, in the sense of how an individual perceives him or herself, is *the* basis of personal power.

Identity has to do with how you respond when a stranger sitting next to you on an airplane asks you what you do for a living. Do you silently review the possible ways to answer that before you open your mouth? Do you mentally stutter about whether to say, "I'm a nurse" versus "I work for Beth Israel hospital," or "I teach at Somewhere U.," or "I'm an administrator," or "I work for Yale," or whatever your other options are? If you've been out in the world anywhere, you know that the announcement that you are a nurse is likely at best to provoke a fixed smile on the person who hears it, and at worst, will simply lead into a fumbling pass, or grisly stories of your seat companion's experiences with surgery or bedpans or childbirth. Knowing that such are the likely responses makes one hesitate to announce one's profession, and that makes one feel guilty and pretty soon any possible conversation trickles away into mutual discomfort.

It takes a long while before you discover that your hesitation to announce your identity isn't *ipso facto* evidence of identity conflict about being a nurse. Your listener simply doesn't know what to do with that announcement of identity. Nobody but nurses know what nursing is all about these days, but that's hardly surprising. Very few professions have an automatic and realistic public identity, including medicine. Yet the public thinks they understand what it is to be a doctor, while not knowing how to talk with a nurse on an airplane.

One can have some fun with what the word "nurse" conveys to the stranger in the next seat, and why it is so hard for laymen to respond to the identity. There are some people to whom the word "nurse" conjures up dark and regressive images of breasts and mothers and turns them into instant children, unable to get beyond the intrapsychic experience. There are others for whom the word "nurse" means angel-in-white, and it's very difficult to make light chatter with angels. One could go on and on, but the point is that the guilt one feels about publicly proclaiming one's identity is *not* because one is ashamed to be a nurse or should be. It's because they—the audience—don't know how to respond and that's simply socially awkward. It has no other big meaning.

Holding on to the identity as nurse is perplexing these days as others attempt to erode that identity. In some psychiatric hospitals, for example, nurses are merely "clinicians" or "therapists" without separate identity, which is a truly seductive position, since it seems to connote more authority and power than the word "nurse" does. It amuses me to note, however, that the one professional group which never allows itself to be called merely "therapist" is psychiatrists, who are always "doctor."

Even within the profession, there are attempts to obscure the identity of nurses when arguments begin about whether nurse practitioners or other nurses in expanded roles are really practicing nursing or medicine. A nurse who diagnoses and treats illness is still a nurse, if she feels herself that, and holds to that identity. Indeed, holding to the identity of nurse makes the activities one does nursing, even when they were "formerly medicine."

Identity as nurse is not the same as identification, however. All of us might have trouble identifying with some of the excesses and limitations of the profession, or some of our colleagues, of nurses whose care is poor or whose public image is antithetical. But we don't have to identify with all nurses, with all of nursing's multitudinous programs, planks, or platforms, in order to continue to enjoy an identity as nurse, and it is from that identity, that personal sense of self with a particular label, that power and leadership come.

"Nurse" is not only a perfectly honorable title, but one of such enormity and complexity that it is difficult for any one of us to adequately describe even to the most fascinated seat companion what all of modern nurse-work is about. And nurses are changing rapidly, from the missionary, self-abnegating, altruistic, and undereducated to the assertive, proud, aggressive, and powerful and we find those changes difficult to explain. With all the changes in the profession, in the care of patients, in interprofessional relationships and public image, it is not surprising that we find our identity slipping. But if we are to be leaders, to take leadership to reform the health care system (since there really is no other task), as individuals we might well spend some contemplative time making sure that identity as nurse is firmly glued into place as a personal definition from which we can then confront the various pulls for identification.

LAW 2: EVERY ONCE IN A WHILE, LOOK UP.

This law takes some explaining.

The conductor, Toscanini, was well renowned for his ability to memorize every detail of the score of a symphony or a concerto, and to conduct great orchestras without any music in front of him. This prodigious feat of memory stayed with him even into advanced years, but there were occasions when he was conducting when he would forget a phrase or an entire section of the music and miscue the orchestra. But he had conducted the NBC symphony for so long that the orchestra knew the music as well as he did, and played it as it should have been even when his cues were wrong.

One day late in his life, he was conducting the orchestra playing something big and uplifting, with lots of horns and drums and entrances of whole sections of the brass. He conducted at great speed with large gestures as well, and in the middle of one section signaled for the trumpets to come in. The trumpets knew they weren't supposed to come in just then, so they didn't. Toscanini looked dismayed and angry and in eight more bars gestured again for the trumpets to enter. Again, because that wasn't the way the music was written, they didn't. Finally, in a flurry of arm waving and with increasingly savage looks, Toscaninni cued the trumpets one more time and one trumpet let off a loud, and misplaced blat.

The symphony concluded and after Toscanini left, the concertmaster met with the orchestra. "Why," he said, "why, when you knew the maestro sometimes forgets the music, why did you ruin the performance by not paying attention to the music?"

From the back of the room, a disgusted voice said, "Some fool looked up."

Sometimes we need to look up from the daily, routine pressures of work to see what is really going on.

The most stunning example of "looking up" is happening right now. As you may know, the Carter administration (following the logic of previous administrations) believes there are too many nurses and federal funds should be withdrawn from nursing education. Among the arguments administration spokespersons make for this oversupply is that of the 1.4 million nurses in this country, at any one time, only 70% of them are employed. This is taken as evidence that nurses aren't really working at the jobs the federal funds trained them for. The implication is that nurses are lazy (just sitting home raising kids), or disaffected from their profession (and thus, nursing shouldn't get any more money if it's that unpopular). Yet, recent research by some nurses who looked up and designed studies to help other nurses look up, stops such arguments with a bang.

Data reported by Mabel Wandelt show that the problems of nursing shortage in institutional care are not problems of nursing, they are problems of poor working conditions, little authority or autonomy, eternal battles with administration and physicians, rotating shifts, poor fringe benefits, no allowance for part-time work, child care, or other forms of humane employment conditions long a part of industry. Wandelt's data say problems of nursing shortage are not problems of low pay, though that is important. More crucial to the nurses surveyed were the conditions of work. Nurses, having looked up, are no longer willing to be treated like cattle, moved from shift to shift without reason, made to feel guilty for wanting every other weekend off, made to feel pushy for wanting to know at least a week in advance what shift one might work. Nurses have come increasingly to realize that institutional care depends upon nursing responsibility, but that nursing authority does not match the responsibility.

Many years ago I worked with some nurses in a small psychiatric hospital to assist them to develop some nursing standards for admission of patients, and for nursing participation in milieu activities. It became obvious early on that nothing could happen in the nurses' discussions until they could all get together in the same room at the same time. They couldn't, because of shift coverage, and in this particular institution the need to staff both the evening and night shifts with R.N. complements meant that at any one time, one-third of the nurses would be engaged in direct patient care, unavailable for group activity. Mind you, at this point in the discussions, the issue was simply to get the nurses together, to find out whether there was even concensus on agendas, to get to know one another—this was not even political organization, and certainly not an attempt at unionization.

The solution? The nurses approached the medical director through the director of nursing and simply told him that next Tuesday at 2:00 P.M. all of the nurses needed to leave the wards and could he please arrange for the residents to cover. He thought (and he was right) that it might be good experience for the residents to do that, so it was arranged and the nurses began to work fruitfully on their agendas.

Looking up means learning that there are real reasons, if not rational ones, why things happen the way they do. If an institution is short staffed, there are real reasons, usually buried in administrative policy, or regulatory agency pressure, or unwitting personnel decisions, not in nursing sloth. Until it is possible for institutions to accurately record the actual costs of nursing care, as opposed to the cost of administration, or mortgage amortization or housekeeping, supplies, utilities, and xeroxing, nursing will continue to feel the burden of the pressure to contain costs, since nursing service is the largest non-capital part of any institution's budget.

There are also real reasons why such research to establish direct costs of nursing has not been done. Apart from very complicated methodological issues, it must be clear to administrators that if ever they could say out loud what the costs of actual nursing are, versus other costs, the nurses would rise up in fury to see how their salaries relate so little to patient charges, and how costs for non-nursing services (and thus, charges for them) have risen at a pace far faster than nursing wages.

LAW 3: SOMETIMES IT'S GOOD TO BE A PROBLEM.

Florence Nightingale is known in nursing for her books on nursing and on hospitals, for her invention of epidemiological statistics, and for the creation of modern nursing. Yet she was, in her time, a troublemaker. In an early book, little known until feminist literature tracked it down, Ms. Nightingale rails against the emptiness of Victorian womanhood in a bitter statement as radical as any statement of women's issues these days. In *Cassandra,* written after her first visit to Kaiserwirth, she castigates a society that would think so little of its women as to confine them to their houses and their needle work, even preventing women from reading the news of the day, and certainly not taking advantage of the intellect as obvious in the female as in the male. Her mission to the Crimea can be seen as trouble-making, as it certainly was to the Army surgeons who refused to let her and her band of 38 nurses into the pest house that the army hospital had become. Her work was not that of the visionary and self-sacrificing lady; it was reform of the military health system and she accomplished that with courage and militancy, not with soft voice and fainting spells. In a great many ways, nursing as we know it today was founded on trouble-making.

Sometimes it is necessary to be part of the problem in order to make it clear what the problem *is*. So much of what nursing does so well with patients and with the systems in which we work is invisible simply because it is done so well. If a post-op infection is prevented, there will be no thanks to the nursing that did it. If the food is hot and delivered on time, nobody will know how much screaming to the diet kitchen the Head Nurse had to do to make it happen. The doctor who pushes the elevator button on his way to his busy rounds has no way of knowing that the fact that the elevator gets there, takes him upstairs and closes softly behind him is due to some nurse in the night getting the maintenance folks there to fix it. If a hypertensive patient does not stroke out early because a nurse practitioner has helped him alter his diet and exercise program, titrated his medications, and supported him through a change in lifestyle, nobody even notices.

It is one of the frustrations of good leadership that the leader who anticipates problems and solves them will never be applauded by the followers because no problem happened. An oncology nurse specialist friend of mine knew from her role as representative of nursing on certain medical committees that nurses were soon going to be asked to give experimental drugs under medical protocols, but also that the nurses would be the ones to try to revive patients who succumbed to the drugs, or to try to elicit consent from patients who had no way to understand what they were signing off on. This nurse worked through the medical committees to design some rules to govern the responsibility of nurses for the giving of experimental drugs, and prevented untold problems for the nursing staff. But the nurses had no way of knowing what she was doing, or how their lives were made easier by her efforts.

It's very hard to measure something that *doesn't* happen—all the attention goes to the things that do.

I've come to look forward to the days when nurses will be sued in their own names for malpractice. Not that I want nurses to lose those cases, or to be punished for honest error. But there is something quite pernicious in the current state of malpractice law (as made by lawyers and courts) that has a lot to do with the extent to which nurses and nursing realizes its power and authority.

The current state of malpractice law, according to Angela Holder, who appears to be an acknowledged expert, makes one realize how little law has to do with the reality and how much with a certain kind of politics. Holder cites case after case in her first book of instances of error committed by nurses where the nurse is not thought to be liable at all, and the doctor is sued. My favorite is an old case in which the nurse gave an IM injection and the needle broke off in the patient's arm. The nurse was not even named in the suit, the doctor was, and the court held that it was *his* responsibility since he had ordered the medication to be sure that it was given correctly and without error. What is probably more to the point is that the nurse had no financial resources that would make it profitable to sue her (since malpractice suits are by definition for damages, usually financial). Yet the court's opinion has the effect of defining the legal responsibility of a nurse for her *very own act*—giving an IM injection—as being in somebody else's territory.[4]

There is not yet any settled malpractice against nurses in expanded roles, nurse practitioners, nurse-midwives, etc. That bothers insurance companies a whole lot since they worry about the amount of risk inherent in the expanded practice of nursing and, thus, how much premium to charge to an institution or individual. Yet it is known that the reasons for malpractice suits to be brought have not so much to do with errors of omission or commission as they have to do with interpersonal relationships with the patient and communication with families. Nurses happen to be very good at that; indeed, it is the essence of our practice. In addition, nurses in expanded roles, or any nurse, must be Caesar's wife, better than anybody at everything, else the wrath of the administrator or the physician come down on her head. So it is hardly surprising that there has been no litigation to affirm malpractice allegations against nurse practitioners or nurse-midwives, but again, that absence prevents us from having the opportunity to have new laws made which might help us define and justify the scope of our practice and our responsibility. So long as the law treats us as not responsible, we are invisible.

There is at least one hopeful sign. Some enlightened lawyers are now realizing that in certain kinds of malpractice cases, the testimony of nurses as expert witnesses is called for. In Connecticut, the largest malpractice case ever in that state has been settled for $3.7 million. The State Supreme Court upheld the lower court's decision and that decision turned on the expert testimony of nurses who said that the hospital nurses had *not* provided care which met professionally accepted standards of practice in this instance. A lawyer friend of mine who does a lot of defending of malpractice claims for his clients, which include hospitals (though not the one in this suit), said this was the first instance he could recall of a malpractice case which rested on the testimony of nurses as expert witnesses.

However, one of the nurse experts told me that while the physician who preceded her on the witness stand was allowed to testify about nursing practice, her testimony about the *medical* practice in this case (the medication orders and seclusion orders particularly) was stricken from the record.

LAW 4: TOOT YOUR OWN HORN.

This law follows from the ones before and is simply a variant of "the squeaky wheel gets the grease," or being a problem versus being invisible. But there's another message here as well.

If the public, exemplified in the stranger on the plane, doesn't know how to talk to a nurse, it's their own ignorance, not *our* lack of data. Our professional literature is very moving but we tend to put down the stories of "my patient" or the clinical examples published in our mass circulation materials. The lay public has no access to those articles and it should. But even more importantly, nursing will exert leadership, become more powerful, to the extent that we make known what nursing is about, how it is done, and what we think about it, and what it all means for our patients and for us.

There is a tendency in nursing to think that the only things worth writing and speaking about are the political forces, or the quasi-intellectual forays into conceptualization and obscurantic fog. We are faintly embarrassed to read the testimony of a patient who credits his nurse with saving his life, or making him comfortable, or otherwise having an impact, as if we were suddenly forced out of the closet. Our work with patients is not well described in formalistic jargon, so patients tend to describe our impact in simple words: "She was so nice to me," and that seems unprofessional to we who have studied psychology and communication and everything else to make that niceness professional.

Since the one-on-one human encounter that is nursing care is so private and personal an experience for the nurse and for the patient, we should not be surprised that it is so difficult to talk or write about. We have an investment in continuing to be perceived as nice, yet we have a competing investment in telling the world that nursing is much harder and more complicated than that. We want to share our triumphs, but to do so would be to invade the patient's privacy, so intimate is good nursing. *Yet we must do all that,* for it is sharing reports of nursing practice that makes us all comrades in arms despite divisions of place of work, specialty, gender, degrees, geography, or belief.

Our nursing literature is not impoverished in reports of excellent patient care, humane encounter, or great skill. If there is a general deficiency in not only our literature, but the way we approach reports of patient care in peer review sessions, clinical conferences or other forums, it might be in the extent to which we do not elaborate the thinking that goes behind the activity called nursing. Nursing is an exercise of the intellect. Because the responsibility of nursing is so huge and so complicated, nursing draws on bodies of knowledge from any number of places, including personal nursing experience. How that mental maneuvering is translated into patient care is the core of nursing, yet it is not often discussed, even in the most evocative of patient care presentations.

Selecting among the possible explanations for behavior, the competing bodies of fact or theory to bring one's learning to bear on patient care is as central to thoughtful practice as clear communication, respect for another's dignity, humane approaches, or warm hands. Our literature is full of reports of situations in which nursing worked or perhaps didn't work but all too often, these reports leave out the reasons *why*. Questions of why something works or not are questions of theory or abstraction, and it is abstraction from the clinical event that makes situations comprehensible and allows learning to be passed from one instance to another.

Our intellectual history as nurses mirrors the intellectual history of women to the extent that women are thought not to be bright enough to invent new concepts, play with theories, think logically, or use abstraction. Great strides are being made in nursing these days to overcome this stereotype and think seriously about the principles that guide us, but as yet these efforts are not often translated into reports of clinical work that one can learn from, part of the reason may be that the work of abstraction is not being done by people who are close enough to practice to make it make sense.

Direct patient care as human service is so central to our social mission that it is easily ignored while we toot the horns of power or concept or administrative theory. So we undervalue direct service, ignore its potential as power, base, even ignore clinical work as knowledge and thus, prevent ourselves from falling in love with our own work.

This Law should really be worded, "Toot your own horn. If you don't, nobody else will." Brag. Write. Speak out. Demand to be *heard* when you think you've done something terrific. Ask other nurses to tell you about a patient, like the one you're worrying about, that they did a really good job with. Invent occasions for praise, and learn to take it gracefully when it's deserved. Fish for compliments. Make it your business to remind the busy physician that the reason his patient is ready to go home now is because the nursing staff have worked with him and his family so he can. Volunteer to present your work to case conferences, clinical rounds, peer review, or other settings.

Like the stranger on the plane, we won't as nurses learn truly to value the work of nursing until we know more about it and we won't know more until we manufacture occasions to hear or read about what nursing really is all about.

LAW 5: NOBODY OWNS KNOWLEDGE AND WORDS WILL NOT SAVE US.

There is an impressively strong movement within nursing to recapture the sources of power and leadership which some think we have lost to others. One way that movement takes form is the intense struggle to define what legitimately belongs to nursing and thus, what belongs, by exclusion, to others. There is the belief, apparently, that if we could only get the right words to say what nursing is and what it isn't, we could then erect fences around that territory, claim it for our own, and shoot any rustlers who cross the boundary.

The search for turf is a peculiar and a particular problem with nursing because our potential, and even actual turf, is so huge. Nursing has the responsibility (forget for a moment the authority) for practically all of the person's encounter with the health care system, whether it's direct hands-on care, or manipulation of the environment, or teaching the patient to work the system.

The problems with nursing's territory are political problems and will be solved, if they are, by political means, that is, exchanges of power. Nursing is not well served by thinking that naming all "nursing phenomena" (a task which will occupy us for a millenium) will make it possible for us to say, "That's nursing and everybody else keep your hands off."

The effort to make the process of thoughtful nursing more thoughtful is to be applauded. That nurses have a special interest in patients' reactions to illness and hospitalization, that nursing has a tradition of dealing with the whole patient in the context of his illness and life situation are hardly disputable. But to say that either is *all* of nursing, or that encompassing all of nursing's rightful territory with a set of new labels will make nursing's political problems go away is simply naive.

There is floating around, a draft of a paper being prepared by an ANA Council on the scope of practice of nursing. The paper says a number of controversial things but one of them is that nursing is limited to diagnosis of human responses to illness; diagnosis of disease is the physician's territory. The paper goes on to make some exceptions for intensive care nurses who can "diagnose" fibrillation, and take action, only to have the physician come in to validate it, of course.

What is suspect about this example and this paper is that it represents an awfully unsophisticated knowledge of practice. In the first place, fibrillation is not a disease—myocardial infarction is. Thus, following the logic of the paper and hewing to the notion that nursing does not meddle in diagnosis of disease, the nurse who labels a phenomenon "fibrillation" is still practicing nursing and doesn't need a physician's validation. Even that assumes, of course, that the mere act of labeling is practicing nursing, or medicine, or any other discipline.

There appears to be a trend in the same nursing diagnosis literature that makes nursing diagnosis out of symptoms of what are already well-established conditions. That would seem to me to be counterproductive to the long term future of nursing and its expanding boundaries. If a nurse can enumerate, as nursing diagnoses, all the symptoms of something, why should she wait for somebody else to add them up and attach another label which then is outside her purview. For example, one sees examples of nursing care plans in the literature in which nursing diagnoses are listed as "secondary to" some other label. For instance, a psychiatric nurse has written a whole bunch of nursing diagnoses for a paranoid schizophrenic patient that include things like "alteration in communication secondary to paranoia" which means the patient is suspicious and talks funny. It also is characteristic, indeed, symptomatic, of the "disease" that paranoid schizophrenics have difficulty communicating. Why, then, is nursing diagnosis of this kind even needed? Because nurses aren't supposed to read the medical literature and know the symptoms of a condition?

To follow that theme further, if a nurse working in primary care notes in the history and physical examination that a patient has burning on urination, urgency and frequency, flank pain, and cells in the urine sample, surely she can as easily come to the conclusion that there is a urinary tract infection as anybody else. Just as surely, it would be very poor patient care to make up a nursing care plan for each of the symptoms, yet that is the logical extension of some of the nursing diagnosis work in situations such as these where a disease is present.

Perhaps nursing diagnosis can go the furthest where there is disease, but where the patient's needs transcend either disease symptoms or secondary effects.

For example: A patient has been hospitalized on the same unit twice in the past 6 months for what has variously been thought to be subacute bacterial endocarditis, cellulitis, or FUO. She is back again for a course of IV antibiotics, and other than running a low grade fever, she feels okay. The nurses know her well, know that it is difficult for this Italian grandmother to be away from her family for so long, to be bored by having to lie in bed for days on end when she feels okay, and to be scared because her diagnosis is still not clear. The evening nurses bring in, on their own time, and with their own money, a pizza for this patient and her roommate to share. I defy you to put into nursing diagnosis language what this lady's problem was. Yet you *should* write a nursing care plan that would include pizza, prn.

All of this nursing diagnosis stuff isn't all that serious. Because nursing diagnosis is so young as an intellectual movement, it has in it still some moments of conceptual hilarity.

A nurse practitioner saw a patient who complained that her skull was growing outwards. Sure enough, it was, and the nurse practitioner examined her, determined the proper x-rays and other tests to order, got the results, referred the patient to a neuro-surgeon and in the fullness of time the patient had a craniotomy to remove a non-malignant meningioma. The nurse practitioner visited the patient on the surgical ward, and checked the chart. A student nurse, new to nursing diagnosis perhaps, had written the care plan and the very first nursing diagnosis for this patient whose head is covered with ace bandages, who had undergone four hours of tinkering with her brain, who had tubes and wires from every orifice, was "potential alteration in comfort." In the first place, that is simply a bastardization of the English language in this case: there's no potential there, the patient probably hurts. Secondly, while comfort is no doubt important in all patients, one could guess that in this patient, it is not the central issue. Finally, whatever happened to the perfectly useful English word "pain" as a nursing diagnosis. Is that too medical?

The process of diagnosis and the act of labeling are supposed to enable us to communicate better. But invention of a new language hardly accomplishes that purpose. At best, it gives us airs and affectations; at worst, it sets up false intellectualisms that may not even follow the rules of logic or language.

I do not object to nurses diagnosing anything, whether it's human responses to illness and hospitalization or physical or psychological disease. There is nothing especially sacred about diagnosis as a process. What might be sacred is the base of knowledge from which a diagnosis might spring and the extent to which different professionals are differentially prepared to attach diagnostic labels to objectively determined phenomena. What I object to most strongly is the notion that simply creating new names for things that already had perfectly good names will somehow fix nursing's political territorial problems.

On the one hand, it is simply unlikely that if nursing declares that human responses are its singular territory, anybody will listen and obey. We as nurses haven't paid attention to anybody else's boundaries, including medicine's and psychology's and social work's, so why should we expect anybody else to pay attention to ours? On the other hand, to set up a way of thinking that simply institutionalizes what is already wrong is simply regressive. That is, nurses already cross the boundaries, with knowledge aforethought, into the practices of medicine or social work or psychology, or respiratory therapy, or hospital administration. When we do it, it's because we know what we're doing and issues of patient care cannot await somebody's definition or respect someone else's prior claim. If it is within the coronary care nurse's responsibility to diagnose fibrillation and do something about it (while waiting for the doctor, perhaps), then isn't it nursing? What is the doctor going to do, tell her it wasn't fibrillation, it was something else? Not if she knows what she's doing, and not if he's smart and not if they both share an interest in saving the patient. Who owns the right to labeling is irrelevant.

Nursing will not be saved by empty intellectualism which does not pay attention to the reality of clinical work, which already has distinctive language. When we undervalue nursing we are forced to think that unless we invent or otherwise put together new words, we won't know what we're doing, or be able to defend it. We know now what nursing is, what it does best, where its focus is, even where its flexible boundaries are. But we distrust the fact that those ideas are best expressed in lay language—common English without surplus meaning and somehow that doesn't seem good enough.

LAW 6 is a different kind of law: EVERYONE ELSE IS MORE SCARED THAN YOU ARE.

Nursing operates often from a posture of subservience, struggle, obsequity, and awe at the power of others who seem so overwhelming. We worry, with reason, about job security if we were to challenge and we are achingly aware of interprofessional and administrative battles.

In crouching around the fires of our own insecurity, we forget that marauders outside are under pressures of their own that are acted out on us.

It is very hard to be a physician these days. The poor boys are under fire from everything from the Federal Trade Commission to consumer groups, from the Department of Health and Human Services to local medical societies, from the excesses of individual physicians within the system which color the public's view of doctors, from universities, Health Systems Agencies, the Internal Revenue Service, the public press, and the organized nurses. The vision of the doctor as a god is gone but the physicians who were socialized to think of themselves that way are still with us, and very nervous. It is not comforting to think of losing one's hard-won power, which is what is confronting physicians. It's not nice to think about having to change one's code of ethics, as the AMA did this summer, to explicitly recognize the contributions of other professions, and swear physicians to cooperation when they are used to control. It's not easy to have court decisions come down, as one did in Virginia, which stated that psychologists were as reimbursable as psychotherapists as physicians, absent any data that physicians were any better at it. And it must be quite unpleasant to psychiatrists to have Congress question and debate right now (as it is) appropriations for a huge study of the efficacy of psychiatric therapy so that Congress can decide if it should be paid for *at all* with public funds.

Nurses who work in teaching hospitals forget often that the house staff, who are the ones who cause them the most trouble, are operating out of fear, if not out of exhaustion. The life of the resident physician is truly the pits and it is no wonder that they pass along the slights and cruelties of their situation to nurses. The internal politics of medicine are such that any physician in training, or junior faculty member, is mostly concerned about protecting his or her future and will, therefore, fight off anything that might get him or her in trouble, including bad reports from nurses.

Hospital administrators are running the most scared, under the gun of cost containment, and under the pressures of lay boards and physician power figures. A hospital administrator's life is not a happy one. He is in a business that has a market factor, but he does not control the market or the resources. He has no credibility with his professional staff because he usually has never laid his professional hand on a sick person, and his efforts to make his institution managerially sound are likely to be laughed at by nurses and physicians who think "management by objectives" is for the intellectually unable. Hospital administrators get all the flak from the lay community for beds not made, for lab tests lost, or surgical mistakes, or cold dinners, or hot ice water, and they can't do a thing about it.

Social workers are nervous that their profession is suffering under the onslaught of, among others, nurses. Physicians' assistants are clearly a dying breed as their own dependence and lack of mobility paralyzes them.

Respiratory therapists, physical therapists, occupational therapists are coming to realize that the incursions their professions once made into nursing's territory will no longer be tolerated as nurses now know how to do those therapies, well and cost-effectively.

Knowing others are more miserable than you makes it possible to confront the daily fights more securely, and to interpret the behavior one sees as a nurse and has to deal with, with new eyes and ideas.

Sometimes it pays to be paranoid, sometimes it doesn't. One symptom of paranoia is ideas of reference, and in nursing it is all too easy to think that the excoriating issues that come down on us have anything at all to do with nursing. More and more it seems to me that nursing is emerging as very strong in its sense of identity, in its influence, in its authority, and what we often feel is backlash. We must be doing something right for that to happen!

LAW 7: NURSING ISN'T WHAT IT SEEMS TO BE.

There is a lot of thoughtful debate in nursing on the extent to which nursing is an art or a science, or an applied science, or some kind of amalgam of all of the above. This debate is more important than it looks on the surface, for the kind of definition eventually arrived at will, in many ways, determine what nursing's scope is, what are its prerogatives, and what it should look like in both education and practice.

I suggest to you today that nursing is neither an art nor a science, but is a *craft.* This thought has been simmering away for a long time in the back of my brain, but was brought to consciousness by an article in the *New York Times* Sunday Supplement in early September. In the business and finance section that day was a story about the Steinway piano company and its new manager. He was most articulate about the product—the Steinway piano— that is the purpose of the company and how a company designed to produce such a valuable product ought to be managed.

The product of nursing is nothing so tangible as a 10-foot long concert grand, but the notion of nursing as a craft is no less appropriate. The "product" of nursing is patient care. That is, the product of nursing is a *process,* not a physical thing, not an outcome measurable except as process. That product is no less beautiful, nor less finely tuned than a Steinway piano, just harder to get one's hands on.

Nursing is a craft in the sense that fine crafts, like piano making, combine both the art of the wood worker with the science of sound production. The newspaper story quotes a wood carver as saying that his art or skill will never be amenable to mass production or automation, so carefully must it be done, so individually, on each piano. A sound technician may take 250 hours or so to delicately file off the hammers to make exactly the right sound for a piano, making distinctions between sounds that escape even concert pianists. The manager of the plant and the subject of the story clearly understands the nature of a business dependent on fine craftsmanship, and thus, pays attention to his craftsmen as they ask for a new tool to make their work better, but not necessarily faster. The manager heeds the advice of the craftsmen to buy a huge new piece of equipment to bend the wood for the grand piano's exterior case, and replace cumbersome hand bending, but he does not interfere with the slow pace of exquisitely tuned production. The standard of excellence, on which the name of Steinway was established, rules; efforts to make the company adhere to modern management efficiency programs dissolve in the manager's respect for the craft.

Nursing is a craft too in almost exactly this sense. It cannot be hastened, or done with lesser-trained people, if its quality is to be maintained. Nursing works with the art of intuition and observation, at the same time needing the sciences of physiology, pharmacology, and patient care. Nursing is in part technical skill, as is a craft, in part art, as is the eye of the woodworker, in part science, as is the work of the piano technician, but nursing's value, like Steinway's, is not restricted to either art or science.

Yet nursing is a practicing profession, not one dedicated simply to the development of new knowledge for others to use. And at the same time, it is more than merely a set of activities that can be defined and thus taught and passed along to lesser-prepared individuals as tactics or skills or strategies. To be done well, nursing must be done by those who know the whole of it, the art and the science, put together as craft. For the product of nursing is also esthetic as is the piano, both in the way it looks and in the way it sounds.

Nursing has much more in common with the crafts of the world, and with the performing arts of drama or music, which are themselves crafts, than with the traditional sciences or the traditional arts. Thought of in this way, nursing begins to make sense by analogy and it begins to be clear why it is so frustrating to try to explain nursing by any convenient stereotype of art or science. When nursing is thought of as a craft, it begins to be possible to talk about it even to laymen, for the craftsman's terminology can be used, and even laymen understand the difference between the potter and the painter. The tools with which nursing works, in observation, intuition, in communication with patient or family, in equipment and procedure, become the craftsman's potter's wheel, or the awl or carving knife, or ceramic oven. The material on which nursing works is not clay or wood, but rather human problems and potentials. The product is not a vase or jar or piano, but rather a solution, a metaphysical event, an anchor point in a life experience which has no physical properties but is nevertheless real. And our senses tell us when it's right.

Nursing is too big and complicated to be subsumed under any particular way of thinking about it, and that's part of our problem in explaining it, in using its power, in relating nursing to the larger world. Yet that, too, is reality and anything less than an appreciation for that complexity demeans our work and our issues.

Finally, **LAW 8: NURSING IS DANGEROUS.**

It might be possible to do several minutes here on how dangerous it is to be a nurse these days, and that might be relevant also. But the sense in which I mean this Law is that nursing is dangerous to the rest of the world, particularly the world of health care delivery.

Nursing, despite its image, is inherently radical, and getting more so by the day. The values that are nursing's are the values that make people nervous, for they are the values that cannot be questioned as right: responsibility, authority, and accountability in coherent relationship; individual power and control over one's own life; reward based on merit as opposed to position, gender, or other external signs; rationality and participation in decision making as opposed to automatic investment of power in defined authority; intolerance for discrimination on the basis of sex, race, economic status, or anything else; respect for individual difference.

Nurses will no longer tolerate working conditions that do not allow for the fullest and best practice of the profession. Nursing will no longer accede to demands for productivity when that means decrease in quality of care. Nurses will no longer allow others to divide us. Nurses no longer automatically believe that the hospital administrator or director of nursing knows best, that the physician is god, that the nurse must leap into the gaps in the system to make it better for everybody. The health care system has run for a long time on the energy, personpower, and altruism of nurses, and like the characters in the movie "Network," we aren't going to stand for it any more. Nurses have realized that our best source of external power will come from the excellence of our care which teaches the public, the consumers, what nursing is and can be.

Nurses are especially dangerous because we know how the whole system works. We are the only people there all day, every day, night, and weekend. We know where the bodies are buried. But we are also dangerous because we know how to use that information, not to foment riot, which we could do, for that would not be good for the people whom we serve. As we come to understand the nature of our profession, its place in the larger scheme of things, we identify channels through which to work to make change, and it is already happening. We are all the more dangerous, therefore, because we are so numerous, so pervasive, so firm in our knowledge, and so *impatient.*

Linda Aiken, outgoing President of the American Academy of Nursing, has provided a way to think about the agenda for nursing for the '80s which I like a lot. She said in her Presidential address in Dallas earlier this month that nursing is after nothing less than a renegotiation of the social contract of nursing with the public, with other providers, and with the administrative structures in which we operate, including the external bureaucracies of Congress and the federal system. The notion of "social contract" provides, for me at least, a way to harness energy toward something. Nursing's contract has been, for the 100 years plus of American nursing, to serve without question, without pay, without reward, and without visibility. That must change.

Nursing's contract with institutions has been to be there always, to make the system run, to keep costs down and care up, and make everybody from the housekeeping staff to the physicians happy. That too must change. Nursing's contract with the public has been to be nice and clean and pleasant, to complain little and confront not at all, to be the image of all that is caring and comforting but never to be smart or aggressive or intellectual or powerful. That must go.

I began with a hint that the picture of nursing as leaderless was wrong. It is wrong in many ways, but the simplest of them all is that there is more leadership in nursing, in nurses, by our sheer numbers than there is in any other field. Counting only those defined as leaders by position of defined authority, there are more team leaders, head nurses, supervisors, directors and assistant directors of nursing, primary nurses, faculty, deans, directors of nursing programs, nursing home administrators who are nurses, executive directors of voluntary public health nursing agencies, nurses in private practice, nurses on hospital boards and committees, nurse practitioners, clinical specialists, nurse-midwives, charge nurses, presidents and officers of nursing organizations, health systems agencies, health departments—the list could go on—there are more nurse leaders than there are power figures in any other profession.

The mantle of leadership is on *all* of us; we don't even have to fight for it. Will we wear it with comfort? Will we wear it invisibly, as the Emperor with no clothes? I think not, but it is your mantle as well as mine, so you tell me.

ENDNOTES

1. The story of BI has been told recently by Dana Beth Weinberg (2003) in *Code Green: Money-Driven Hospitals and the Dismantling of Nursing,* Ithaca, NY: Cornell University Press.

2. Cohn, J. (2001, May 28). SICK: Why America is losing its best hospitals. *The New Republic,* pp. 20–25.

3. Fagin, C.M., & Diers, D. (1983). Nursing as metaphor. *New England Journal of Medicine, 309*(2), 116–117; *American Journal of Nursing, 83*(9), 1362.

4. The notion of nurses under the law has been beautifully described by Mary Chiarella, using Australian legal documents. She treats the law essentially as narrative, building a case for the invisibility of nursing in the law. Her book (which is her doctoral dissertation for a PhD in law) breaks important new ground but it has not been advertised, reviewed, or otherwise marketed in the USA. See Chiarella, M. (2002). *The Legal and Professional Status of Nursing.* Sydney: Churchill Livingstone.

BEYOND CHICKEN LITTLE

This was the Jessie M. Scott Lecture for the American Nurses Association, in Anaheim, California, June 16, 1986. Now there's a truly ironic story here.

Jessie Scott had been Director of the Division of Nursing in the Bureau of Health Manpower in the Health Resources Administration in Washington, DC for many years. When she retired, the ANA honored her with an award—the Jessie M. Scott Award for contributions to nursing research. The award is presented along with other ANA awards on the first night of the ANA Convention, in a gigantic ceremony. The recipient then has to give a speech sometime in the following days of the convention. The Connecticut Nurses Association, led by my friend and former student, Linda Schwartz then President, had nominated me, much to my shock and chagrin.

See: here's the story, which Linda and CNA had no way of knowing.

In the early 1970s, Jessie and others had managed to convince their agency that nursing ought to have "capitation" monies for nursing education, as medical schools had. We weren't then in a real nursing shortage, but medical schools had been richly rewarded with amounts of about $2500 per medical student for years. Capitation funds came with very few strings and could be used to pay for the hard-to-fund administrative support for any educational program.

Finally, through Jessie's and others' efforts, nursing got capitation funds, but they were only for entry into practice programs and the amount was something like $250 per head.

This was about the time the Yale School of Nursing was mounting our program for college graduates to enter nursing. Being a young and fearless dean, in a school that always needed money, we applied for these funds to support the first year of our combined basic nursing/graduate program. After all, our students were entering nursing, weren't they? And, funny thing, we got the money. It was pretty pitiful since we were only then admitting 12 to 18 students.

But the trick was, our peculiar program which took college graduates without any prerequisites into a 3-year sequence in which the first year was basic nursing and the second and third, the advanced practice master's level specialty of the student's choice, and had the students sit for RN licensure at the end of their second year—well, it meant that in the second year of this program, there would be students who had come from other disciplines into nursing and were not licensed and students who were already nurses, licensed, in the exact same courses and clinical experiences. And I apologize for the length of that sentence.

The fact that in this second year we had licensed and unlicensed students called into question our eligibility for the much more important federal funds for advanced practice training. Once I realized this, we never again applied for capitation funds; we had them for only one year.

But our application put Jessie in a terrible spot that I knew nothing about. The funds that had come to support nursing capitation had come out of the medical education funds and the possibility that they were being used to educate nurses as NPs who might compete with physicians was a political no-no.

All of that heated up under Jessie's feet. For reasons I do not know, the regulations that descend from funding bills in nursing had never been written for public comment before. Now, Jessie and her staff were pressed to devise the regulations for the advanced practice funds and needed to wall off this little incursion of our program type. They wrote one paragraph into the regs that essentially said that funds from the advanced practice training sources could not go to programs in which not all of the students were "nurses," meaning registered nurses. I know now, but didn't then, that Physician Associate programs were eyeing this big pot of money for advanced practice primary care training.

Paragraph 3 (c) became the focus for a letter-writing campaign against these funds being used for the training of "non-nurses." As it happens, only Yale's program was affected. So we generated our own letter-writing campaign. Yale's General Counsel, the inestimable José Cabranes helped us orchestrate the letters as well as helped us understand what the ground rules were: letters are sent, somebody logs them in a grid, so many for, so many against, and whatever side gets the most letters, wins. I sent a faculty member to DC to copy the letters (they are public) and she came back with a sack full of Xeroxes of hand-written letters clearly done as part of a class assignment at a bachelor's program outside of DC which shall be unnamed here. Our count exceeded theirs.

Eventually José had to call the General Counsel of the Bureau and then threaten the end of civilization as we know it in what I have come to call the "asbestos telegram" to Dr. Henry Foley, Administrator of HRA at the time. "The proposed regulations, if adopted, will do grave and irreparable harm to one of America's leading nurse training institutions and the nation's first collegiate school of nursing. Accordingly, if the proposed regulations are adopted, Yale University will take such legal action as may be appropriate in the circumstances to restrain DHEW from accomplishing the unwarranted, discriminatory and unlawful designs of the Bureau of Health Manpower."[1] That caused the offending paragraph to be rewritten and reinterpreted, and just to be sure, José got our Congressman, the late Robert Giamo, to read into the record in the House what is called a "colloquy" to nail down the interpretation that we crafted. The funds were to support nursing education but the intent of the legislation was not to deny advanced practice funds to programs which happened to admit persons who were not then licensed as nurses.

This was my metaphorical doctoral education in policy, legislation, regulation, and politics. And, from my point of view, my enemy was Jessie Scott. And I was hers, I thought.

Of course, it was never personal, but that didn't help how it hurt. Many years later, when she could, Jessie told me the Clue about the medical education funds and it all fell into place.

So I am about to receive the Jessie M. Scott award and that's the context.

I wore a white dress with a Yale blue blazer and I tried to honor Jessie as well as others in my brief acceptance remarks. The whole thing was videotaped and the subsequent speech was audiotaped and I sent them both to Jessie—a peace offering and an expression of shared understanding. I did admire Jessie—she was a tough lady and she advocated for nursing with great grace.

Speaking to an ANA audience in these years was a fun challenge. The audience, especially for a named speech, would be huge and varied. They're in convention assembled so the mood is celebratory. Valuing and honoring nursing is the strategy to bring nursing—disparate, internally divided— together. For at least the hour and a half this speech took.

Chicken Little was an alarmist. He was walking in the yard one day when an acorn fell on his head. "Oh my, the sky is falling," he said and as you recall, he went off to tell the king about it. On the way, he collected a number of his barnyard colleagues, all with cutesy names—Ducky Lucky, Turkey Lurkey, Goosey Woosey, and so on. They all believed the sky was falling and they all joined the parade to tell the king. Pretty soon, they came upon a fox, who asked where they were going. When he had heard the story, he smiled foxily and told the birds that he knew a short cut to get to the king, and they should follow him. They did and he led them straight to his lair, where he had several gourmet dinners of chicken, duck, and goose. And the king never knew the sky was falling.

There are lots and lots of alarums we hear, which is why I began with Chicken Little. This morning I wish to talk a bit about alarums as acorns, then take us beyond them to certain themes that seem to me more valid predictors of the future, and end with what are less alarums than clarion calls for changes in nursing practice and education, our image, and our credit. You will have to decide whether I am Chicken Little or the fox or some other animal.

A quote for you:

> To attempt to give nurses instruction as to the reason why (in
> reference to the details of management and treatment) would
> be, in the majority of instances, to inflict a heavy task upon
> them and to lift them more or less out of their proper sphere,
> possibly at the risk of withdrawing them from due attention
> to their less intellectual but equally useful functions.[2]

That's from 1906.
Another one:

> Nursing is not, strictly speaking, a profession. A profession
> implies professed attainments in special knowledge as distin-
> guished from mere skill; nursing is an honorable calling,
> nothing further, implying proficiency in certain more or less
> mechanical duties; it is not primarily designed to contribute
> to the sum of human knowledge or the advancement of sci-
> ence. The great and principal duty of a nurse is to make a
> patient comfortable in bed, something not always attained
> by the most bookish of nurses. Any intelligent, not necessar-
> ily educated woman can in a short time acquire the skill to
> carry out with implicit obedience the physician's direction.[3]

That was 1908.
And another one:

> "Look at this chart, this patient is going to a Nurse Clinic.
> Can you imagine, they're even letting nurses write in the
> charts now."[4]

That was 1966.
And yet another one:

> "My, God, you mean it's legal for nurses to use stethescopes?"

That was 1976.
And another:

> We are not talking about a turf battle, we are talking about
> public health. Does the Legislature want nurses to practice
> without a doctor's supervision? This issue is not payment of
> any alleged services provided, but rather whether or not you
> want RN's...having the privilege of making independent
> medical decisions.[5]

That was 1984.
A pessimist, an alarmist, a Chicken Little might take the 80 years' worth
of these kinds of quotations as evidence that nursing's sky has been

falling for a very long time. But that's ridiculous, even for a Chicken Little. The sky can't fall that long. More to the point is the fact that these perceptions of nursing are simply incorrect, wrong, delusional and can be—have been—destroyed by fact.

It is useful sometimes to remember some facts, some historical themes and trends, for it is all too easy for nurses to feel victimized by constant criticism in a random world. The world may not always be rational, but it is not random.

The "trained nurse" is responsible for the creation of the modern institution called Hospital (and also, of course, the Nursing Home, Home Health Care Agency, and Mental Hospital). Until surgeons could be assured that placing their patients in a common place to recover from surgery would not be putting them in jeopardy, surgery was done on kitchen tables in homes, at great inconvenience and under questionable conditions. When hospitals began to be organized under nursing services, instead of the dubious stewardship of untrained laypersons, physicians quickly recognized the convenience of being able to see recovering patients all at once, in the same place. Similarly, the nursing services provided quality control over patients' diets, cleanliness, the sterility of operating suites, with greatly improved patient recovery statistics. Physicians could spend much less time worrying about details of patient management, and thus see many more patients in office practice, relying on hospitals to provide operating facilities, expensive equipment to be shared among many, and relief from night calls and house calls.

The major treatment for disease in the early part of this century was nursing; the tools of the physician were opium and amputation. The cure for typhoid fever, for instance, before immunizations and antibiotics, was entirely nursing care: alchohol baths to lower the temperature, fluids to treat the dehydration. Nursing used to concentrate on helping the patient recover from the interventions of surgery. The surgeon amputated, and the nurse controlled the bleeding, prevented infection, and prepared the stump for rehabilitation.

World War II changed nursing forever. And what is happening now dates particularly to that period. Public health and sanitation had already begun to wipe out diseases that had formerly occupied large proportions of hospital facilities. Sulfa and penicillin and later the other antibiotics began to offer cures to what formerly could only be treated. Antisepsis carried to the battlefield improved surgical technique, and the capacity to transfuse or provide plasma on site all improved mortality statistics. And psychiatry discovered ways to manage the emotional stress of battle and return soldiers to the line quickly.

The war also created a nursing shortage in this country, and that created a whole host of auxiliaries to nurses and later, different forms of nursing education. And very shortly after the war, the Hill-Burton Act provided funds to build hospitals and the Veterans Administration increased vastly, and all of that required more nurses.

And the discoveries of science increased the complexity of patient care and medicine, for as more and more became known about the body and how it works, specialization in medical-surgical nursing and pediatrics began to grow to join nurse-midwifery and psychiatric nursing as special areas of practice. Federal funds began to support nursing education, to help fill the nation's need for nurses. Nursing education itself changed to include more science, then more nursing theory, as nursing's intellectual base was built.

It is simply a fact that the coincidence of timing with a short supply of nurses and a hugely increased need held us back for some time, for the need was so desperate, and we had little choice but to fill it.

We weren't just standing still, however.

There always has been, and perhaps always will be, a shortage of nurses, of more or less magnitude. But number-counting does not always reveal it. The advances of clinical science and nursing science, which cannot now be stopped, will always contribute to a nursing shortage, because what those advances do is create more work. When nurses know more, we can do more, and we find more that needs to be done.

The Institute of Medicine, assigned by Congress to advise the administration on the proper role for federal funds for nursing and nursing education, provided convincing evidence that while the supply of nurses might have been marginally adequate (in 1980), the demand had vastly increased. In part this is due to the enormous (and sometimes questionable) dependence upon intensive care. What is intensive about intensive care, of course, is nursing. And intensive care units eat nurses. As changes in the way funds flow to hospitals have changed practice patterns so that hospitals may now be used more appropriately for people who really need them, the burden of work on nursing has also increased. ...

One could take the nearly constant reports of resistance to nurses in expanded roles as alarums. Arkansas tried to restrict the practice of nurse practitioners by demanding physician supervision, signed protocols, and a ratio of no more than two nurse practitioners to one supervising physician. That move failed. In Tennessee, it took the nurse practitioners and physicians 5 years or so to finally agree on proper credentialing that shared the authority between the Medical and Nursing Boards. In Massachusetts, the nurses successfully fought off a very wrong-headed move of the Medical Association to restrict their practice and cause them to wear name tags specifically identifying their responsible physician. Indeed, the State Government slapped the doctors' wrists for going beyond their authority in proposing this regulation.

North Carolina was the first state to have a nurse practitioner licensure law (and a registered nurse licensure law, for that matter). It provides limited prescriptive authority, with each nurse's formulary subject to approval of a joint medical/nursing board. An issue now in North Carolina is for nurse practitioners who work in non-traditional settings, for instance, a mental hospital, to have the authority to prescribe and monitor psychotropic drugs. But we must not forget that simply wanting to write prescriptions in one's own name is not the issue. The issue is that the people we must care for need not to have their care even more fragmented than it already is. Patients need to have medicines. Nurses know which ones they need.

In New Jersey, a nurse practitioner was sued for practicing medicine without a license. The suit was brought by the Medical Board, not by a patient. Her alleged offense was recommending a mammogram. The case was thrown out. What was really at issue was not the performance of the nurse, it was the fact that she worked for a new HMO which had taken business away from the local medical practitioners.

You should all know the Missouri case. There two family planning nurse practitioners were alleged to have practiced medicine in examining women and then prescribing birth control and fitting diaphragms. It is not coincidence that the suit was instigated by, among others, the brother of the president of the State Medical Society. The Supreme Court of the State of Missouri upheld the nurses' practice. While the Missouri case was being decided, a nurse practitioner in Ohio was sued on a similar basis. There, the story was even uglier, for that suit was brought by a physician who had sent his own secretary to see the NP, to collect evidence that she was practicing family planning. When the Missouri case was settled and the decision announced, the Ohio suit was dropped.

The report of the Graduate Medical Education National Advisory Committee (GMENAC) in 1980 predicted that by 1990 there would be an oversupply of physicians and thus the numbers of nurse practitioners and nurse-midwives should be held to then-current training levels. That recommendation was never enforced, despite efforts to cut training budgets. Further, the report has been called into question on any number of grounds, not the least of which is that in studying non-physician manpower, the GMENAC committee changed the rules. When they studied physicians, they studied supply. When they studied non-physicians, they studied demand, and that is not considered kosher. Further, it is often ignored that while GMENAC did project oversupplies of physicians in some specialties, it projected an undersupply in general practice—primary care—which is, of course, the advanced nursing specialty of adult nurse practitioners.

There is now legislation mandating third-party reimbursement for nursing services in Medicare, Rural Health Clinics, Champus, and Medicaid, all federal programs. Third-party reimbursement is now legislated in 14 states. Eighteen states have legislation authorizing certain nurses to prescribe, and one survey shows nurses are routinely recommending over-the-counter and prescriptive medications in 46 states. ...

We overcame the alarums about the safety of nurse practitioners and nurse-midwives (and nurses of all kinds) with a huge body of research literature. There are now, by conservative count, over 1,000 research articles about nurse practitioner practice with very little inconsistency in the conclusion that safety is not at issue. Reviews of the nurse-midwifery literature, presented in testimony before a Congressional Subcommittee, point out that there has never been an instance of a study that showed nurse-midwives to have a negative effect, and considerable evidence that nurse-midwifery care is highly effective and even cost effective. We have overcome nearly all of the political alarums as well, with well-organized political strategies. It should be noted that we have never lost a legislative skirmish, even when we have had to carry them to higher courts.

The new battles are economic, but even there the progress is extraordinary. The main reason is because in the economic arena, there are different actors. Besides physicians who really do not control the funds, there are administrators, managers, insurers, and the Federal Trade Commission and they are mostly on our side. HMO's have long realized that when they are in a position to substitute nurses for physicians, which is after they have established a market and a track record, they will. Nursing homes are reading the research that shows the difference geriatric nurse practitioners can make in the well-being of their clients. School health services are turning to nurses again. And on and on.

The newest alarum, the threat to malpractice coverage for nurses in expanded roles, must be seen for what it is as well: an economic issue. It really isn't that nurses are so much more likely to be sued, or make insurance companies vulnerable. This issue is perhaps really two; first, even Congress has now recognized that the liability insurance game needs considerable cleaning up. When everyone from the Boy Scouts, to the circus, to local restaurants, to nurse-midwives has trouble getting liability insurance coverage, it means the problem is not us, it's them—the insurers, and perhaps the whole inflated legal system that has grown up around personal injury cases.

It is also possible that in the more narrow health care field, the challenge to malpractice coverage of nurses is a part of the growing competition of nurses with physicians. One way to stop the competition, of course, would be to remove personal liability coverage.

The ringing of this alarum fades a bit when we realize that the issue really isn't *us*. Defining the problem as a political and economic one makes it possible to attack it by political means and economic data, and that is what is happening right now. Clearly this is not a death knell.

There is one final alarum to address, and it is the one we hear the most often and the loudest: that nursing is so divided that we can never move forward or get together on anything important and that therefore, we are doomed. This allegation ignores some pertinent facts.

We have been arguing, debating, among ourselves in nursing since Florence Nightingale's feuds with Mother Bickerdyke. We have debated modes of education, the wisdom of licensure and certification, professional organizations, credentialling, economic and general welfare, men in nursing, standards of practice, interprofessional relationships, the price of subscriptions and membership in professional organizations, endorsement of candidates for public office, whether to wear uniforms and caps or not, scope of practice, entry into practice, titling, federal support, and a National Institute for Nursing in NIH. And probably other things we have mercifully forgotten.

Some of these have not even been our own battles, for it has been in the interest of others to keep us divided. After all, nursing is the largest of all of the health professions, and if we ever got together on the same thing, we would be quite intimidating. Some of these issues have been more apparent than real, and they died quietly away. But we might be advised to recognize that there is a distinction between political issues and professional ones. In a group of people now 1.9 million strong, it would be amazing if there were not internal differences. We live in different parts of the country, we come from different backgrounds, including educational ones, we have chosen different areas of practice, we do not all belong to the same political parties or even political persuasions, we have the same variation in beliefs and values that the population itself has. Why we should have to adhere to a standard of agreement higher than is expected in any other body is an interesting question.

What those who criticize us for divisiveness miss in the nursing dialogue is that the arguments we have, the distances and debates, are over means, not ends. What binds us together is the commitment to the value of excellent nursing practice and to the public evaluation of those who perform it. What binds us together and transcends all of the superficial divisions, is what it is like to do the work.

Nursing, it is said, is a set of simple routine activities for which a minimum of training is required if the nurse is just a good person—a nice, kind, motherly person with a big heart and warm hands. To produce nurses, the legend goes, just take nice people and turn them loose.

People think they know what nursing is. Mothers without 4 years of nursing school tend their sick children and literally nurse the babies. Everyone at some time "nurses" a cold (and sometimes "doctors" it too). Yet nursing involves far more than either the title would indicate or the lay activity would suggest.

Nursing puts us in touch with being human. Nurses are invited into the inner spaces of other people's existence without even asking, for where there is suffering, loneliness, the tolerable pain of cure, or the solitary pain of permanent change, there is the need for the kind of human service we call nursing.

The intimacy that is the core of nursing gives us a peculiar aura. Some people are embarrassed in the company of nurses. We are supposed to be dignified over vomitus, uncringing at the sight of blood, calm as we debride the decubitus, pack the wound, give out the bad news. Nurses must hear, but never tell, the secrets of the dark side of the soul, the hates and jealousies, the anger and violence, the cursings at fate, the bargains with God. The terrors of psychosis, the joy of a peaceful and happy birth, the erosions of poverty and discrimination that turn a body thin and sour-smelling are part of the nurse's world, all day, every day.

Nursing is so personal a service, so private an experience, so invisible alone in a room with a patient that no one will ever know it fully except the individual nurse. We do for others what they would do for themselves in the privacy of their own homes. Because nurses have never had the prerogative of omnipotence, we find it comfortable and natural to be with the patients as human beings, without social distance. The tradition of nursing care is lodged in an explicit value—that it is our job to help others do what they would do for themselves if they had the strength, will, or knowledge. And, when recovery is impossible, to assist others in the ultimate act of dying, dignifying the individual with all his personal history, idiosyncracies, needs, values, and desires.

Some of what we do looks so easy to the untrained eye. How could putting a bedpan under someone take 4 years of college? How could feeding a helpless, aged woman take a degree? How could mixing a formula, taking a temperature, asking about a health history merit a curriculum? By itself, any task is more or less simple; but nurses must do all of these and many more complicated ones, and do them with grace, the reassuring illusion of speed, and some purpose and plan in mind.

When done either superbly well or dreadfully badly, nursing seems so simple, for what is invisible in any human service is the thinking behind the act. Nursing requires the use of all the visual, aural, tactile, and psychological senses; they detect the data upon which one acts. The intellect sorts and classifies, questions and predicts, for it is imperative to the practice of nursing that we understand enough of how the human body responds to illness and treatment that we may distinguish what is okay from what is trouble, what requires our skill and what requires the talent or training of others, what is normal and what is anomalous. A good deal of what is now social work, respiratory therapy, occupational therapy, physical therapy, psychiatry, and medicine began as nursing.

The activities of nursing that directly connect the nurse and the patient are crucial, but what is less often understood is the extent of nursing's entirely separate but equally compelling responsibility: no less than managing the whole experience—the entire environment—of the health care system. The nurse is in charge and must make it work in the service of those who need and want it. It is the nurse who must see that the room is warm and the ice is cold, the dinner is served properly and on time, the doctor is called and informed, the family is comforted, the lab gets its results back on time, X-ray pays attention, the floors are swept and the costs—always the costs—are kept down.

And here the bells begin ringing again, but they are not alarum bells. Rather, they are bells singing in a new future for us, if we hear them right.

There is an interesting and subtle change in the nursing literature that I have been tracking for some time. It has to do, I think, with a growing recognition of the power of clinical wisdom not only to effect change in the health or illness status of patients, which we have long recognized, but to effect change in systems of care—a kind of change that takes us beyond the invisibility of nursing's service.

The power of clinical wisdom is increasingly being seen in reports of how and what nurses think. We see it in many ways. It used to be that the lectures in schools of nursing or in conferences of nurses were given by physicians, and then a nurse would come in at the end with an "implications for nursing" session. Now, one sees conference programs and curricula in which nurses do not only the implications, but integrate them with the physiology or pathophysiology, knowing that these are sciences of the body and how it works, not the sciences of other disciplines. The clinical case reports carried regularly in the large circulation nursing journals now begin with the primary nurse presenting the case, and perhaps (and not always) commentary somewhere along by the physician. Meanwhile the primary nurse has consulted with a psychiatric liaison nurse, or a social worker, or a respiratory therapist or someone else, but it is clear, the management of patient care is the nurse's.

And we are seeing in the nursing literature much more about what nurses observe and conclude in their practice. How nurses detect that patients in intensive care are about to go bad, or that a given patient will make it or not is now being addressed as a serious matter of clinical scholarship, not simply of nursing intuition or tradition. How nurses find out what outpatients really want and need when they drop in to clinics is now a whole trail of inquiry. How, and what, nurses diagnose hits the literature in nearly every issue of every nursing publication and some of it is splendid stuff. ...

Increasing attention to clinical wisdom—to what might be called "second opinions of nurses"—is one theme in the nursing literature.

The "second opinion" analogy is used deliberately, and deliberately as an analogy. Second opinions, in medical practice, are advisory to the primary caregiver, and nearly any human being is more likely to listen to advice than direction. More important, second opinions, especially when they disagree with the first opinion, are occasions for legitimate discussion (and in the case of surgical second opinions, for questions of reimbursement). Second opinions are requested by the patient, not the clinician.

Suppose we were to adopt the concept, the language, this way of talking about nursing's contribution to case management. We might not use the actual process, or we might. What we would do is make real and legitimate our interest, and of course, we would document it in the chart. The model is already there for us to borrow. It would be lovely to get rid of the famous doctor-nurse game and for us to stop pretending that we have no opinions and judgments.

A second theme is even more pronounced. One sees in the nursing literature another kind of "second opinion" work—nursing's increasingly obvious acceptance of the responsibility for the appropriate use of technology and treatment.

When intensive care units came into being in the 1960s, initial attention focused on their life-saving capacity, and surely that was well documented. But toward the end of the '60s, and later, there began to appear in the literature some questions about just how the technology was being used. One nurse, for example, who had been in a master's program for a year, returned to her prior job in an intensive care unit for the summer between her years in school. Having been away for a while, she was struck with how incredibly noisy it was. Things clanked and people talked in loud voices, and machines hissed and gurgled. She wondered just how much sleep and rest patients were getting in this unit, for clearly they needed it. She studied that and found that patients went uninterrupted for an average of only 9 minutes a day, clearly not much more than a cat nap. Her findings came to the attention of the chief of surgery who was administratively in charge of the unit (because she brought them to his attention), and the protocols for monitoring and the rules for noise control were changed.

A more recent example: A nurse-midwife became interested in just how the clinical decisions to artificially stimulate labor in women who were past their E.D.C. were made, because as a midwife, she was getting pressure from her medical backup to use labor stimulation when she felt, on her own clinical judgment, that it was not needed. She reviewed the literature and did her own retrospective data collection on a group of patients cared for in a low-intervention nurse-midwifery service. She found that the conventional obstetrical advice about how long a pregnancy lasts, or ought to last, was founded on sand.[6] That is, there is much more variation in pregnancy dating than had been pulled together before. Further, she found that the consequences of allowing a pregnancy to continue normally past the 42 week point were not bad. She, too, brought her findings to the attention of the obstetrical service and the protocol for stimulating labor was changed.

Another one: A clinical nurse specialist whose thing is diabetes was called upon to consult with the nurses in the high-risk perinatal service about patients who presented with gestational diabetes. She noted, from her knowledge of diabetes, that it would be important to treat patients with gestational diabetes, which is temporary, with a kind of insulin that would not build up a sensitivity. It happens that there is a fairly high incidence of insulin-dependent diabetes that develops later in these women, and it would not be a good idea to treat them in pregnancy with a kind of insulin that would make their later requirements for insulin go up. The perinatal nurses and the clinical specialist also brought this one to the attention of other clinicians, and the practice protocol was changed.

Other examples: a recent article about the MUGA scan, a very high technology diagnostic procedure usefully discusses the technique itself and what it shows.[7] What is more interesting is that the article explicitly indicates the nursing responsibility to be sure that the pre-scan orders are correct, and that the MUGA has been ordered for things it is likely to be able to accomplish. A similar study of obstetrical ultrasound by a nurse showed that of the data examined, a very large proportion of ultrasounds for IUGR were ordered incorrectly.[8] That is, ultrasound for pregnancy dating must be ordered in a certain time frame, and with a certain interval between scans. This study, too, explicitly put the authority for monitoring the use of this technology in nursing's hands. And yet another study examined the preoperative preparation of patients for surgery which would invade the colon. In addition to providing very useful advice on emotional and physical patient preparation and teaching, the nurse-author specifically details the antibiotic preparation that should precede the surgery, citing the experimental literature on its beneficial effects, and enjoining surgical nurses to be sure it is done.[9]

Now these items seem to me to represent a long leap from the days, and they are not long ago, when a nurse was sued in Idaho for just such "interference" with the practice of others.

Let me turn up the volume on the bell—again, not an alarum bell—a little more. There are four things that are happening in nursing just now that clang a changed future.

First, the responsibility, authority, and accountability of nursing is finally coming together. The examples I just gave are the tip of that iceberg.

One of the effects of a nursing shortage was to create a method of assignment of work called team or functional nursing. It was thought that if one could divide up the work and concentrate certain tasks in certain worker categories, it would be more efficient. The problem was that dividing up the tasks also divided up the people—that is, patient care was fragmented and nurses were not particularly happy spending a day doing nothing but blood pressures or medications. In contrast, case assignment and primary nursing are not administrative solutions, but professional practice solutions to the delivery of care, based on the notion that one nurse in charge of one patient can deliver better care.[10] It turns out that that care is also cheaper, and it turns out that morale is improved when primary nursing can be practiced (which, of course, means when there are enough staff).

What is important in primary nursing is not only that the schizophrenia that used to characterize functional nursing is gone, but that the nurse is able to use her or his complete scope of practice being identified, and therefore accountable for it. And with the authority, based on more intimate knowledge of patient need, to assign the work for others at other times of the day. And with the authority to determine, in the interests of the patients, the interventions of others. It is a useless and draining exercise for nursing to have the responsibility, but not the authority or the accountability without the responsibility. When those three come together, the work role becomes coherent and the potential impact not only on patient care but on system reform is revealed.

Intensive care is intensive nursing care. There, the nurse's role has long contained more authority. There is a fascinating new study that shows just how important that is.[11] Researchers at George Washington University have been studying intensive care for some time. They are particularly interested in defining which patients it is really good for, and under what conditions. They have a measure which they call APACHE, used to define the physiological status of patients in intensive care, and shown to be reliably predictive of mortality. Their most recent study took a national sample of intensive care units, and using APACHE to control for the severity of the physiological condition, they compared mortality rates among the units. There were some units in their sample with mortality rates quite below the average for the group, in spite of having patients who were just as compromised. And there were some with higher mortality. They found that the variable that most explained the difference was whether or not the head nurse of the ICU had the authority to admit patients and close beds. Where she or he did, mortality was much less. Where nurses and physicians fought over turf or did not communicate well about patients, mortality was higher.

The literature on the effects of the authority and accountability of intensive care nurses and of primary nursing now joins the literature on primary care nursing—the work of nurse practitioners—and the nurse-midwifery research. It should be clear that the same issue appears in all of these instances. When nurses have the proper scope of practice, the authority to practice it, the accountability for our own actions, and the responsibility to make it work, it can be demonstrated (and has been, over and over) that care improves and probably costs decrease. The incredible waste of nursing talent attributable to limited practice roles and lack of professional autonomy can be shown to be inefficient and ineffective.[12]

There will be much for nurses in different practice roles, bound together by this shared authority, to learn from each other, and we are doing that too. A recent anecdote from a graduate student illustrates the point. This student is between her first and second years of a family nurse practitioner program. She is working this summer as a staff nurse in a rehabilitation unit. There, in the course of being primary nurse for a patient, she had cause to do something she has done throughout her first year of education in primary care: write a consultation request for a physical therapist. In primary care, physical therapy honors her request, even as a student NP. But she discovered, when called on the carpet, that primary nurses may not write consultation orders, only physicians may. That's nonsense, for the level of responsibility of the primary nurse is precisely the same as it is for the NP.

Nurse practitioners have told me of instances in which visiting nurses were prohibited from accepting changes in telephone orders from them, even, when they were the primary caregivers for patients at home. That will have to change, and will when nurses get together and realize what the commonalities of practice are.

So the increasing coherence of responsibility, authority and accountability is the first difference-making theme.

The second is that nursing is rediscovering the nature of the work. The examples given earlier about clinical wisdom and the wise use of technology fit in this category. In addition, nurses are building up a body of literature and experience on alternatives, especially non-invasive substitutes for high technology, or expensive care. ...

Pat Benner's path-breaking work on how nurses become experts and what expert nursing consists of is an example of rediscovery.[13] And there are now many more reports of the carefully analyzed clinical case in the nursing literature, cases that provide us with new ways of thinking about, conceptualizing, nursing's work. Surely setting up standards of care, whether they are professional organization platforms or local institutional generic nursing care plans are examples of the rediscovery of nursing's work. Reading some of them is a mind-boggling exercise for one who left the med/surg world some years ago! The quality and amount of decision-making now required of nurses is extraordinary and extraordinarily visible.

Which leads to the next theme of things that are making a difference: documentation.

Nursing has been invisible in part because our work is so private, but also because it is so little recorded in places where the information can be saved. Again, nurse-midwifery provides a nice example, for nurse-midwives have kept records of services delivered, and outcomes, for years and years as part of their own professional code. When it came time to argue for reimbursement, or change in credentialling law, the data were right there, and were used. Now that there are computers to help, it is possible to record at least the quantity of nursing—in time, or number of patients seen, or visits—in a way it was not before. Even the eternal forms nurses have filled out for years at least once a day, on "patient acuity," forms used to calculate staff needs for the next day or shift, can be remembered by machines, and those data are priceless. When nurses begin to write discharge summaries that are retained in the permanent chart, we will have moved a step further. The discharge summary or clinical abstract will then become available for inclusion in the mass data systems that now provide standard hospital statistics. One problem with nursing's invisibility is simply that we have not had data in the form in which it would be made useful, and collecting it anew for each challenge to our practice has been tedious and difficult. Now that we are recovering the work, it is possible to produce the kind of information that can be entered into mass data systems, to lurk there until it needs to be called upon. And that is coming very soon.

I said a minute ago that the patient acuity information collected routinely for staffing hospitals is priceless. Actually, it has a price and an increasingly definite one. And that is the last theme I wish to present today. For the final difference that is going to matter to nursing is that nursing is now *claiming credit*.

Now credit, like it or not, is an economic term. It connotes value, which is usually, but not always, monetary. We claim credit when we can attach to the work a value that is measurable. Good works alone, or warm hands just won't do it.

About 2 years ago there was an article in *Harper's Magazine* by a resident physician, David Hallerstein.[14] The article was a clever approach to teaching the public about why medical care costs what it does. What Hallerstein did was take a real hospital bill and publish it, annotating it as he went along to explain what the items on the bill meant.

The bill came from an unnamed New York City hospital, and it represented 24 days of care for a patient, Mrs. K. Mrs. K spent 24 days in an intensive care unit, in which she eventually died of some nasty chest condition, it is not clear what, for the identifiying information has been removed. The bill shows all the drugs, procedures and treatments she had, and buried each day among the gantrisin charges, trach sets, and chest X-rays is a line called "room and board," with a price, $500 per day.

Now this is intensive care, remember. Buried in the $500 per day is the cost for nursing, along with the so-called hotel costs. It has been estimated in one study that nursing is about 50% of the room and board cost in intensive care. (Actually, a more recent study with a better definition of nursing care costs puts the figure closer to 65%, but we'll be conservative here). For 24 days, then, at half of $500 per day, nursing cost Mrs. K. (or her insurer, for she had insurance coverage), $6000, of a total hospital bill of over $46,000. That figure, $6000 for 24-hours worth of intensive nursing care per day turns out to be about $10.40 per hour, the best bargain in town. Now that is what Mrs. K was charged, not, of course, what the nurses were paid because she really did not get 24 whole hours of one whole nurse every day.

But nursing was invisible in this bill.

Economic invisibility—the invisibility that comes from not being measured—means that it is not possible to attach a value to nursing, a value that is recognized by conventional societal norms.

All that is about to change, within the next 2 years, by my best guess. There are already a small group of nursing studies that have attached dollars to nursing within and across DRG's. Now there are really two issues here. One is the professional policy issue that wishes to unbundle and make visible, for nursing's political purposes, our work. That is separate from, but quite related to the public policy issue, which is attaching appropriate dollars to services rendered, whether they are hospital services, medical services, or nursing services.

When DRGs were invented, it was for the explicit purpose of providing a tool for better management of institutions, by defining, using data which were available, the product of an institution.[15] It is not possible to compare institutions, nor to determine efficiency or effectiveness, without a definition of what the work of the thing is, whether it is Chryslers or patient discharges. DRGs were intended to be a management tool, but the Health Care Financing Administration (HCFA) adopted them as the basis for prospective payment.

It was known in the beginning, by the developers of DRGs that the information on which DRGs were formed did not include data directly relevant to nursing resource consumption, that is, nursing time. Thus, one of the inventors has observed that it is strange to find that nursing care, one of the most studied of all hospital services, is the last item to be added to the DRG costing model.[16] Indeed, while prospective payment fixes a price per case, which differs among DRGs, nursing care within that price is still based on a per diem figure as if every patient required the same amount of nursing care every day. Which is, of course, nonsense.

In fact, it can be hypothesized (and even demonstrated with data) that there are at least five distinct patterns of the deployment of nursing time, and they vary by categories of DRGs. The typical elective surgery pattern, for instance, starts at some mid-range, increases on the day or so following surgery, then drops back to a minimum level for the rest of the stay. The typical pattern for reconstructive surgery (such as hip replacement) starts at a mid-level, has a little blip on the day after surgery, but remains essentially flat. Patients leave the hospital with a similar dependency in function, it's just that now the original problem has been fixed but complete healing has yet to take place. The pattern for terminal illness (absent palliative care) starts at a relatively low level of nursing intensity and rises in an ascending curve in the last days of life, which may also be spent in intensive care. The trauma or emergency admission typically starts high and gradually falls off, but never to the bare minimal level, for those patients continue to have problems which require nursing assistance. And then there is a pattern that is characteristic of the very old and ill, or patients with comorbidities and complications, which has spikes and valleys throughout the stay.

Sovie, at the University of Rochester, did the largest study to date on nursing intensity and DRGs.[17] She had data on some 456 of the then 467 DRGs and attached nursing intensity not only to DRGs but to costs of care. The implications from her study have already been translated into practices at Strong Memorial Hospital. Now, patients are being billed directly for nursing service, based on the level of care provided each day of stay. Further, Sovie was able to identify certain patterns of care by unit that made management sense. For example, on one unit, some nine DRG's accounted for over 80% of the patients. That suggested to her that generic nursing care plans could be written, to be emandated by the primary nurse, and the saving in time alone would provide one more staff member.

The nursing management literature is becoming increasingly optimistic about the possibilities for nursing under prospective payment and DRGs. The nursing clinical literature has yet to quite catch up, but it will soon.

HCFA has funded a very large study which will be completed this summer, with the explicit purpose of figuring out a way to weight DRGs for nursing intensity. I am privileged to work on that project. While I cannot provide a full report, because the study is not yet completed, I can tell you a few things.

First, it is very clear that it will indeed be possible to calculate a way to allocate to each DRG a nursing weight, to determine which are the most nursing-intense. That means, among other things, that it is already possible to figure out which DRGs are the heaviest consumers of nursing time, and it should not surprise you to find that they are also the high volume Medicare DRGs—the diseases and dysfunctions that appear in the elderly, the chronically ill, and the generally debilitated. These are not necessarily the "sickest" patients, not the craniotomies from head injury, or the terminally ill. What takes nursing time is not necessarily the severity of the illness (as compared to other illnesses, or as compared to other stages of the same illness). Skin ulcers, for example, are in the top 20 high nursing intensity DRGs.

More importantly, if it is possible, as it will be, to weight DRGs by nursing intensity, then it is possible to convert those weights into dollars—proportions of the room and board rate, proportions of the hospital bill. For another part of the project will report a costing model for nursing.

When it is possible to determine how much nursing a patient received by day of stay, by length of stay, by pattern of care, by patient discharge, or however else the data might be accumulated, then it is possible to determine accurately the costs of nursing. Now that might not be thought to be in our interest, and some of us have worried about whether it was wise to separate the costs for nursing from the costs of everything else.

What is obvious, however, is that if the costs can be defined, then so can the income generated by nursing. For when nursing is broken out of the routine room and board cost as an income generating service (which it is, of course, remembering that the reason for the existence of the modern hospital is to deliver nursing care), then nursing becomes not a cost center, but a revenue center, in accounting terms.

Revenue centers are attributed the income they make, and here we get to the crucial point: *revenue centers get to decide how to spend it.* No management system in the world can accommodate a revenue producing department that is not allowed authority over its revenue because no manager would work in such a situation.

So now nursing is a revenue center in institutions (and it is inevitable that the same general methodologies will be applied to long term care, outpatient care, and eventually home care). The nurse manager, then, is in a position to estimate income by nursing case mix (that is, the pattern of nursing intensity over the casemix of DRGs). The manager is then also in a position to determine how to allocate the resources to deal with the anticipated case mix. That suggests to me that the wise nurse manager will decentralize decision making so that the clinical wisdom, of which I spoke earlier, becomes available for decision making. It is really only the nurses at the unit level who can make clinical sense of the case mix data. For example, and this is a fairly trivial one, if the unit is a surgical one, and the pattern of nursing intensity for the DRGs commonly housed on the unit is determined, and if it is as I suggested, with a peak on the second day and a gradual decline, then it would make sense for nursing to spread those peaks out over the entire week, instead of on Tuesdays and Wednesdays as they may be now. A head nurse who argues such a change will have a great card to play, for it is in the institution's interest to provide nursing resources to meet patient need, and if a way to do that more efficiently, without increasing costs, just distributing them better, is found, no administrator in her or his right mind will reject them.

The prior research and the present project already have demonstrated the vastly increased options nursing has when we have data—information about patterns and systems of care.

But to return to the money issues, when nursing in hospitals and other facilities becomes an income center, then nurse managers will simply have to have control of the budget. It will require the talent of a prepared nurse, not a non-nurse administrator, to figure out how best to use the resources, since only nurses know the clinical exigencies behind the numbers.

When nursing has the budget, the income, then nursing is valued in a way we can never be without the money. But the value of nursing will not simply be administrative; it will be in valuing the work itself. Nursing will no longer be fixed at so many hours per patient, but rather will be determined on the basis of patient need, and billed as such. It will be the working nurses who determine patient need, and who will argue for more time when the need is measured and apparent. It will also be working nurses who will invent newer ways to do better care more efficiently, whether it means having staff specialize in particular kinds of patients, or reassigning patients from one part of the unit to another to save steps or equipment or time, or changing the paper forms, or the practice protocols, or the standing orders or the interprofessional relationships that slow nursing down. That kind of work will require not just warm bodies, but superb nurses, clinical wisdom, clinical leadership. ...

And that, my friends, will mean that hospitals will increasingly look carefully at the kind of person they employ, and that will mean a close look at nursing curricula. For hospitals will be interested in having the best possible nurses, the ones who know not only the clinical work, but the hard conceptual work and the systems savvy, for only that combination of knowledge will suffice. And that, of course, will mean a major revolution, perhaps overdue, in nursing education, to return us to a serious study of practice and the phenomena thereof.

Nursing is already something like 50% of the room and board bills to patients and their insurers, and somewhere around an average of 30% of total hospital charges. That is the single largest non-capital chunk of hospital budgets. And hospital care is the single most expensive commodity in health insurance. And the federal government is the single largest insurer. The federal government wishes to be a "prudent buyer" for its money, hardly a questionable desire. When the federal government, in the form of HCFA, decides to support research to allocate nursing within DRGs, there is some good reason to guess that it will happen. And many other things will flow from that.

Nursing is claiming credit, then, in the four ways I have discussed. All four are related, but claiming the money is the most important. With that claim comes a kind of professional authority, accountability, and responsibility we have said we wanted all along. It is about to come to us and I think we are ready. We have been building toward this eventuality for years and years.

The possibility for nursing to return to the central role we once had, when nursing's service was indeed the service on which patients depended, is not only good, but nearly guaranteed. That possibility should override many of the things that now separate us, or distract us. Nothing would be more important than for nursing to claim the credit due for good work done, a credit now about to be defined in money, and of course, with money comes the image of nursing as professional service.

I will end then, if you'll forgive me, with a light analogy. There is a lovely song in the musical comedy, *Kismet,* part of which goes like this:

Why be content with an olive
When you could have the tree?
Why be content to be nothing
When there's nothing you couldn't be?
Why be contented with one olive tree
When you could have the whole olive grove?
Why be content with the grove
When you could have the world?

The world of nursing, of health and illness care is about to return to us. And I don't know about you, but I'm tired of the olives, especially the pits.

ENDNOTES

1. This was a telegram (remember them?) so all of this was in capital letters which read now, in emails and other contexts, as shouting. Cabranes to Foley, Mailgram March 1, 1978, 11:30 PM Est.

2. Kalisch, B., & Kalisch, P. (1978). *The Advance of American Nursing.* Boston: Little Brown, p. 150.

3. Kalisch & Kalisch, *ibid.,* p. 153, quoting W. Gilman Thompson (April 28, 1906). The overtrained nurse. *New York Medical Journal, 83,* 845–849.

4. Lewis, C. (1982). Nurse practitioners and the physician surplus. In Aiken, L. (Ed.). *Nursing in the '80's.* Philadelphia: Lippincott (pp. 254–255).

5. Hartford Courant, 1984.

6. Nichols, C.W. (1985). Clinical management of size/date discrepancy. *Journal of Nurse-Midwifery, 30*(1), 15–24; Nichols C.W. (1985). Postdate

pregnancy: Part I: Literature review. *Journal of Nurse-Midwifery, 30*(4), 222–239.

7. Funk, M. (1983). Preparing the patient for a MUGA scan. *Critical Care Nurse, 3*(5), 57–61.

8. Goodhart, L.J. (1976). The effect of modern technology on clinical practice: Ultrasound in obstetrics. Master thesis, Yale University School of Nursing, New Haven, Connecticut.

9. Sanford, Rhea (1986). Family participation in care—hospital to home. Unpublished Master's Thesis, Yale School of Nursing.

10. Manthey, 1980, *ibid.*

11. Knaus, Draper, & Zimmerman, 1986, *ibid.*

12. Diers, D., & Molde, S. (1979). Some conceptual and methodological issues in nurse practitioner research. *Research in Nursing and Health, 2*(2), 73–84. Diers & Burst, 1983, *ibid.*; Molde, S., & Diers, D. (1985), *ibid.*

13. Benner, P. (1984). *From Novice to Expert: Excellence and power in clinical nursing.* Menlo Park, CA: Addison-Wesley.

14. Hallerstein, D. (1984). The slow, costly death of Mrs. K. *Harper's,* pp. 84–89.

15. Fetter, R.B., Shin,Y., Freeman, J.L., Averill, R.F., & Thompson, J.D. (1980). Case Mix Definition by Diagnosis-Related Groups. *Medical Care, 18*(2) supplement, entire issue.

16. Thompson, J.D. (1984). The measurement of nursing intensity. *Health Care Financing Review,* annual supplement, pp. 47–55.

17. Sovie, M., Tarcinale, M., van Putee, A., & Stunden, A. (1985). Amalgam of nursing acuity, DRGs and costs. *Nursing Management, 16*(3), 22–42.

Nursing and Shortages

The passage of legislation that created the Prospective Payment System (PPS) for Medicare, those prospective payments based on Diagnosis Related Groups (DRGs) revolutionized not only the way hospitals were to be paid but the way they would need to rethink their work.

But when DRGs came in, organized nursing reacted with "death of civilization" arguments, not realizing that this way of thinking about production in hospitals would be a huge boon to nursing. (I didn't Get It either, for a while, nor did the DRG boys).

When I left the deanery at Yale in 1985, just when PPS was being phased in, Professor John Thompson asked me to work with the DRG boys to extend their research into incorporating nursing intensity (acuity) into the PPS system. I was on an extremely steep learning curve, on the bleeding edge of public policy. Oh, wow, was this fun!

It was also the time when DRGs were being considered for adoption in other countries, especially Australia, about which more later.

The incentives under PPS were to decrease length of stay since Medicare was now going to pay by the case, not by the day. Cases were going to be defined by DRGs, and the payment was going to be pinned to the length of stay (LOS) on a national average.

Length of stay dropped like a rock. The leisurely workup, the long recovery period just disappeared.

Some thought that this would mean that we wouldn't need so many nurses because there wouldn't be so many patient days and hospitals began to weed staff. What nobody realized is that if you cut off the "easy" patient days at the beginning and end of the patient's stay, it concentrates the "sick" or "hard" nursing-intense days and that's what happened.

*This pitched the USA into a nursing shortage different from previous ones. The issue was no longer supply but **demand**. Linda Aiken and Connie Mullinix did an important bit by cutting to the economics: oligopsony (the notion that only a few large employers—hospitals—control wages). And they*

214

fed in the demographics of nurses and the relationship between economic trends and nurse employment, a phenomenon nursing had long understood as the "refrigerator nurse." That is, where nurses are free to work or not, they will work to provide their families with whatever they need. And when the family doesn't need, they will stay home.

The late Carolyne Davis, RN, Ph.D., then head of the Health Care Finance Administration, called together an invited conference to put together the best thinking about the nursing shortage and I was asked to do the keynote, I suppose on the strength of my DRG affiliation.

I remember this speech as coming one day after I had come back from Australia and I was seriously jet-lagged. I remember writing the end of the speech on the plane from New Haven to Washington, DC. I remember what I wore: basic black with a great black and blue scarf. I remember being energized by this occasion. And then I don't remember much else.

But when I reread this for this book, it seemed prescient and obstreperous for the same issues are with us now.

If my assignment is to provoke some thinking about how nursing education and nursing service might address the nursing shortage issue, then perhaps the most provocative thing I could do is define the problem. And, where possible, define also where the problem comes from. For unless we understand that, any solutions will be band aids over a gaping wound.

I begin, then, with a redefinition.

What we have here is not a shortage of nurses. The ratio of employed nurses to population is higher now than ever—533 FTE per 100,000.[1] There are more hospital nurses employed—over 90 per 100 beds (which is, of course, less than one FTE per shift per bed). As a proportion of total hospital personnel, registered nurses now number 58%.[2] A higher percentage of registered nurses are working, full or part time—nearly 80%. And further, the number of beds and the number of patient days is *lower* in 1987 than in 1982.

In 1983, the Institute of Medicine declared that the supply of nurses was marginally adequate and thus the federal role in supplying nurses could end, and that responsibility be turned over to the states. That's only 4 years ago. Only 3 years, ago, in 1984, the vacancy rate for hospital nurses was the lowest ever.[3]

I suggest that what we have here is not a shortage of nurs*es*, it's a shortage of nurs*ing*. The problem isn't supply, it's demand. And to document that, it is only necessary to show one set of figures. (See Table 1.)

These data are from the 35 general hospitals in Connecticut for the past 5 years.[4] They show that while there has been an overall decline in the number of patient days recorded on "routine care" floors, the number of patient days in special care has actually risen. Routine care days declined 23.1% over the period; special care days increased by 8.4%. Put that together with the AHA data which have been used to define the current shortage. Those data

TABLE 1 ADULT MEDICAL SURGICAL SERVICES ROUTINE AND SPECIAL CARE DAYS ALL CONNECTICUT GENERAL HOSPITALS FY 1982–1986

FY	Routine Days	% Change	Special Care Days	% Change
1982	2,477,557	+0.93	173,324	+3.93
1983	2,431,631	−1.85	178,330	+2.89
1984	2,273,474	−6.50	183,637	+2.98
1985	2,067,421	−9.06	183,892	+0.14
1986	1,880,413	−9.05	183,544	−0.18

suggest that the hardest jobs to fill are not the intensive care unit jobs, they are the general medical/surgical nursing positions. It's not that patients are sicker. Disease hasn't changed all that much, nor has invasive and heroic technology. What has changed is that there is a much narrower range of sickness to be cared for, and the range is all at the high end of the curve. Patients are simply not being admitted for rest cures any more, or diagnostic workups, so that the proportion of "sick days" in the hospital is higher, and so is the demand for nursing care. The statistics on which the IOM based its conclusions are simply painfully out of date, and did not anticipate what would happen with Prospective Payment. Indeed, any statistics that do not consider case mix, whether defined by DRG or nursing intensity will miss the point: the work has changed.

So, in spite of the fact that there are fewer patients to care for, and that there are more nurses to do it, there is a perceived shortage. This is a shortage of nurs*ing*, not of nurs*es*.

A NURSING SHORTAGE

There is a point to this redefinition besides word play.

To define the problem as a shortage of nurses is to suggest the easy solution: produce more. That isn't even all that hard. Federal dollars did it before, they could do it again. Throw some money at student aid, throw some incentives in the form of capitation for increasing class size—it's all been done before, with great success. Schools hungry for the dollars get creative about recruitment and publicity and pretty soon, we have fixed the warm body problem and we can go on to other things.

But the problem defined that way means it is just a warm body problem, fixed by more warm bodies. That definition converts nurses back into widgets, interchangeable parts in a massive machine, to mix a metaphor.

To redefine the problem as a shortage of nurs*ing* opens up the possibility of examining instances, causes, and consequences differently, and perhaps coming to different solutions. The solution to the warm body problem is all too clear and is basically uninteresting. The solution to the shortage of nursing, however, leads us to contemplate not only the shortage of nurses in hospitals, but the shortage in every other part of the health care system. There is a much wider range of variables to consider including barriers to practice, economic, and social conditions, and especially, the nature of the work.

NURSING TODAY

First, let us consider what nursing is. It is a great deal more than merely a, forgive the expression, manpower issue, which is what the present construction of the problem as a shortage of nurses suggests.

Nursing is, and always has been, two things: the care of the sick (or the potentially sick) and the tending of the entire environment within which care happens. Nursing is not merely health promotion—lots of people can do that, including lay persons. Granted, caring for the sick is a difficult business, and it is shared in complicated institutions with other professionals in a delicate balance of power. There will always be hospitals, there will always be mental hospitals, and nursing homes, and home care agencies, and rehabilitation hospitals, and children's hospitals and we are deluded if we think that the greener pastures of outpatient work or health promotion or ambulatory care (where, by the way, people are very sick) will be where nurses of the future will work. Nursing is care of the sick.

The reason for the existence of the modern organized health care system is to provide nursing care. If surgery could be done safely and economically on the kitchen table, and if people could survive it, it would be. If diagnosis and management of serious medical illness could be done in office practices, in 8.5 minute visits, it would be. If the chronically mentally ill could be taken care of at home, and protected from the world and from themselves, they would be. If the demented, the frail, the paralyzed, the very old could be cared for at home, they would be and it would be a whole lot cheaper—because public policy would not contemplate channeling the money to family home care givers—they're supposed to want to do it anyhow.

The reason for the existence of the modern hospital, mental hospital, nursing home, home care agency is to provide nursing care. Hospitalization is a call for nursing. The modern hospital, as a place of treatment rather than custodial care, owes its history to the discoveries of science—antisepsis and later asepsis[5]—and the creation of the trained nurse. When surgeons learned that patients could survive their treatments if they were all placed together under controlled conditions of hygiene, light, air, nutrition, it became necessary to have people there to tend to them. Fortunately, Florence Nightingale had started St. Thomas' school of nursing in London (17 years before Lister started his hospital) and the modern hospital was born, catering not only to the orphans, pensioners, and poor, but to those with means too. As it later came to be a place which housed the resources physicians needed for diagnosis and treatment of disease, and where the watching and monitoring and ministrations called nursing could be provided, nursing became not only central to the hospital, but the very reason for its being.

There is no such thing any more as "general" or "generalized" nursing. All nurses are specialists.[6] That's simply the way the health care system is organized, and there is a reason for that. The amount of knowledge that it takes to deal with all of the possible things that can go wrong with all of the human body's systems, fluids, parts, or cells simply has to be broken into parts so that it can be apprehended. The organization of the health care system is not just a fiction of the politics of organized medicine—it's the way the human body is organized or the way living is. The afflictions of children are different from those of adults, which are different for different ages of adults as well and it simply makes intellectual sense to organize efficient health care delivery systems around the bodies of knowledge required.

When a nurse takes her or his first job, the process of specialization has to begin. Surely, specialization can change, but within a very short working time, nurses have to know a particular field in some depth, which means the depth of knowledge in another area is lost. That's okay; with nearly two million nurses out there, there ought to be enough to go around, no?

Well, no, actually.

The hardest nursing job is the general medical surgical position and it is not surprising that those positions are the hardest to fill, according to the AHA data. It may be that these positions lack the glamour of the special care unit, or the emotional pull of pediatrics or psychiatry. But it may also be that the amount of knowledge needed to care for people in these kinds of units is an enormous and unappreciated challenge.

In one typical university-affiliated hospital, data from two similar general medical units over a 3-month period showed, for about 500 patients, 109 different DRGs. These are DRGs, not diagnoses, which would have numbered in the thousands.[7] Not only do nurses have to learn (and relearn constantly) how to care for people with that many different things wrong with them, but they need to learn how to work with the 17 house staff, the 40 or so attendings, the four chaplains, the six social workers, and all the families as well. And, of course, patients' particular sets of nursing needs probably come in easily 109 different categories, which do not match the DRG labels.

Surely intensive care is hard work—after all, intensive care is intensive *nursing* care. But intensive care is much more predictable and governed by tested protocols and procedures than is general medical/surgical nursing. What makes nursing difficult is the vague, risky problems—the patients whose aneurysm might burst but hasn't yet, the uncontrolled hypertension, the potential bleeding or infection or confusion or fall. In intensive care, there are a limited number of other professionals and they're by and large the same faces. And the knowledge base in intensive care is a whole lot more firm—we know much more about the physiology and complications to be monitored and we know more about how to do that. No wonder experienced intensive care nurses say "You couldn't pay me enough to do general med/surg anymore."

We forget sometimes, that one of the things that has produced the reality of nursing these days is that, slow as it has been, nursing has moved into the educational environment. Even diploma school curricula are no longer confined to repeated and routine practice of procedures, if they ever were. We are an educated society and even when fancy psychological theories, or even fancier immunological ones are not explicitly studied in schools of nursing, they appear nearly daily in the newspaper and magazines we cannot avoid.

As nurses have gotten better educated, our capacity to find and understand problems in patient care has grown as well. Part of what makes for a shortage of nursing then (not nurses), is that there is more work to do because our own science and education has made it so. Before Dumas,[8] preoperative preparation was a shave and an enema. Before Elms,[9] admission to the hospital meant locking up the patient's valuables, introducing him to the roommates, pointing out the solarium, and charting vital signs. Before Ford,[10] outpatient nursing was measuring height and weight and changing the paper on the examining table. Before Igoe,[11] school nurses were mainly good for getting you out of gym.

So there is a shortage of nursing because there's a lot more to do. Part of that is a function of changes in the use of hospitals stimulated by Prospective Payment in part, but it was already beginning to change before that.[12] But the larger part is that the nature of the work itself has changed over time, without much attention or applause.

And finally, the nature of nursing has changed, now with some consciousness, to encompass the second of nursing's social mandates: the tending of the entire environment within which care happens. Nurses are the ones who must see to it that everything else functions, every other department does its job, or must fill in when they aren't there, especially in small community hospitals. How do we know this? Because we are the ones who get yelled at when it doesn't happen.

Registered nurses are the most versatile of employees. We can do everything aides and LPNs can do (and ward secretaries, interns, and ancillaries as well). Whether institutions have indulged in downward or upward substitution, the effect on registered nurses is the same. If there is more ancillary help—aides, technicians, etc.—nurses have to supervise them and that's work piled upon work. If there is a high proportion of RNs, there will also be fewer of them, and each one's job is bigger with no helpers.

The tending of the entire environment is something we have not particularly prepared or educated nurses for, except when we socialize our young into nursing and teach them how to get along with others. We have particularly not paid enough attention to teaching nurses how the world operates, the laws of the jungle, how and why decisions are made the way they are, and especially, where the money and power are. And why.

But nursing is two things: the care of the sick and the tending of the entire environment within which that happens. The "product" of the hospital is the episode of care; it is not the hours of nursing, the tests, x-rays, meals served, pounds of laundry changed and washed.[13] A patient is discharged when the care is finished; the cure may never happen.

Thus another thing that makes nursing very hard work is the constant feeling of incompetence, of being victimized without knowing what one has done to deserve it, of having no advocates, no place to turn, no help in making things happen. The imbalance between the authority, responsibility, and accountibility of nursing is stunning and draining.

No wonder there's a shortage of nursing.

THE NEW SHORTAGE

But everyone seems to agree that this shortage is different, and most people attribute that to the diminished number of people coming into the field or indicating an intent to do so in national surveys. This is the widget definition and while it applies to the future, it does not explain the shortage now. The new shortage is attributed to the lack of a significant economic incentives, meaning increased salary with a BSN or even a decent salary, and the increasing tendency for college students to seek money over a chance to serve. Somehow, the working environment itself escapes attention.

Without disputing the truth of either of these attributions, there is a question here that needs answering: whose problems are these? Or, in the words of the conflict resolution folks, who owns the problem?

There is an implicit message given out, particularly in the mass media, that these issues are problems with nursing, that somehow we caused them. The negative public image we have is our own fault.

In a paper presented last summer to an invitational conference on the shortage sponsored by Sigma Theta Tau, Myrtle Kitchell ("Kitch") Aydelotte listed nine liabilities of the nursing profession.

The first four blame the victim:

- a public image that augurs against recruitment of intelligent, ambitious, and motivated individuals
- a lack of an adequate number of nurses who can engage in self and institutional governance
- the inability of the profession to clearly articulate its economic value
- the failure to place high value on ... the staff nurse ... position[14]

The list says we are ugly, timid, confused, impoverished, and elitist. I don't believe that.

Let us distinguish between two things: the working conditions—demand and turnover, and turnover is the problem, not retention in the profession;

nurses are not leaving nursing in droves—and recruitment. For there are different solutions depending upon how the problem is defined.

But first, let's talk policy.

THE SHORTAGE AS A POLICY ISSUE

It is of interest that this conference and the one the NCNR had last week are being held at the federal level, and that in many states there are Governor's Task Forces or other bodies deliberating about the nursing shortage. That implies that there is something about a shortage of nurses that is an issue of public, governmental, policy interest.

A shortage of warm bodies, a shortage of nurses, is arguably a public policy issue. (So is a shortage of physicians, also addressed in earlier times as a public policy issue, but that's another story). It is not the government's business to worry about manpower except perhaps in the context of defense policy. But it may well be a matter of public policy to worry about a shortage of nursing, if access to care, quality and cost—the policy issues—are compromised. So let's redefine the problem.

Public policy in the United States regarding health care has not exactly been either clear or coherent. But policy analysts, including Paul Starr,[15] have simplified things for us. Health care is a matter of public policy because of its relationship to economics. If people are not healthy, they do not work. If they don't work, they don't produce. Or, if they don't work, they don't have money to spend, which amounts to the same thing. Production is what makes the capitalist world go around.

But remember, the reason for the existence of the modern hospital is to provide nursing care. When that care is not available, the capacity of the hospital to produce is compromised. Sure the hospital loses money, and so do physicians, but neither of those is a public policy issue. Access to care is compromised, and so is quality and the cost/quality equation goes out of balance. *That's* the policy problem.

One study, referred to earlier, of two similar general medical units examined the effects of short staffing. One unit was short of staff, using the hospital's own definitions and the other was adequately staffed, again using the hospital's own definitions. For the most frequently occuring DRGs, average inlier length of stay on the short staffed unit was 1.28 days longer than on the other unit. When only the six most frequent DRGs were examined, the average length of stay was significantly longer on the short staffed unit in two of them. The hospital used a simple four-level measurement of nursing intensity, with level one being the lowest. The data show that nearly three-quarters of patient days on the short-staffed unit were in category 3 or 4 (73.4%) while only a little over half (56%) of patient days on the adequately staffed unit were in the higher intensity categories. The complications recorded were higher on the short-staffed unit and were generally preventable—generalized infections and UTIs were the highest volume complications.

Another study says that when there is a shortage of nursing, nurses retreat from practicing the full scope of possible service, and they provide only minimal, safe care, in their own definition.[16] Patients, or their insurers, still pay the same, however.

The cost of nursing shortage cannot really be determined in the fullest sense. Lost days of work because treatment is delayed is surely a "cost", if not to Blue Cross. And lost income to physicians is surely a cost as well. The cost to hospitals of closing beds is serious since the fixed costs of the institution continue, even if salary costs do not. And hospitals do not decrease the number of administrators when the number of nurses goes down. The costs of keeping the institution open by using agency personnel is not only in the absolute dollars paid, which are considerably more than would be paid to the same number of employed staff (if they could be found)[17] but the psychological cost to the employed nurses who earn less and work harder has to be factored in as well. I know of no study that has looked at a comparison of lost revenue from closed beds versus the incremental costs of raising salaries to staff the entire institution, and such a study ought to be done.

This same study I've been citing examined the costs of short staffing on these two medical units. The major cost—revenue loss—to the hospital occurs because of lengths of stay beyond point at which the price of care is federally set. The study concluded that the total differential net revenue loss to the hospital (annualized) comparing the short-staffed unit with the other was $152,920, and this is only one unit in a hospital which has about 480 beds.

The shortage of nursing is, of course, not just in hospitals. A particularly flamboyant example of the expensiveness of a nursing shortage is upon us right now, and it also represents a failure of public policy.

The new law to regulate nursing homes has just been passed as part of the Budget Reconciliation Act. It is an unusual piece of legislation in a number of ways, not the least of which is in the detail of its prescriptions, unusual in law, more usual in regulations. The new law calls for serious attention to patient's rights, including rights to information and informed consent, the right to have one's own physician in attendance, and the requirement for regular periodic assessment and care planning. According to the New York Times, the law is projected to cost an additional $832 million, primarily for compliance, to be shared by nursing homes, the Government, and some patients. Buried in the law is the prescription for 24-hour licensed nurse coverage, and 8 hour per day, 7 days a week Registered Nurse coverage, surely a very minimal requirement you would think wouldn't have to be legislated.

The *New York Times* report[18] of the law notes that the nursing home industry has been subject to study and investigation for years, with continuing problems of quality (to say nothing of continuing scandals). The new law applies not only to nursing homes, but to home care, although the reporter acknowledges that home care has escaped the criticisms of nursing homes.

The reporter fails to make the important connection: nursing homes are staffed primarily by unlicensed personnel and it is no wonder, therefore, that there are problems of quality. It has been observed that it may be precisely this lack of professional personnel that makes the nursing home industry the most regulated of all sectors of health care. Home care, however, has been staffed by registered nurses and directed by registered nurses, and it is not surprising that there are quality differences.

The requirement for more licensed personnel in nursing homes was initially resisted by the nursing home industry on the grounds that (a) it was too expensive, and (b) there weren't any nurses to be had anyway (partly because the pay is so poor). The present law passed with a coalition of nursing home administrators on board. Why? The basic problem is levels of reimbursement and nursing homes have felt, with some justice, that the reimbursement system was tilted toward hospital care. This was one way to argue the reimbursement levels up. My colleagues in home care say that they have no problem at all with the new provisions in the law—they are already exceeding the minimum standards set. One might wonder whether it might not have been a better use of federal funds to take the $832 million and throw it at upgrading nursing positions in nursing homes. There is little question that such a move would be effective in raising quality, as well as cost-effective.

The policy issue was defined here as regulation; the perceived problem was control. The real policy problem—the value problem—is that the elderly or the chronically mentally ill (who comprise a large number of nursing home patients) have to be kept invisible. The new law amounts to punishment of nursing home administrations with a swift kick at federal reimbursement rules rather than an acknowledgement of a concern for the elderly and sick which might suggest professional nursing care as a solution.

The shortage of nursing is a policy problem of another kind in the mental health system, especially the public system. In Connecticut, which may be a bit worse than some other states, there has long been a cap on admissions to state mental facilities because the staff was inadequate to handle admissions. So mentally ill persons, including substance abusers, have been backing up in community hospital emergency rooms for years. The cost of their care in the E.R. is enormous, and the care itself is enormously trying for the nurses who work there. The mental health system devised an emergency and crisis intervention program to ease the problem, but all it did was create yet another fragment to an already uncoordinated mental illness treatment system. And the revolving door continues to revolve.

The reluctance of policymakers to consider what the nature of the work is, in nursing homes or in mental hospitals, leads to a definition of the problem that is simply incorrect. In neither case has the definition of the problem been framed so that innovative solutions could be sought; regulation has been the only answer, and regulation is always expensive. And in neither case (nor in the case of hospitals, for that matter) has the real nature of the institution been considered.

The reason for the existence of the modern hospital is to provide nursing care.

If nursing manpower is arguably a policy problem, then why are we here?

I suggest that the shortage of nursing—not nurses—does indeed come in part from the items Kitch Aydelotte listed, as well as some others, and that the part of the problem that is the policy problem is the extent to which nursing has been *prevented* from being part of the solution and instead has been labeled as part of the problem.

BARRIERS

There has been a long systematic and successful attempt to keep nurses away from the money. In a capitalist society, money is a way of keeping score—the more you have or control, the more you are valued. The fact that nursing salaries are what they are, that the range of salaries is so restricted that nurses reach the peak of the scale after about 7 years of working, the restrictions on direct payment for services rendered, are not the fault of nursing. We are up against an intricately complex system of historical decision and rule, social power, and professional boundaries. But there is a simple way to think about it—define the situation differently.

The reason for the existence of the modern hospital (etc.) is to deliver nursing care. That being the case, the barriers in the way of nursing's capacity to do that become a policy problem. And when those barriers fall, and are advertised to do so, the problems with the public image of nursing as a recruitment problem will fall, too.

A colleague told me that his answer to the question about why there is a nursing shortage is simple: "Who wants to join a powerless profession?" After I took my hands away from his throat, I thought about that.

All of the data about nurses leaving the field, or leaving a particular job, for that matter, point to the same thing: lack of authority over one's own practice, lack of autonomy and professional recognition.

All of the data about what makes particular hospitals attractive places to work[19] and all of the data about job satisfaction say the same thing: authority over one's practice, autonomy, and professional recognition. Simply: the right to decide for oneself. *That* is the power we seek.

That power comes, however, not from argument, or position title, degrees or credentials, or professional association position papers. The power comes from having a desired resource, and these days, that resource is money.

Aydelotte says one of the problems is the nursing profession's inability to say how we contribute financially to institutions. But that is not *our* problem, we didn't create it. There has been a deliberate attempt to keep nurses away from the money. It goes back to the 1930s when Blue Cross was negotiating contracts with hospitals.[20] It was then in the interest of the hospital (because they would make more money in those post-Depression days) to lump nursing's services in with the room and board costs of the institution so as to be able to charge Blue Cross more. It's no more complicated than that, and not even political.

But time passed, and different forms of reimbursement sprang up, and government got into the act and there was lots of money around and nobody particularly cared what anything cost. People forgot how to do cost accounting because nobody was paying any attention to the money anyhow. So year after year, hospitals added increments to their overall budgets and there would be some negotiation over the rates to be charged and everybody lost sight of what the relationship of cost to charge really was. And nursing was still buried along with brooms, breakfast, and the building mortgage. A nursing service administrator was "given" a budget and it often included not only the nursing salaries and fringe benefits, but other things like small capital expenses— IV poles—and supplies and xerox costs. The nursing budget often became the dumping ground for other expenses that the accountants didn't know where to put, or later, when rate setting came in, the nursing budget was a convenient place to hide non-nursing expenses since everybody knows nurses are so expensive anyhow and there are so many of us and nobody looked inside the nursing dollars.

And when people worried at all, it was about what nursing cost, since it was always such a big chunk of the hospital's budget, often the largest single chunk. Not many people were thinking about what nursing generated for the institution or, heaven knows, about the fact that if you believe that the reason for the existence of the modern hospital is to deliver nursing care, nursing generates it *all*. There was hardly any thought about the fact that there was no way to manage the institution for quality or anything else because there was no way to link the services rendered to the services needed by the people served. Hospitals were organized to deliver meals, or laundry, or x-rays, or visits, or whatever and great hordes of managers were needed to sit on top of those departments.

Head nurses were berated for approving overtime (money is a way of keeping score) but given no credit when they stopped unnecessary tests or procedures, or got the x-ray department to schedule the patient earlier rather than later, or reduced duplicate tests, or untangled bureaucratic nightmares, or found lost charts. Nursing was defined only as time (and thus dollars), not as service. And because nursing was only a cost, a budget to be kept within, it had no power at the policy table. It only drained institutional resources, not made them.

In a conference last year on the nursing shortage, I said something of the same thing and then argued that the very first priority nursing must have to fix the nursing shortage is to go for the money. I meant unbundling nursing from other costs and other ways of attributing costs, and relating nursing time directly to patient requirement and need, and to institutional need, too. Then, billing patients or their insurers for those validated costs, and then collecting the money for the service, or billing other departments when we do their work.[21] It's not a difficult idea, and it's not even difficult to do in these days of computers.

If you know the cost of something, you can attach a price.
If you know the price, you can charge for it—bill.
If you bill, you can collect.
If you collect, you have generated revenue.
They who maketh the money geteth to decide how to spend it.

In other words, control of the resources generated by nursing gives nursing the control over our own practice, for we then have a way to negotiate using the same coin of the realm everybody else does.

The important point, however, is to be able to attach nursing services (and their cost) to patient requirements, which vary from patient to patient and day to day. This is basic to a variable billing system and cannot be replaced by global notions of nursing department budgets, which only allow a nurse manager to say how much it costs to treat a patient on the average (you just take the nursing budget and divide by patient days) but do not allow the manager to link costs to case mix to particular patients. Thus the only thing the manager can manage is the global budget, not the patient care itself, which is where the action really is.

To truly manage such a system will mean that institutions will have to decentralize because management of individual patient care requirements must be in the hands, ultimately, of those who deliver the service. Those who are closest to the expense need to manage—not "control"—it. When institutions decentralize, individual control over one's own practice is no longer an ideal, it is a reality. And we will have achieved the authority and professional credit we have said we wanted. It is possible, with the luck of idiosyncratically visionary management, to achieve such control and credit without having the money too, but it's a lot better with it. Money is a way of keeping score.

Money is something everybody understands and it gives us a way of talking about the work that is clear to the lay person, including the potential recruit. To coin a cliche, money is power, and having it means that nursing is no longer the "powerless profession" nobody would wish to join. Money keeps the score of nursing's role in health care delivery—a measureable, quantitative, powerful index. Money managed in the service of others, committed to resources required by the enormous scope of human problems we deal with makes nursing visible and attractive even to those yuppie college kids who want to make money as a career goal.

Now, I said something like this at this other meeting referred to before, but I had to leave the meeting a little early to catch a train. After I left the room, another participant in the conference, an Executive Vice-President and Dean of a Medical Center said, "I think that Donna Diers' point to go for the money is the worst position to take. ... That is not the image of nursing that should be projected to the American public as its central issue. ... I am speaking ... to public policy and going for the money is the wrong public policy. ..."[22]

Well, balderdash.

To be charitable, he may have thought I was suggesting going for *more* money, that is, increasing health care expenditures, and in a cost conscious environment, that would be foolish. I was only arguing, actually, for nursing to have the credit—an economic term—for what we already do. Now, I would add an additional agenda.

There is a myth floating around that there is not enough reimbursement money coming out of Washington, and so states are being pressured to take more of the responsibility, primarily by increasing the rate ceilings. But at the same time, the next phase of DRG-related work is commencing and people are beginning to use the DRG data system to probe more deeply into where the money is and where it goes altogether. We already know that Medicare Part B is the fastest growing part of the health financing system. Now, institutions are monitoring physician practice patterns for their use of ancillary services, as well as length of stay, and are producing reports showing how each physician stacks up against his or her colleague specialists, treating the same DRGs. I have seen some of these data coming out of one state-of-the-art management project and they are stunning. There are millions of dollars tied up in ancillary services and extended lengths of stay—dollars already being spent—which could be turned to other purposes, including nursing. To the extent that nursing is implicitly, if not explicitly, charged with tending the entire environment, we are in a position to contribute to the cost savings in these areas, and we should be able to claim some of those savings to enhance nursing's functions.

I submit that not only is going for the money the best possible way for nursing to rid ourselves of the "powerless" notion, but it is the best possible public policy. The policy issue here is quite simple: money ought to buy something of value. Until we know what nursing costs and contributes, by patient, by day, by stay, we have no way of participating in decisions about whether that's the right amount, too low, or too high. We cannot be creative about using nursing resources. We cannot really develop the knowledge about what in nursing works or not. We cannot negotiate our resources, decide to spend now to pay off later, or make rational changes in staffing or other costs. And most importantly, we cannot calculate the benefit of nursing's service, because the value of nursing or any other service is always a tradeoff between cost and quality.

The operational barriers to attaching dollars to nursing service are already down. The public policy issue is that nursing may need the help of legislation or regulation to make it happen, over the sloth or resistance of administrators or others. Now that the government has taken the position of being a "prudent buyer," we are in a position to help—to be part of the solution, not part of the problem.

We may need the help of public policy to straighten out things that are not really policy issues in other parts of our field as well. Among the things that make nursing appear a powerless profession are the continuing well-advertised attempts to control our practices through regulation and other means. Third-party reimbursement and prescriptive authority, for example, are not really public policy issues. But we may have to turn to legislation to make them happen because negotiation with those who resist because of economic competition is unlikely to prevail.

Public policy as law and legislation runs behind the clinical reality. Things have to change faster in the real world than the law or legislation can keep up with. Thus, nursing has often turned to public policy when issues were not necessarily matters of policy concern, to fix into place clinical realities. *Bernardi v. Community Hospital Associates* made hospitals liable for the acts of their employees and recognized that nurses are indeed employed by hospitals and liable for their own acts.[23] This not-very-novel interpretation, however, brought nurses out of the employment relationship to physicians, which had created the *respondeat superior* ("captain of the ship") doctrine so politically abominable to nurses. *Darling v. Charleston Community Hospital* made hospitals liable also for the acts of physicians to whom practice privileges had been granted, and interfered with the conveniently casual relationship physicians had to institutions, which they treated like their workshop. *Sermchief v. Gonzales* brought modern nursing practice to public view, rejecting the claim that family planning nurse practitioners were practicing medicine without a license.[24]

Sometimes legislation has to be passed to clean up what cannot be cleaned up by negotiation. Wherever the educated talents of nurses are constrained by artificial barriers in law, regulation, interpretation of statutes, or common practice, there is a shortage of nursing.

A WIDER VIEW

Since the data upon which the allegation of the present nursing shortage is based came out of hospitals, it is assumed that the shortage is restricted to hospitals. But that's wrong.

I have already alluded to the shortage of nursing in nursing homes and in the public mental health system. There is also a shortage of nursing in specialist practice.

One of the dumb things that happened just before Prospective Payment went into effect in 1983 is that some hospitals, anticipating budgetary shortfalls, began to freeze nursing positions and then eliminate them. Some of the first to go were the clinical specialist positions, partly because administrators, including nurse managers, could never figure out what these people did, and partly because (once again) there was no way to cost out and evaluate their services. This was a dumb move for a number of reasons, but I will deal with only one of them.

The data on why nurses leave positions or leave the field lists a number of "dissatisfiers." Salary is first, but number three is "lack of support on the part of hospital administrators" and number four is "insufficient opportunity for furthering professional education" and number seven is "lack of support on the part of nursing administration" and number nine is "insufficient in-service education" and number eleven is "lack of competent support personnel."[25]

Nurses want to get better at the work. We really do not consider ourselves robots putting the same piece of equipment together day after day after day. I said earlier that all nurses are specialists these days. And the most highly trained are the clinical nurse specialists—nurses who have made a life work out of coronary care or oncology or pediatrics or psychiatry or whatever. The role of the clinical specialist addresses all of the dissatisfiers listed. The clinical specialist runs interference, and because she or he has the power of knowledge, the clinical specialist is in a position to provide the managerial support nurses say they want and need. The clinical specialist is the built-in inservice person, especially when she or he collaborates in the care of particular ill persons. Clinical specialists have access to libraries and secretaries, and they have to keep up with the literature and the changing science. They have *time,* which staff nurses do not, to read or write or think something through, to serve on the interdisciplinary committees for DNR orders or Baby Doe regulations. Clinical specialists are the support personnel to the nursing staff—not the ones to run errands and deliver things, but the ones to help the nursing staff with their work. They are not like the industrial line foreman whose role is controlling. They don't do staffing and discipline and punishment. The clinical specialist should be the clinical leader, and if that role is also combined with clinical management, so much the better.

The presence of clinical leadership makes the work of nursing more satisfying, the data says, and satisfied nurses stay. Where there is not that kind of clinical leadership, there is a shortage of nursing.

And again, this shortage shows up in nursing homes and in public mental health. Kane's work in nursing homes is convincing evidence of what can happen when gerontological nurse practitioners are allowed to work to the full scope of their practice.[26] McBride's study of the clinical nurse specialist in a state hospital shows what can happen when that role is instituted.[27]

Nurses want to continue to grow, to keep up with new knowledge, to be where the action is. In medicine, that creates academic medical centers and geographic full-time attendings, and hospital practice privileges for clinical faculty of the medical school. The equivalent in nursing might be the clinical nurse specialist position, which attracts nurses to institutions and keeps them there.

Speaking of doctors...

When the GMENAC report came out in 1980, there was another dumb interpretation that is connected to the nursing shortage. That report, as you know, predicted that there would be a serious oversupply of physicians in 1990, and the word went out that somehow that meant that at least some jobs for nurses were going to be scarce. Potential nurse practitioner students heard the word over and over: the docs would take over the jobs and there would be no room for them.

Two recent studies suggest that the GMENAC predictions were off considerably, and that the problem is not nearly as serious as once thought.[28] But the studies also show that the problem of oversupply of physicians continues to be serious in the high-tech specialties; that's where the money is. Newly minted doctors are not rushing to rural practice or family practice, general internal medicine, or pediatrics. Those aren't where the academic or financial rewards are. In the meantime, as more and more things that used to be treated in hospitals are now dealt with in outpatient facilities, the need for primary care has only grown. As people are discharged earlier from hospitals, the need for skilled home care is there. As handicapped children have joined the educational mainstream, the need for skilled clinical services in schools is there. As more and more babies survive newborn intensive care with developmental disabilities and handicaps of various kinds, the need for experienced nursing to prepare these children for school has exploded. As the conditions of jails have been exposed, the need for more than just a once a week physician visit is there. As the terrible problem of AIDS came to consciousness, the need for nurses has become obvious—there is no cure to be had. As "managed care" has come to be a new reality, the notion of nursing in such systems, especially HMOs, becomes essential. And as outpatient surgery booms because there aren't enough nurses to staff the inpatient surgical services—well, need I go on? The notion[29] that physicians will somehow turn into nurses to fill these gaps is just silly.

In all of these areas there is a real, demonstrable shortage of nursing. And it is compounded by restrictive laws and regulations with old-fashioned interpretations of what nurses are and do. Four years after *Sermchief v. Gonzales* was decided, we still have state boards of nursing and attorneys general believing that listening to heart sounds is the practice of medicine, or that calling a red throat "pharyngitis" is illegal for nurses to do. Or that only physicians can recertify the need for nursing home care (when nurses have been figuring out how to get their services to Medicare patients on home care for years).[30] Or that a physician must be physically present when a nurse-midwife delivers a patient in a hospital. Or that regional anesthesia must be administered by an anesthesiologist, while a nurse anesthetist can only "top off" the spinal or the epidural.

What we are dealing with here, of course, is not safety. These restrictions on the practice of nursing are there for one and only one purpose: to protect the physician's billing opportunities. Surely that should not be a priority for public policy, much as some recent interpretations of law or regulation would make it seem so.

The present nursing shortage is only going to get worse, and not just because of the numbers-in-the-pipeline problem. Already, we know of the enormous growth in home care and nursing home care and unless policy dictates that the scandals of the nursing home industry infect other areas, more nurses will be called for. These will be specialist nurses—nurses with particular learning in geriatrics, psychiatry, intensive care. I know of one home care agency in Connecticut that hires nothing but nurses with 5 years of intensive care experience; that's how sick patients are now at home.

The AIDS epidemic is going to get worse. The demands upon nurses will only grow and the demands will be both in and outside of the hospital. Again, specialists will be needed—specialists in oncology, in infectious disease, and especially in mental health and substance abuse.

"Managed care" means nurse-managed care, whether the organization is technically a nursing center or not. "Case management"—the magic solution to the problems of uncoordinated care—is doomed to failure unless the case managers are skilled at whatever they're managing, which is (or ought to be) patient care; primary nursing has taught us that. Case management is too important to be turned into baby-sitting.

And there will be new jobs, specialist jobs. Every new high-tech service that opens up will have to have a senior nurse running it (a bone marrow transplant unit is my latest local example). Nurses like those kinds of jobs—they stretch our learning and the opportunity to participate in a new and exciting field as a colleague is very seductive. These new positions will take nurses away from general medical/surgical practice, which is where they are most needed. Discharge planning departments are entirely nursing and always will be; they will have to change from the dumping ground for nurses the institution is letting work off their retirement to places of creative planning and community connecting.

And there will be new academic opportunities as well. Schools of public health, of health management, of hospital administration, even schools of medicine are already coming to realize how much they need the contribution of nurses to the teaching of their students and to the findings of their research.

And funny thing, there is about to be a new shortage of physicians. The restriction on importing foreign medical graduates (FMG) has already produced one anecdote; one policy type suggested that nurses move into the perceived gaps in pathology, psychiatry, and pediatrics where FMGs used to go. He hasn't yet talked to nurses about this, and we may well wish to resist doing others' scut work.

The shortage is of nursing; the shortage of hospital nurses is just the tip of the iceberg. But at least it poked nursing onto the policy agenda. Now we have to stay there, and now we have to change the agenda from quantity to quality.

A WARNING

Under conditions of a shortage, the temptation is to make do, to fill in the gaps with overtime, to stop doing nonessential things. Immediately after World War II there was an immense nursing shortage, as hospitals were built under Hill-Burton funds, as the Veterans Administration developed, and as the nurses in the military came home to raise families. It was also a time of technological and scientific advancement, which increased the amount of work to be done. I do not think it is an accident that this period represents a very low point in nursing's professional development and in the development of our science and service. There was just too much to be done, and education, research, thinking disappeared first. We should not allow that to happen again.

This time around, the perception of the nursing shortage may be different because what is happening is not just overtime, it is closing of beds. We are saying "no" and turning from Pollyanna into Lysistrata. It is very difficult to say no when the demands get too heavy because we create an ethical dilemma: patients need care, so how can we refuse to be there to give it? What patients need, however, is *good* care, and patients are not well served by a strung-out, burned-out staff of nurses. Again, if the problem is redefined, it is easier to deal with. *Our* responsibility is to deliver good care. The administration's or hospital's responsibility is to provide the resources to do it; it isn't our problem. Surely we cannot abandon patients and walk off the job precipitously. But we can make clear what the conditions are under which we will continue to work, and if they are not met in a reasonable length of time, then actions must be taken to stop the flow of patients in, even if that means canceling surgery, closing intensive care beds, closing the emergency room to walk-ins, or whatever. Saying no is clearly the better short-term solution and it gets nursing a certain amount of attention. It makes possible some negotiations we have not had the chance to do before. It makes administrators and professional colleagues believe finally what Knaus, Draper, and their colleagues have shown: that where nurses and physicians work as colleagues and where the authority of the head nurse to close beds is supported, mortality rates in intensive care drop.[31] Surely such cooperation and its effects extends to other types of institutional care settings.

This a time for creative grappling with basic problems, the problems of control and power.

Which leads to the question, in whose interest is it to have a nursing shortage? Organized medicine is already basking in the publicity that there are more college students intending to be physicians now than intending to be nurses. The response of the American Medical Association to the nursing shortage is instructive. The AMA Board of Trustees has recommended:

1. Support all levels of nursing education, at least until the crisis in the supply of bedside care personnel is resolved.
2. Support government and private initiatives that would facilitiate the recruitment and education of nurses to provide care at the bedside.

3. Support economic and professional incentives to attract and retain high-quality individuals to provide bedside nursing care.
4. Support hospital-based continuing education programs to promote the education of caregivers who assist in the implementation of medical procedures in critical care units, the operating and emergency rooms, and medical/surgical areas.
5. Cooperate with other organizations concerned with acute and chronic hospital care to develop quality educational programs and methods of accreditation of programs to increase the availability of caregivers at the bedside and to meet the medical needs of the public.[32]

It doesn't take much of an intellectual leap to read into these proposals the serious concern of organized medicine that their billing opportunities (especially in the high-tech, high income specialties) not be interfered with; that "caregivers" at the bedside don't have to be nurses and might actually better not be, for they can be created, trained, and controlled by medicine, exactly as P.A.'s are; that what the AMA wants is widgets—at the bedside—not the uppity nurses in specialist practice or management who might ask trouble-making questions.

We should resist the oh-so-logical notion that one way to fix the nursing shortage is to break the job down into definable tasks and then assign them out according to levels of personnel. Task discrimination works only downwards and it is dangerous. If certain tasks are defined to be able to be done by lesser-trained personnel, that will mean eventually that registered nurses *shouldn't* do them, and that will turn the job of the RN into a manager of personnel. People become nurses because they want to nurse; writing the care plan and then turning over the care to others is not what's fun (writing the care plan is a great pain, as a matter of fact). Breaking up the work of nursing this way in order to compensate for a lack of manpower is a slippery slope upon which we should not set foot. What is slippery isn't task discrimination, it's defining certain, things as "not nursing." If it's not nursing, then we have no title to supervising it, assigning it, or taking the credit for it. We ought to be careful to retain title to all of nursing's work and not define out those things that are not, that can be done by others not even minimally trained in nursing, because that category of work will only increase and so will the workers: they're cheaper. And even if others create new categories of personnel—"obstetrical technicians" is one I heard of recently—we will still end up supervising them because we're the only ones who are there all the time to watch the work. We might as well own it.

Where there is work that clearly is not patient care, we should argue for support staff to do it—fetchers and carriers, secretaries, clinical medical librarians, clerks, housekeeping folks, and so on. And we should expect that these staff functions will assist the work of the institution, which is nursing. And if *we* have to do it, we ought to get the economic credit.

Which leads us to another point that is really not our business today to decide, but it at least ought to be acknowledged.

We had better pay attention to the boundaries and fences nursing is in the process of constructing between and among us for they only break what could otherwise be a very powerful occupation into smaller, weaker units. I refer particularly to the entry issue. We might take a lesson from medicine here. One way in which medicine has made itself into the sovereign profession it now is, is to claim all the turf for itself. Medicine scooped up pharmacology a long time ago; it has claimed administration by requiring physicians on boards, or AMA approval of programs or other things. It has claimed insurance as physicians dominated Blue Cross, controlled Blue Shield, and invented Part B of Medicare. It has sometimes even claimed nursing. Listen to the language of the Medical Practice Act in Michigan:

> Practice of medicine means the diagnosis, treatment, prevention, cure or relieving of a human disease, ailment, defect, complaint or other physical or mental condition, by attendance, advice, device, diagnostic test, or other means, or offering, undertaking, attempting to do, or holding oneself out as able to do, any of these acts.[33]

Nursing—all of it from basic hygiene to the most complex clinical decision making—belongs to us and we should not sell off any of its parts to anybody else.

The perception that something is broken in nursing and has to be fixed by changing standards for entry into the field raises a question: Whose perception is that? Why can't there be several ways to enter the field? The discrimination in levels of competence, then, should be done in the clinical arena and not automatically on the basis of educational credentials. One of the ironies in nursing is that there are no reliable data about the differences among graduates of different kinds of educational programs. In fact, it embarrasses some that diploma graduates still tend to have the highest scores on the NCLEX examination despite its intention to test the kind of nursing process thought exclusive to BSN education. One thing we simply do not know, no account for in these proposals, is who the diploma or associate degree graduates were before they were nurses. It has been estimated that perhaps 30–40% of associate degree graduates were college graduates before, and it is not surprising that they perform as well as new BSNs.

What is the problem here? The present multiple-entry system has been in place for some time and it's working. If it ain't broke—and the data that it is broken are lacking—don't fix it. Particularly if in fixing it, we begin to impose artificial limitations on people's abilities to give human service. Licensure has only the most tenuous relationship to competence.[34] There ought to be ways in which people can enter the field and then progress in it, either through an educational or a clinical ladder, based on ability and desire, not on artificial distinctions. The present obsession with entry seems only to alienate nurses from nurses, an odd stance to take just at a time when a coherent statement about nursing might be in order. Surely there should and could be differentiations among nurses, and those should be made in clinical institutions. Other than a few random, and not well designed attempts to differentiate on the basis of education, that is not being done, and for a very good reason: it won't work. The clinical world just doesn't break up that way, as it also resisted the style of practice imposed by the "integrated curriculum" and as it resisted confining nurse practitioners to the care of the "worried well," patients with minor, acute, or stabilized chronic illnesses. Mildred Montag has observed that associate degree education has turned out differently than it was planned, and that there are things in the ADN curricula that were never intended to be there, when production of the technical nurse was designed.[35] But they *are* there, and they are working.

What needs to be fixed is the extent to which educational programming cuts off opportunities for continued growth and development, either in employing institutions that limit the upward mobility opportunities by defining steps by degrees, or in educational institutions that need to collect a lot of tuition and so require repeated, and wholly unnecessary, experiences.

Some labor economists have thrown another wet towel at us. Some argue that so long as "nursing" encompasses what they call the "most menial" as well as the most advanced activities, it will be hard to argue that salary ceilings should be pinned to the most advanced tasks. Rather, they say, the top salary will be fixed to the median level of task performance. This argument deals with the nurse as employee—as widget—and is as clinically ignorant as the integrated curriculum. Surely experience and knowledge ought to count, and the work of practice ought to be divided into chunks that reflect that. But the chunks are unlikely to be tasks, and they might not even be people. And we will drive ourselves mad trying to figure out which patients, by disease or service or location, are the "hardest" to care for and thus ought to be recompensed the most. The hardest to care for may be the wandering Alzheimer's patient in a nursing home, now turned over to the least well prepared, cheapest staff.

We are just now being able to *find* nursing as researchers begin to examine "nursing intensity" using real data and real quantitative methods. We have never known before, except intuitively, what kinds of patients take the most nursing effort and what kind of effort they do take. We are just beginning to discover the relationship, or lack of it, between nursing's resources and other resources, and the possibilities of understanding nursing's work are mind boggling.

As data systems evolve to include nursing, as time, task, diagnosis, or indicator, we learn more about the work. For example, when DRGs are ranked according to nursing intensity, it is no surprise that among the most nursing-intense patients are those with multiple trauma or head trauma. But it *is* a surprise to find that among the most nursing-intense also are children, the elderly, especially patients with stroke, and those for whom the treatment itself has caused dependency. We have found that depression is a variable highly associated with nursing intensity[36] and so is immobility. We have noted patterns of nursing intensity across days of stay, patterns which have implications for numbers and kinds of staff, as well as management of services at the unit level.

It is way too early to predict how this information will be useful to us because we are very new to it. The point to be made, however, is that now it is possible to even *have* information about nursing and how it works that we never have had before, and we can use that information not only to deal with shortages, but to make the best use of all of our resources, short or not. We are beginning, therefore, to move away from mere rhetoric to actual facts about how the health care system operates.

IMPLICATIONS

For the next 2 days you are going to have to come up with some recommendations, some aimed at the Division of Nursing. I'm glad I get this place on the program and then go home because I'm not at all sure where all of this analysis logically leads. Any paper about the nursing shortage runs out of steam when it comes to solutions.

Some nursing organization, or a combination of them, ought to tackle immediately the public image problem and simply hire the best possible firm of people who do image-making for a living. If an advertising agency can kill new Coke in the service of selling old Pepsi, they can surely help us out. In fact, the Governor's Task Force in Maryland has suggested exactly that, and requested that the Governor use his influence to get advertising agencies to contribute the work *pro bono*. We should draw upon the data we have about potential nurses and about what we're told are the public perceptual barriers here. Nursing is a primarily female occupation. So? Advertise it that way to the feminists. Nursing is dangerous (you can get AIDS). So? Advertise it that way to the adventuresome. Nursing is hard work, hard physical and intellectual work. So? Advertise it that way to the smart ones. Expand our sights beyond the high school age group and tap the untapped resources: women whose children are old enough so that they can think of new options, hospital volunteers who might now wish a professional role, retired policemen and firemen. We might even give up our historic sexism and try to recruit men. That would certainly enlarge the pool.

But if we are to recruit people seriously into nursing, there has to be something there that will be satisfying, both in the educational programs and in the work environment.

The exciting and creative things in nursing these days are happening in practice, not in nursing education. That's a reversal of order, and caused in some part by the creative and innovative things that happened in nursing education 20 or so years ago. Thus the necessity to marry education and service seems obvious. Only now, I think service may help education more than the reverse. I am distressed when I hear that nursing service managers are approaching schools of nursing with peace offerings and white doves, as if the schools would solve their problems. That's again the widget definition and we must go beyond that.

We should take our guidance from as sure and clear an understanding of what nursing is these days as possible, from the work of the profession. Ask some staff nurses sometime what would make their working lives better and the answers will be rather simple: safe parking, tuition reimbursement, enough supplies and linens, shift differentials, a sensible shift rotation, perhaps even participation in making scheduling decisions. Many of the solutions to improving the working environment are simply, or complexly, managerial.

We do need good nurse managers. Not nurses with MBA's—you can hire an accountant or financial manager or marketing assistant. What we need are nurses who know the nature of the work, know how to distinguish between responsibility, authority, and accountability, know how to argue effectively from data, nurses who know that the reason for the existence of the modern hospital is to deliver nursing care. Educational programs, including joint degree options with schools of business or health management, could be encouraged, with the requirement that there be serious clinical specialty preparation as well. We need nurses who are prepared to analyze systems and policy, for knowing how the world operates is the ultimate empowerment. Educational efforts in this direction could be supported, but again, only when there is a clinical base from which to operate.

Creative approaches to nursing education, at any level, can be invented, where there is real understanding of the work of nursing. Undergraduate students are being prepared for the role we might understand as primary nurse. Why not involve selected primary nurses in the educational enterprise, with really truly faculty appointments and prerogatives. Primary nursing can be lonely; having a student around gives the nurse a chance to share the workload and the wisdom, and somebody to talk to as well. One could probably figure out a way to supplement the salaries of six or eight primary nurse-faculty for what it costs to hire one full-time assistant professor, and one could get a lot more mileage.

Ways to accelerate basic nursing education are not difficult to think of either. Surely students can be tested for competence and then not asked to repeat experiences they already have had. College graduates or RNs from diploma and associate degree programs can be sped along faster than high school students. Upgrading RN's does not solve the quantity problem, but taking the wider view of the quality issue, equipping nurses for leadership and change justifies the effort.

While it is not really the responsibility of the federal government, especially the programs of the Division of Nursing, to fix the working environment, there are times, and this may be one of them, when the carrot of the federal dollar should be acknowledged. Under the excuse of federal funding requirements, a lot of change can happen, especially if projects are set up as research and demonstration or experimental programs. Schools of nursing may take advantage of this stimulus as well, and attack some of the problems in nursing education, such as the inability of universities to count faculty practice as intellectual work, or the requirement of questionably essential curricula just because we've always done it this way. Part-time study can be supported if requirements for full-time enrollment in order to qualify for funds are adjusted. The temptation to create new nursing programs should be resisted, especially when their major function may be to sustain a faltering community college or small liberal arts college.

Special projects designed to bring the resources of educational institutions and clinical institutions together can be supported. Not just joint appointments and faculty practice arrangements, but other ways in which the resources of both can be shared. Schools of nursing have nurse-researchers—can they be involved in studying turnover? Quality assurance? Develop information systems? Can they provide inservice education and staff development? Can they serve as systems consultants, helping nursing staff grow in their understanding of the value of the work?

Clinical institutions have people who know how to do the work. Can they not participate in the educational enterprise as faculty, as curriculum consultants, as partners?

The long-term solution to nursing shortage problems will remain in changes in the policy arena. Can we not begin to work on that now with cleverly constructed experiences for nurses as legislative interns, as consultants to policymakers, as members of policy and planning groups whose placements are orchestrated under special training projects?

A long time ago, at Duke University, there was a lovely project in which a group of newly minted BSN graduates negotiated to have their very own hospital unit to staff and in which to practice to the fullest scope of their training. Could not such contracts for service or other institutionalized formats be devised now, as a way to demonstrate nursing at its best, and in its best management?

I'm not sure that nursing services need more funds in the form of federal dollars. Rather, I think nursing services need help in capturing the money that they already earn, and in negotiating to trim back funds now going in other directions. There is a lot of money in health service delivery; there isn't, however, in nursing education. Whatever incremental funds might be used to target the nursing shortage ought to be carefully screened for the "widget factor" and not aimed simply at churning out more numbers from the same tired curricula into the same exhausted work environment.

Aiken and Mullinix have five recommendations to deal with the nursing shortage. Three of them have to do with salary scales, shift differentials, and fringe benefits for experienced nurses, all of which are problems internal to the service setting, solved by administrative activities that do not need to be supported by federal funds. Or at least Division of Nursing funds. But perhaps there are ways HCFA could be encouraged to use its power to attack the nursing shortage creatively. There are two explicit suggestions, both of which have been made to HCFA without apparent success.

First, HCFA could mandate the collection of nursing resource data from all hospitals, at least for Medicare patients. This would mean that they could require hospitals to break out nursing costs separately and they could require two very simple additions to the Minimum Data Set: number of days in special care units, and number of days at each of, say, five levels of nursing intensity.[37] These two bits of information, combined with the information already collected, will expose nursing resources, by DRG, and allow reasoned consideration of whatever proposals to use resources better are invented. Without data, we just spin our wheels.

The second suggestion comes from Ed Halloran.[38] He has argued, effectively, I think, that hospitals could and should treat the costs of nursing education (which he defines in service terms as portions of head nurse and clinician salaries) as "R and D." His own figures for University Hospitals of Cleveland show that by the most generous calculation, nursing education costs were about 5% of the nursing service budget (or about 1.5% of the total hospital budget). Any company which produces anything invests between 6% and 8% of its resources in R and D, and many invest far more than that. For a hospital, nursing education is indeed R and D—creating a workforce— while it can be argued that paying for medical education under Medicare does not enjoy the same policy position. Regulations could be written to allow, or even require, hospitals to budget these kinds of R and D expenses.

Aiken and Mullinix argue that the work requirements of nurses should be restructured, and they specifically target the lack of support personnel and lack of computerization in nursing. Certainly computers could take over some of the routine memory functions nurses now carry, and that would allow us to spend our resources more wisely. And certainly educational programs to make nurses computer literate could be supported. But what nurses really need is not simply the skills of the light pen and the screen menu. What we need to know is how to collect and then use the data that can now be accumulated with ease with computers. We need to have nurses who are able to translate patterns of care or other information into management and clinical strategies. And even before that, we need to have nurses who can contribute to the creation of information systems, so that our own variables do not get lost in the program. We should learn from the fact that it is only very recently that we have even unbundled nursing enough to find out how very valuable that capacity is, and we should be preparing practicing nurses and nursing students to make use of information now.

The fifth recommendation from this report is the development of more effective collaborative models of physicians and nurses. Surely there are opportunities here, but it would be hoped that such collaboration does not wait until the physicians are attendings. Why not a course on nursing for medical students? Let's teach them all those technical things we end up teaching them anyhow, and let's sell CPR too. As a matter of fact, what about special educational programs for non-clinicians in schools of business or public health or management, places that train the people who will eventually sit at the same management table as nurses? We could easily expose these students to what nursing is, teaching them something useful to them as citizens, like CPR, and begin to build a network of sympathizers.

Long-term solutions to the nursing shortage will depend also on having nurses in key places in the policy and public forums, including as journalists. Would it not be possible to support nurses seeking degrees or experiences in public policy, in journalism, in business and management as well as in nursing?

I am with Virginia Henderson in thinking that the way to change the public's image of nursing is to deliver good nursing care. But it is well-nigh impossible just now, in many places. We even know what many of the solutions are and it wouldn't take much data collection or literature review to find out the rest. Many of the solutions are not appropriate targets for federal activity and ought simply to be fixed at the local level.

The nursing shortage is code for something else: an intense examination and reformation of an obese and ineffective health care system. The USA spends more per capita and as a percent of GNP than any other industrialized country in the world, for questionable return. Our infant mortality places us about 17th among the developed countries. Our life expectancy is exceeded by Japan and Portugal, among others. Our death rates from trauma are higher than Australia, which has draconian penalties for speeding, running stop lights, and driving while drinking.

The "nursing shortage" is in danger of becoming a fad, a new obsession. Obsessing about numbers conceals the real problems of the workplace, the money, and nursing's less-than-visible role in the minds of others. Nevertheless, the present crisis gives us an opportunity to discover what nursing really is and does. That visibility alone will be a recruitment device.

The nursing shortage is not our fault, and we must get over that notion first. Nursing is just fine; the working conditions are not. This shortage or any other future one will be attacked by solving the *real* problem, and releasing the talent and power of our numbers. We may actually not need more.

ENDNOTES

1. Prescott, P. (1987). Another round of nursing shortage. *Image, 19*(4), 204–209.

2. Aiken, L.H., & Mullinix, C.F. (1987). The nursing shortage: myth or reality? *New England Journal of Medicine, 317*(10), 641–646.

3. Aiken, L.H. (1983). Nursing and nursing education: public policies and private actions. *American Journal of Nursing, 83*(10), 1440–1444.

4. Thompson, J.D., & Diers, D. (1988). Management of nursing intensity. *Nursing Clinics of North America, 23*(3), 473–492. Connecticut was one of

the first states to develop statewide databases, under Prof. John Thompson's leadership. CT data have been important in policy discussions since the late 1960s.

5. Thompson, J.D. (1984). The uneasy alliance. In D. Yaggy & W. Anlayan (Eds), *Report of the Duke Conference.* Cambridge: Ballinger.

6. Diers, D. (1985). Preparation of practitioners, clinical specialists and clinicians. *Journal of Professional Nursing, 1*(1), 41–47.

7. Flood, S.D., & Diers, D. (1988). Nurse staffing, patient outcome and cost. *Nursing Management, 19*(6), 27–33. This article had not been published when I gave this speech.

8. Dumas, R.G., & Leonard, R.C. (1961). The effect of nursing on post-operative vomiting. *Nursing Research, 12*(6), 12–14.

9. Elms, R.R., & Leonard, R.C. (1966). Effects of nursing approaches during admission. *Nursing Research, 15*(1), 39–48.

10. Ford, L. (1982). Nurse practitioners: history of a new idea and predictions for the future. In L.H. Aiken (Ed), *Nursing in the '80's* (pp. 231–248). Philadelphia: Lippincott.

11. Igoe, J. (1980). Changing patterns in school health and school nursing. *Nursing Outlook, 28*(6), 486–491.

12. Thompson, J.D. (1985). Prospective payment and the role of hospital care. *Health Matrix, 3*(4), 31–36.

13. Fetter, R.B., & Freeman, J.L. (1986). Product line management within hospitals. *Academy of Management Review, 11*(1), 41–54.

14. Aydelotte, M.K. (1987). State of the profession and strategies for the future. In *Arista '87: The Nursing Shortage.* Indianapolis: Sigma Theta Tau Int'l.

15. Starr, P. (1982). *The Social Transformation of American Medicine.* New York: Basic Books.

16. Prescott, P., Dennis, K.E., Cresia, J., & Bowen, S. (1985). Nursing shortage in transition. *Image, 17*(4), 127–133.

17. Prescott, 1987, *ibid.*

18. Pear, R. (1988, January 19). New law protects rights of patients in nursing homes. *New York Times,* p. 1.

19. American Academy of Nursing (1983). Magnet Hospitals, Kansas City, KA: Author.

20. Thompson, 1984, *ibid.*

21. Diers, D. (1987). Strategies for change (transcript of conference). *American Journal of Nursing, 87*(12), 1645.

22. Stemmler, E. (1987). In *Strategies for Change* (transcript). *American Journal of Nursing, 87*(12), 1657.

23. Hogue, E. (1987). *Nursing and Legal Liability.* Owings Mills, MD: Rynd.

24. Wolff, M.A. (1984). Court upholds expanded practice roles for nurses. *Law, Medicine and Health Care, 4,* 26–29.

25. Wandelt, M.A., & Pierce, P.M. (1981). Why nurses leave nursing and what can be done about it. *American Journal of Nursing, 81*(1), 72–77.

26. Kane, R.L., Jorgensen, L.A., Teteberg, B., & Kuwahara, J. (1976). Is good nursing home care feasible? *Journal of the American Medical Association, 235*(5), 516–517.

27. McBride, A.B., Austin, J.K., Chesnut, E.E., Main, C.S., Richards, B.S., & Roy, B.A. (1987). Evaluation of the impact of the clinical nurse specialist in a state psychiatric hospital. *Archives of Psychiatric Nursing, 1*(1), 55–61.

28. Clare, F.L., Spratley, E., Schwab, P., & Iglehart, J.K. (1987). Trends in health personnel. *Health Affairs, 6*(4), 90–103; Misek, G., & Karnell, L.H. (1987). The surgical resident pipeline. *Health Affairs, 6*(4), 119–127.

29. National Health Policy Forum (1987). Briefing paper: The nurse shortage: supply and demand, pay and power. George Washington University, NHPF, Washington, DC, #469.

30. Mundinger, M.O. (1983). *Home Care Controversy—Too Little, Too Late.* Rockville, MD: Aspen.

31. Knaus, W.A., Draper, E., Wagner, D.J., & Zimmerman, J.E. (1986). An evaluation of outcomes from intensive care in major medical centers. *Annals of Internal Medicine, 104,* 410–418.

32. American Medical Association (1987). *Nursing education and the supply of nursing personnel in the United States* (Report of the Board of Trustees). Chicago: AMA.

33. Andrews, L.B. (1983). *Deregulating Doctoring.* Emmaus, PA: People's Medical Society (p 21).

34. Johnson, S. (1983). Regulatory theory and prospective risk assessment in the limitations of scope of practice. *Journal of Legal Medicine, 4*(4), 454–464.

35. Montag, M. (1983). An honest difference and a real concern. In *The Associate Degree Nurse: Technical or Professional.* New York: National League for Nursing.

36. Talerico, L., & Diers, D. (1988). Nursing intensity outliers. *Nursing Management, 19*(6), 27–33.

37. Sovie, M.D. (1985). Establishing a nursing minimum data set as part of the data requirements for DRGs. Nursing Minimum Data Set Conference. University of Wisconsin-Milwaukee School of Nursing, May 15–17; Thompson, J.D. (1985). The nursing minimum data set. *Ibid.*

38. Halloran, E. (1984). Nursing education activities of University Hospitals of Cleveland and their financial implications. Unpublished communication to Carolyne Davis, Director, Health Care Financing Administration.

WHOA!

When DRGs were going to be imported to Australia, there was the same knee-jerk response as organized nursing in the USA had. The Aussie nurses, led by Debbie Picone, now Deputy Director General of Health for New South Wales, seized the agenda. Debbie visited the USA and Yale and our friendship began then. "Then" was about 1988. She went on to the UK, which was then contemplating some form of DRG-based funding. Debbie was on a "study tour" and the report she brought back to Australia informed the nursing research agenda there—to create nursing cost weights for DRGs, something we have not done in the USA. Debbie became Ms. DRG down under.

The first time I met Debbie was at a conference held in Sydney at the Royal Randwick Race Course, a wonderful venue for a conference, sometime in the late 1980s. Not too long after, maybe a year, Prof. George Palmer of the University of New South Wales invited me to spend 3 weeks in Sydney to go around to hospitals and talk about DRGs. I learned many years later that my task had been to "put a human face on DRGs." It would have been nice if someone had told me that because my experience was being driven by a lovely young woman, Debbie's research assistant, in a tiny MiniCooper all over Sydney, to audiences whose composition I didn't know, to talk essentially all day about casemix and applications thereof, a field in which I thought of myself as a novice. It was an exhausting and exhilarating experience and I'm told it made a difference.

This piece was an editorial published in the Australian Nurses Journal (1991, 20[10], 8–9, used with permission) and the result of a meeting convened by the Australian Nurses Federation (ANF) on Debbie's suggestion. She and I flew to Melbourne together for this. It was a session with the nursing leadership of ANF, which, like all nursing organizations in Australia, has no USA equivalent.

This little editorial cut right to the crux of the dilemma Australian nursing found itself in.

Some idiot American healthcare consultant (well, I do know her name and she built a whole reputation on this stupidity) advised the government that if they were going to adopt DRGs for payment then they would have to adopt a management model that had physicians as budget holders. The Johns Hopkins Hospital (which is singular in the US context—there is no other US hospital organized the way Hopkins is) was held to be the shining example of a "matrix" management structure with "product lines." What the consultant didn't tell government was that the Hopkins model spectacularly failed, especially as concerns nursing, and that the Hopkins nurses eventually created quite an interesting contractual model of their own. The nurses organized (not in a collective bargaining sense) as small firms who proposed staffing standards and quality standards to the physician budget holders. In effect, they said, "This is what we promise to deliver for N dollars. If we deliver under what we have proposed as budget, we get to keep the difference. If we go over budget, you have every right to contract with someone else." (An empty promise—who else was there?—but a great bargaining strategy.) Well, they delivered under budget for the first 3 years in the test product line, but did they get to keep the money? Not hardly.[1]

I think my work in Australia helped nurses in New South Wales develop a way to participate in policy, through Debbie's research and our advocacy. My contemporary work there builds on this, to try to make real what this editorial proposes: DRGs as information system for clinical management.

The Aussies pronounce it Whoa-ah—two syllables.

Robyn Parkes (Executive Director of ANF at the time) asked me to write something about the lessons Australian nursing might learn from the United States about DRG-based casemix stuff. Sorry to tell you: there aren't any! See, the problem here in the United States, and perhaps in Australia as well, is that casemix *management* has been confused with casemix *funding*. And hardly anybody is paying any attention here—and perhaps there—to casemix *management*, which is where the action is.

DRGs were originally invented for quality control, a piece of contemporary history that is lost in the politics of funding. The notion was that it is not possible to detect differences in outcomes unless one can have a definition of more-or-less homogeneous cases. Apples and oranges, or kiwis and bananas, or whatever your metaphor, are not comparable entities. One can compare one apple to another apple—or cases in one DRG to others in the same grouping—but without this kind of case definition, to extend the food analogy, it all converts to mush.

That aside, DRGs were also invented to provide a data system. No more, no less! That they were adopted by the US government as a basis for prospective payment under our Medicare is an accident. They were quite simply there at the time. That DRGs were attached to funding here, and are soon to be in Australia, messes up people's heads.

DRGs do not prescribe a management structure. What they ought to prescribe, but haven't been used for, is a management *information* structure. That information should be as useful to nurses as to physicians and administrators. But the issue of who ought to be In Charge is a political one quite apart from DRGs.

I am given to understand that some sort of "Johns Hopkins" management structure is thought to be advocated in Australia. That model puts physician specialists as budget holders of services (medicine, neuroscience, surgery etc.) But note that Johns Hopkins is and has always been a very physician-dominated place. And the physicians are *fulltime* (in appointment, if not in time commitment), not VMOs (Visiting Medical Officers, like community physicians in the United States). Hopkins is not a matrix management structure; the illusion of physician managers is just that. In fact, the administrators are in charge. And in further fact, the nurses at Hopkins have organized their own quasi-contractual arrangements to control nursing practice themselves and sell it as a package to the service chiefs.

Nobody, certainly not in the United States, is using the DRG-based information systems to advantage. Everybody is trying to best them, contravert or play the system. But ours is a private health care system and government has limited power to fix it. So Australia shouldn't turn to the United States for instruction in how to deal with a DRG-based budget system.

The academic notion of a "matrix management" system, which is what Hopkins is supposed to be and isn't, had a good deal of appeal. In such a system, the clinicians—nurses and physicians—would use the DRG-based information to make decisions about resource allocation, quality of care, standards of practice, and so on. The administrative types would be in charge of seeing to it that the resources, including negotiated support services, would be provided to those nurses and physicians who determine how the resources are used. NOBODY is doing that here.

Management in a DRG context can be implemented in any old kind of structure, provided there is the information available and the will to use it in the service of making the resources do what they're supposed to do—provide an acceptable (efficient and effective) quality of care. We nurses are increasingly the policepersons of the system. DRG-based information gives us a tool. In my own beloved country, hardly anybody is really using the information. Nobody seems to want to *manage*. Everybody seems to want to protect turf.

The reason for the existence of the modern hospital is to deliver nursing care. Medical procedures not requiring heavy support from nursing can be performed outside the hospital. Management of the modern hospital must focus on management of care delivery.

In *Return to Snowy River,* the first really Australian film I know, there is this wonderful scene of the hero riding a horse off a cliff, photographed so beautifully and graphically it makes one gasp. The horse dies, the hero lives.

One wants to scream "Whoa!" as the horse goes out of control. So: "Whoa!" Please, friends, don't do it the way we did.

ENDNOTE

1. Heyssel, R.M., Gaintner, J.R., Kues, I.W., Jones, A.A., & Lipstein, S.H. (1984). Decentralized management in a teaching hospital. *New England Journal of Medicine, 310*(10), 1477–1480; Johns Hopkins nurses earn salaries and pursue autonomy in new "professional practice" units. (1987). *American Journal of Nursing, 87*(4), 713–714, 730, 734.

BETWEEN PRACTICE AND POLICY

The Forum for Contemporary Thought at the University of Virginia is a university-wide event in which schools of the university invite whomever they wish to give a public presentation and to perhaps participate in other events. Anticipating an interdisciplinary audience, I wrote this trying to use nursing to speak to more general issues of practice and University life (delivered November 1, 2001). This was going to be a Very Big Deal—the honorarium was more than generous and they had arranged special accommodations in a building designed by Thomas Jefferson. (Every speech at U.Va. must include some reference to Jefferson). The audience turnout was somewhat disappointing and not nearly as interdisciplinary as I had thought, but that is often a fact of life when the speaker is a nurse. People simply do not have a clue that nurses might know something worth hearing. Oh, well.

I am singularly honored to be with you today in this formidable place. To stay in a building designed by Thomas Jefferson ought in itself to inspire one to loftier ideas and more clever expression. ...

It is surely a surprise to have been invited to speak at a Forum for Contemporary Thought. Such platforms are usually reserved for people who belong to tweedy secret inner circles, people who read and understand *The Economist*, people who are asked to peer into the future and help us get there unscathed, people who live important lives at the center of important intellectual and social issues.

I am a nurse, to the core of my being. Surely a socially useful occupation and surely we have seen interesting times and been part of complex social issues. Today I want to use the point of view that the experience of operational health care provides.

A Forum for Contemporary Thought will already have discovered that some of contemporary thought is revisionist history. And much of predicting the future is just lucky guesswork. Ted Marmor, a distinguished professor of political science and management at Yale, not usually given to confessing he was wrong, has produced a most interesting backward look at predictions he and Paul Starr, another distinguished professor, made about how the American health care system would look.[1] Their initial predictions were made in the early 1980s, looking forward to 1995. As political scientists, their gazes were informed by the crystal ball of both economics and politics.

Marmor acknowledges that their earlier prediction of an increasing role of market forces in shaping American healthcare was mild compared to what really happened. But the vision of huge, vertically intergrated managed care firms never transpired. Indeed, the Columbia HCA/Humanas of the world fell on their economic and legal swords.

The effect of market power to constrain physician practices and incomes, even in the face of increased physician personpower, was their most on-target shot. Their optimistic guess that the increasing number of women physicians would change professional practice did not, they acknowledge, take account of how much occupational socialization would affect women physicians rather than the other way around.

I happened to read this article and hear Ted discuss it as I was pulling together the initial thoughts for this presentation. I was instructed. Mostly I was instructed not to try to extrapolate from today what a dimly seen future might look like. Rather, what I would like to do is to give a few contemporary observations in health care. "Diffident observations" these might be called, stealing that charming term from a critic's review of Paul Simon's lyrics. I've chosen to call these collectively "between practice and policy."

Some definitions are in order.

By "practice" I mean the activities that connect the individual and collective intellect to the world as performance. Teaching is performance. So is brain surgery, litigation, the ministry, management, and nursing. Nursing is two things: the care of the sick (or the potentially sick) and the tending of the entire environment within which care happens. Practice is the art and science of direct patient care and creating environments for care. It is also managing those environments and patient populations for the best possible outcomes in patient state and colleague fulfillment. Practice requires not only what we describe as clinical expertise and specialized knowledge, but also locating that practice in its relevant contexts in organizational design, authority, interprofessional collaboration, regulation, law, and, of course, policy.

By "policy" I mean to include public policy—the acts of government or governmental agencies, and what I am calling for lack of a better label, private policy—the acts of *non-elected* entities including educational and clinical institutions and foundations and even the media. Included in the category of "policy" will be regulation, administrative law, organizational decision-making, and related operational definitions. When I talk about policy today, I mean that to specifically include the notion of *values*.

What is "between" practice and policy is a black box or to thoroughly mix a metaphor, an arroyo, a canyon, a chasm. I do not mean to suggest that there is an opposition of policy to practice, which the word "between" might suggest. Rather, to extend the metaphor, there is a black hole and my theme today is what can fill that hole: data, information, knowledge. I will cast a large net around those concepts, however, for we know now in this postmodern era (whatever that is) that there are lots of ways of knowing.

Today I want to tell some stories, only seven; we won't be here all night. Story-telling, or narrative, is now gaining credibility in venues from the *Journal of the American Medical Association*[2] to *Health Affairs*[3] as "anecdote matters." It is now being argued that a layer of narrative on top of hard science makes both practice and research better and more accessible. So here are the stories.

SCIENCE TO SERVICE

Yale University just completed the celebration of our 300th year. There were many wonderful stimulating events, inviting our community in and showing off with great color and humor. At a formal convocation in which the Presidents of Harvard and Princeton made self-deprecating jokes about the historic relationships among them (Yale's first founders were Harvard men; Princeton's were Yale men), Rick Levin, the President of Yale University made an observation that resonated.

He proposed that the new wave of University investment in science would (or perhaps he meant should) embrace not only the challenge of doing good science, but of translating (his word) the science to service. Not only finding out how things tick (my words) but how to *make* them tick, in different metaphorical time zones and with different clocks.

President Levin has made remarkable commitments to the community in which Yale lives, to the point at which our mayor, running for re-election next week, is pressed to explain his pro-university rhetoric. The old town-gown split has been seriously eroded, to the betterment of both the city and the University. For example, Yale has provided special funds to employees who will buy housing in designated areas around the University and this has attracted over 300 families back to New Haven.

But the science to service connection means more than that. It also means investing in start-up companies that can make the translation from the science to the market. It means putting increasing attention through publicity and targeted faculty recruitment toward research and science which is at the much maligned "cutting edge" of both policy and practice. Sometimes that has meant defending politically unpopular work such as demonstrations that needle exchange programs reduce the spread of the HIV virus. Sometimes, especially recently, that has meant developing showcases for intellectual work that has immediate relevance, such as near-East studies, and studies of terrorism.

I do not mean to suggest that universities give up their right to have their ivory towers of singular contemplative scholarship protected. Rather, I think in many fields we are coming to understand the necessity to develop a new brand of science—the science of application. That is different from the old pejorative "applied science" thought not to have a rightful place in a University. That appellation once served as an excuse for Universities to question whether nursing had a place within their walls.

Contemporary practice professions including politics, according to John McDonaugh's new work,[4] place themselves directly across the divide between science and service, or more generally between theory and practice. If breaching that gap is becoming intellectually credible, I believe we will see an interesting change in how Universities develop their role in the larger society. Especially old private Universities used to sitting on their tax exempt laurels.

The paternalism that used to characterize Universities' outreach might change to (you should forgive me) maternalism. That is, welcoming the outside world in rather than imposing the University's notions on a public assumed to be needy and wanting. I am quite old enough to remember, with nostalgia, the radicalizing events of the 1960s including what became known collectively as the Black Panther Trials in New Haven. One event that has become an unforgettable part of local lore and of national history was when Kingman Brewster, then President of Yale University, on the advice of a senior in Yale College, Kurt Schmoke (later to be a Rhodes scholar, mayor of Baltimore and now Senior Fellow of the Yale Corporation, its governing body) decided that rather than close the University and lock the iron gates to the potential of violent protests that were predicted, he would open up the closed courtyards, and turn loose the University Dining Hall staff to serve beans and rice, salad and Kool-aid to all comers. I was there. The food was quite good, the mood changed from confrontation and anger to dialogue, debate, and a shared sense of being present at a historical moment. The shootings at Kent State, which had happened just days before, were not repeated. The National Guard did not appear on the Yale campus (although they were only a couple of blocks away, right under my apartment window).

When Universities open themselves up, when we welcome challenge and when we do not hide from the world, we begin to make accessible our products of scholarship, science, research, and service. And, creaking and groaning, the world begins to change.

TEST SMALL, MAKE BIG NOISE

The United States is a huge laboratory for testing public policy ideas and, for that matter, for testing health care innovations. We try it somewhere and if it works, it moves into some public agenda. That's what we did with the Prospective Payment System that now funds hospitals—it was tested first in New Jersey—and that's what is going on now with public policy initiatives in nursing workforce matters. But that's another story.

This story is about a little known but potentially incredibly powerful attempt to bring better care and case management to people with insulin dependent diabetes. This one grew up in an unusual test tube—the network of clinics that serve the underserved, the poor, as Community Health Centers, chartered by the federal government.

There is enough science out there now to suggest that there could be standard, aggressive "disease management" for persons with diabetes that, if carried out, could have huge health effects as well as being cost effective through prevention of exacerbations. Diabetes is ubiquitous, especially in the poor, and the prevalence is growing, especially in children. The science now hints at both genetic and autoimmune explanations, which have quite different implications for disease management from simply calling diabetes a chronic illness.

Under a mandate to reduce health disparities, the Bureau of Primary Care invited agencies to apply to be part of a special targeted program which would provide some computer software for data collection and expert disease management guidelines for practice. My friends who work in these agencies believed that this was a new approach to managing diabetes that gave them hope.

The feds enlisted a number of community health centers who all agreed to submit their data to a central depository so that an aggregate sample could be developed. (Most of these community health centers are quite small.) The centers agreed to implement the practice guidelines, and to collect the data. The data collection requirements were made as user-friendly as possible—another innovation in federal programming.

To cut to the chase: the disease management protocol *really* worked. People who had been unable to manage their regimen became able to do so. Some agencies created weight loss programs, cooking lessons, shopping lessons, and a number of other behavior-change initiatives. There was very careful attention to use of different types of insulin for different patients and standard measurement of hemoglobin A1c. Patients got better; clinicians felt proud.

Ah, but then the fault line appeared. Patients who had profited from this scheme occasionally had to be hospitalized for things other than their diabetes. And, oddly enough, the community care was more advanced than the hospital care, even in major medical centers. The community-based clinicians came to realize that when their patients came home from the hospital, their diabetes was again out of control and they had to start over with diabetes management.

Where's the fault in the fault line? First, community care, especially for the poor and underserved, is not in the medical mainstream. It might actually be better than conventional medical center practice but innovations, even federally sponsored ones dedicated to community health centers, do not penetrate the Pill Hills of the world. Second, in the community setting, the diabetes is the center of attention. In the hospital, it's a complication or what we fondly call a "co-morbidity," largely an annoyance on the way to treating the broken hip or the clogged artery. Finally, there is often little coordination of care from the outpatient setting, whether it's a community health center or someplace else, with the inpatient setting.

That last fact has produced a whole new cadre of health care professionals called case managers or care managers and most of them are nurses. Most of their work to date has been helping to decrease length of stay in the hospital by starting earlier discharge planning and assisting in finding places for patients to go after hospitalization if they need more care. Now, it is apparent that at least for some populations, there will need to be created bridges on the front end—from community to hospital. And that is beginning to happen as community health center nurses and hospital based diabetes nurse-educators realize they share the same agenda. And they begin to build the bridge.

DISCIPLINES BETWEEN

"Interdisciplinary" education or activity used to mean getting the geographers and historians together, or the biologists and psychologists, or the doctors and nurses and social workers. Now the rich mix of disciplines produces a whole new stew of understanding.

This story is on me.

I do quite a lot of work in Australia, teaching and consulting about information and operational management and what is called out there, "casemix." Casemix is the application of the Diagnosis Related Groups or DRGs developed in the United States for hospital payment under Medicare, now part of our Prospective Payment System. I worked with the guys who "found" (in their term) DRGs at Yale, and I've extended their work to operations management, quality management, and continuous process improvement.

I started going to Australia in 1986 and spent 8 months there in 2000 (but had to leave before the Olympics started in Sydney. Drat the US academic calendar that starts in September).

In spite of the fact that Australians speak English, or some version of that, the enormous differences between Australia and the United States stunned me. The countries are about the same size; they even share some of the same history, especially in the relationship to England. Both countries have a kind of "pioneer" mentality, conquering new land, finding new opportunities.

It wasn't until I understood something about Australia's ecology that I finally felt as if I had a grip on how and why things happen as they do there, including why the science and service operate as they do.

Tim Flannery's book, *The Future Eaters*,[5] recommended to me by an Australian friend, defined it.

Australia is very old land, probably broken off from what is now Antarctica. It was originally essentially a giant atoll—a ring of land surrounding a huge inland sea. The sea is long ago gone. Now when one speaks of dimensions of Australian land, one needs to put that into perspective. To fly from Sydney to Alice Springs, which is nearly exactly in the center of the continent, takes 3 hours and more and after the first hour, there is no sign of civilization down below. No roads, few bodies of water, the land gets more and more red as one approaches what they call the Red Centre. It would be as if one flew from Washington DC to, let's say, Omaha and then there was nothing until about Santa Barbara, California. Australia redefines the word "vast."

It wasn't obvious to me until I had traveled enough in Australia how important the ecology is to understanding other things. This is a nearly dead continent, ecologically, and various governments have realized that. It is also very far away from anything else and for a long time there was a social protectionist policy that controlled immigration in the service of keeping the population pure. Now, immigration policy is much informed by ecology; there is not a lot of arable land to support a huge population. Australia presently has only about 18 million people, scattered about this vast continent.

Huge hydroelectric systems were built to channel water from rainfall to produce energy. European labor, especially Greek and Italian workers after World War II, came to build the hydro system. The largest Greek population after Athens is now in Australia. Several governments ago, it was realized that if Australia were to enter the global society and economy, producing science and other products, its population base was just too small, so immigration policy was loosened.

I don't think it's a stretch to observe, diffidently, that Australia's decisions to not implement the kind of high tech US-style high risk pregnancy programs might be related to a perception of scarce resources that need to be carefully spent, just as their land needs to be carefully monitored. There is not the rescue of very low birth weight infants there that there is here. Kidney transplants and dialysis are not available as widely as they are here. High-tech care is regionalized. There is considerably more control of physician prescribing by formulary than there is here. The ratio of patients to nurses is generally much higher than it is in the United States, and my observation is that a national characteristic of Australians is that they work *really hard* and play equally hard.

There is a deliberate undersupply of hospital beds in public hospitals, which are the majority of hospitals in the Australia "Medicare" scheme. That means there are sometimes very long waiting lists for elective surgical procedures. Just for the fun of it, I got on the New South Wales Health Department website to find out how long it would be if I needed a hip replacement. Nine months, the answer came back, for a particular physician in a particular hospital.

An odd and interesting spin-off in Australian science is that the population base is too small to support intricate research reviews of the NIH variety in the wide range of specialties and specialty research interests that can now be sustained through Internet capacity, if not on the ground. This has meant, in a personal instance, that a research proposal some Aussie colleagues and I put together could not be reviewed appropriately at the federal level because there were no "peers" to review it. Realizing that, the Aussie equivalent of NIH is now calling for international reviewers when they need to. What effect that will have on the science is yet to be determined.

It would be too bad if international standards of research review diluted some of the innovations in Aussie science. For example, their work in bone marrow transplant and sudden infant death syndrome was very far ahead of work anywhere else in the world. The Aussies are way ahead of the rest of the world in medical record coding specificity, and that coding lies under any integrated clinical/financial information system.

The subtleties of internationalization are not only in trying to understand why the radical Islamic hatred of the United States goes back to the Crusades. If we are to cooperate in building science and service that transcends national lines, we will need to understand more than political science and history. Ecology, we are coming to understand, has a more powerful role on how human behavior evolves than usually recognized. When I think about Australia's ecology and how it has played out in that country's development, the comparison to the United States and our own ecology is patent. Our piece of the planet is excessively well endowed and to those living in deserts and dying continents, our inclusiveness in immigration, our uncontrolled development, seem profligate. Our national exuberance is in part a product of our environment.

REVISING VIEWS OF SILENCE

This story is also about trying to achieve full understanding of complicated things.

Many in this audience will know the story of the Tuskegee study of the natural history of syphilis. It is usually discussed in the context of "informed consent" for the protection of the rights of human subjects in research.

The study was funded and largely conducted by the US Public Health Service, with the Tuskegee Institute as the study site. It enrolled black men with syphilis and assigned them to the then-available treatment or not, then followed them until they died or were lost to follow-up. As an inducement to participate, the men were offered access to Nurse Eunice Rivers' public health nursing services. She was responsible for seeing to it that the men got their blood tests and other measurements. In most of the reports of the Tuskegee study, Nurse Rivers is portrayed either as complicit in selling these men down the river, or as a well-meaning but silent and powerless nurse-tool of the investigators.

Susan Reverby, a historian at Wellesley College and a great friend of nursing, has spent several years trying to unravel the story of Nurse Rivers and the Tuskegee experiment.[6] Using rich historical resources including interviews with people who knew Nurse Rivers, Prof. Reverby concludes that the story is much more complicated. Nurse Rivers apparently assisted some men to get treatment either locally or when they moved out of the South. And she "treated" them with food and vitamins. As Reverby writes, "For Eunice

Rivers, the men were patients, not subjects".[7] She did not see herself as a mindless research assistant. Indeed, she believed that the 1930s treatments were worse than the disease if the disease was not early syphilis or if syphilis was not active.

Reverby's analysis fleshes out the study in its context and Nurse Rivers' context in particular:

> The racism and sexism that provided the underpinnings for medical scientific arrogance has many differing faces, making possible many different routes for resistance, and sometimes escape, for subjects and nurses. [Her story] alerts us to the costs of expecting silence from a nurse and the dangers of an ethic of caring and beneficence when there is neither racial, gender nor class justice.[8]

There is the silence, perhaps, of nursing, but there is the also the silence of public policy and media coverage that is just as pernicious. Bernice Buresh and Suzanne Gordon have produced a very important book, published by the Canadian Nurses Association, which means it is a little hard to come by.[9] The book is *From Silence to Voice* and it is intended to help nurses get "out there" in the public media.

In a section on "being silent", they cite a *New York Times* piece on the refusal of managed care and insurance companies to pay hospitals for patient days during which no surgery, diagnostic tests, or other medical procedures occurred. This should strike you as profoundly silly if for no other reason than it creates incentives to over-test and prescribe. The Greater New York Hospital Association was contesting this practice. Buresh and Gordon point out that nursing was never mentioned. If the hospital association recognized that patients are in hospitals because they need nursing care, whether or not they have procedure and that insurers must pay for necessary nursing care, there was no evidence of it in the story. Instead, the distorted view of the insurers prevailed: patients should just go home if they don't have a codable procedure.

There is silence, and there is silence and we don't own it all.

BEYOND SILENCE

During the dedication of the Vietnam Women's Memorial in Washington DC, General Colin Powell confessed that until he had been asked to part of this event, he had not studied how many women had served in Vietnam or elsewhere. He made a touching speech about how instructed he was to know about the work that (mostly female) nurses had done in Vietnam.

I have a colleague at Yale, Linda Schwartz, who is one of the best politicians I have ever known. Linda is a retired Air Force nurse, retired because on a training mission over Pennsylvania, the cargo door blew off her plane and nearly sucked her and her colleagues out. They survived with quick thinking of the pilot who brought the plane down, but so fast that Linda suffered some neurological damage that you wouldn't know about unless she told you. After that event, she was elected President of the Connecticut Nurses Association, served on the ANA Board and got a doctorate in epidemiology and public health.

Linda studies the health effects of military service in Vietnam, and especially the effects of dioxin—Agent Orange—on women in the military. Most of the women in the military in Vietnam were nurses. Linda's study showed that the incidence of autoimmune disorders, certain cancers, and other diseases were higher in a cohort of military women who served in Vietnam than in a matched cohort of military and civilian women from the same period of time who were never in Vietnam. Part of her study got her into the military archives where she found map coordinates to the sites where Agent Orange had been sprayed. She also tracked down information that showed that our military dumped Agent Orange on our own bases when they needed to get rid of the weight of the chemicals to land the planes. Before Linda's research and political work, women veterans, especially nurses, were not thought eligible for combat-related military benefits because they had not been out in the field. Linda's work showed that the field had come to them. That was what General Powell recognized in his remarks.

In the fullness of time, Linda was invited to go with a group of other veterans to Vietnam and she took with her the maps of dioxin sprayed areas and gave them to the Vietnamese, who are, of course, still living with this poison in their blood and in the soil. This gesture of generosity has paved the way for the new Ambassador to Vietnam, himself a former prisoner of war there, to begin to build connections between the two countries.

Being between policy and practice doesn't just mean doing realistic research on real problems, or applying the findings of research to the solution of public or private policy issues. It means conceiving from the beginning the relationship and working to knit them together.

BACKWARD AND FORWARD GLANCING

I said in the beginning that I was not going to try to predict the future. I lied. It's just too tempting.

Pam Cipriano, your Chief Clinical Officer, contacted me helpfully a couple of weeks ago to suggest I might want to build upon an article of mine she remembered from the mid-80s. I called it, "To Profess, to be a Professional" and I hadn't read it in many years. In that article, published in 1984,[10] I had actually done a prediction:

> Things are about to change for us, not so much in the work... but in the responsibility and authority of it. Without even asking, the health care system is being forced to confront nursing as central, powerful, and reimbursable. ... For

> far too long, nursing [in hospitals] has been buried in the
> hospital bill along with brooms, breakfast and the building
> mortgage. It has not been in the interest of institutions to
> treat nursing as a revenue center and so nursing has been
> economically invisible. ...[11]

At this time, I thought the solution to nursing's invisibility would be to change the way in which nursing services were accounted for (in an accounting sense), using the financial system to fix our problems. I wrote this stuff just as the Prospective Payment System under Medicare was being implemented, and I wrote it just as I left the deanery at Yale to work with the people who invented DRGs, the basis for PPS. Through that work and extensions of it later, I have come to a new understanding of how to "find" nursing and make nursing's contributions visible, at least in inpatient settings. The principles would work in outpatient settings as well, but my personal experience is not there.

Remember: the reason for the existence of the modern hospital is to provide nursing care. If one believes that, then the administrative clinical and financial data systems are available for us to tap. Where I was wrong in the earlier prediction was in thinking that the issue was tracking nursing to patients as individual practice and outcome. That can't be done yet. But maybe that's not so much the point as tracking nursing practice to patient outcomes by nursing unit or service.

Over the last several years, I have had the luxury of working with a talented group of clinical, operational, financial, and technical experts to help create what we call at Yale-New Haven Hospital, RIMS—the Resource Information Management System. Through RIMS we are able to associate nursing to population groups defined by ICD codes and DRGs, and to resources, defined by fee codes and other financial data elements. The secret to this work has been the assumption that because the reason for the existence of the modern hospital *is* to provide nursing care, therefore the outcomes of hospitalization can be attributed to nursing.

One example: length of stay is a powerful variable for health care payors including Medicare. It had been thought that length of stay was entirely the responsibility of physicians, who make discharge decisions. But when we have investigated the effect of nursing innovations on length of stay, it is very clear that while physicians may get patients into hospitals, nurses get them out.

We designed a study to see whether length of stay and mortality were different if patients were on "specialized" nursing units or were "off service" on some other unit.[12] We chose 14 DRGs where there could be an expectation of being cared for on a nursing specialized unit in our hospital. We found that in nine of the DRGs, the hypothesis was statistically supported: patients cared for on specialized units had shorter lengths of stay. In the three where the outcome was in the direction opposite what we hypothesized, we found intriguing clues. One of the DRGs in which patients cared for on *non-specialty* units had a shorter length of stay was DRG 14, stroke. The mortality of patients on non-specialty units was three times higher than patients on their home unit. Patients who die have a shorter length of stay.

We continued this line of inquiry to look at a nursing unit where we could conduct a natural experiment. This unit was a 42-bed orthopaedic/peripheral vascular unit which was destined for architectural renovation as part of a larger hospital project. The PV patients were reassigned to another unit, and the ortho unit became a 27-bed unit. For quite other reasons, we had been tracking the relationship between nursing resources as caregiver hours, patient census, and a DRG-based expert measurement of nursing acuity. The unit at 42 beds had been unmanageable and the nurse manager was thought to be the worst nurse manager in the house. Our data made that clear: the distance between hours of care required by an acuity measurement and hours available as staffing, controlling for DRGs, and census could not be managed. When the unit was changed to concentrate on orthopaedic patients again, with a decreased bed complement, the relationship of nursing hours to patient requirements fell into line. Overtime decreased from 230% over to 30% under budget; patient satisfaction went up 12 points and length of stay decreased twice the amount of the secular trend. The nurse manager became the best nurse manager in the house. We reasoned that when nurses can concentrate on the care of relatively similar patients, they can get good at the work.[13]

We did a similar analysis at the request of the nurse manager of our combined surgical/neurosurgical ICU. She reported that her nurses were telling her "the work is so much harder this year." We took patients who had been on her unit over about an 18-month period and looked at their diagnoses and DRGs, their ventilator use, and a number of other variables she suggested. We could find no particular pattern in patient variables, although length of stay in the ICU did go up over the period.

When we showed her the data, tentatively, because we thought we had not helped her, she understood it instantly. The issue was that these two ICU's had merged staff. The NICU nurses were used to caring for a relatively restricted case mix and when they had to be able to care for the wider variety of patients in the SICU, that's where the complaints were coming from. The solution was not to throw more money and staff at the unit because the work was harder, but rather to understand *how* the work was harder, where, and with whom.[14]

That's what operational management and data mining is all about: understanding the work. The finances are easy; money is just a way of keeping score.

WIDGETS

This is the last story and maybe the most important.

We are about to fall into perhaps the biggest nursing shortage in a long history of nursing shortages. This one will be profoundly different. And if we play it right, we can take the clinical and moral high ground to establish nursing as an essential service and a desirable career choice.

The last big nursing shortage, in 1988, established wholly new understanding of this cyclical phenomenon. Until that point, nursing shortages had been thought to be tied entirely to economic cycles. When the economy was flush, there were shortages because nurses did not have to supplement their spouse's incomes by working. When times were difficult, nurses re-entered the nursing work force. This simple-minded economic perversity was countered by Linda Aiken and Connie Mullinix's definitive paper which, while it used economic trend analysis, reached a different conclusion.[15] They argued that where the workforce is essentially captive to the interests of what they called an "oligopsony" a few very large employers (in this case, hospitals) the employers can conspire, consciously or not, to constrain wages, which will then determine the interest of nurses in employment and their willingness to stay employed.

At the same time, in testimony before the Secretary's Commission on Nursing, John D. Thompson, one of the inventors of DRGs, presented his own data. The data showed that the major intended effect of the DRG-based Prospective Payment System had indeed happened: length of stay in hospitals dropped like a stone. But when he looked at DRG dyads—DRGs that contain the same case types, but split on the presence of a co-morbidity or complication—he found that the ratio of complicated to uncomplicated cases had changed. Furthermore, the case mix index—a number calculated by HCFA to represent the relative case "burden" of a hospital's patients—had risen since PPS had been implemented.

Before PPS there had been the naïve notion that if the easy work-up days and leisurely recover days were eliminated from hospital stays, we would need fewer nurses. In fact, we needed more nurses because now *all* of the days in hospitals were "sick" days. During the same period, the number of ICU beds increased by 300% and ICU's simply gobble up nurses.

The combination of Aiken's work and Thompson's testimony and related findings during the period began to convert nurses from interchangeable widgets to real factors in making hospitalization work, preventing complications, lowering lengths of stay; in other words, the work that nursing has always done, but invisibly.

Aiken has continued that work, of course, and her newest international studies are again opening new understanding of the working life of nurses.[16] Her studies consistently find that what nurses value is respect and authority for practice. In general, the working relationships with physician colleagues and salary are not the most troublesome areas. Nurses report feeling less than valued by *hospital* administration who still tend to think of nurses as widgets.

Last year, I supervised a public health management student, Dea Mannos, who wished to do her thesis on feminist views of the nursing shortage. She is not a nurse (though her mother is) but she is a feminist and a bright, assertive little penny. She interviewed avowed feminists on our campus, most of them members of the Women's Studies program, asking gentle but penetrating questions about the extent to which they could either find feminist explanations for the nursing shortage or feminist initiatives to help nursing out.

To Dea's horror and distress, these feminists had not really thought about nursing much at all. After all, it's a women's profession...not worth noticing. And surely it had not occurred to the respondents that nursing might embody interesting feminist issues, or that feminism might actually be interested in how nursing has dealt with issues of equity or even qualitative scholarship so dear to the heart of modern feminists. Try as she did, Dea could not find in her interview data the tiniest spark of connection between her feminist respondents and nursing. Which made her, and me, profoundly sad.

Here, nurses are not even widgets. We are invisible to a rising body of scholarship and advocacy. The silence of the feminist community about nursing is terribly troubling because it would seem only to reinforce what oppressed group theory identifies as "silencing" as survival technique.[17] If feminism feels it must silence nursing it will not have access to the phenomenal successes of the discipline and the ways in which its future is being created as I speak.

Much of what we used to fondly call "primary care" has already dropped into nursing's hands in peaceful interdisciplinary practice where the old tired worries about whether nurses were maxi-nurses or mini-MDs have just faded away. All—*all*—of the extant literature supports the effect of advanced practice nurses on patient outcomes, patient satisfaction, safety, and effectiveness. That was my prediction in 1980. In 2001, I truly believe that the invisiblity of nurses in hospitals is also about to change as we find ways to reveal nursing's service in administrative data and in narrative reporting. And as we come to realize that the newer challenges for making the health care delivery system work—monitoring payment denials, improving patient safety, initiating clinical process improvement, smoothing bed flow—all require nursing's insights, direction, participation in interdisciplinary practice, and ultimately, leadership.

I am encouraged to see nurses and nursing begin to receive the credit for this central role. Linda Aiken has been careful to put her work in the general health services research literature where it has been respectfully received. The work I have been doing in the last 12 years or so here and in Australia has increasingly been to help nursing develop a language, a set of metaphors, a way of defining issues that make sense to the interdisciplinary world in which we live and work. We are not served well when we depend on our internal private languaging excesses in public discourse. We make much more progress when we can associate our interests with existing agendas; that is the first step in participating in the policy process—getting on the agenda.

And that's the first step across the bridge between practice and policy. The rest of the march is easy.

ENDNOTES

1. Marmor, T. (1998). Forecasting American health care: How we got here and where we might be going. *Jouranl of Health Politics, Policy and Law. 23*(3), 551–571.

2. Charon, R. (2001). Narrative medicine: A model for empathy, reflection, profession, and trust. *Journal of the American Medical Association. 286*(15), 1897–1902.

3. McDonaugh, J.E. (2000). Using and misusing anecdote in policy making. *Health Affairs 20*(1), 207–212.

4. McDonaugh, J.E. (2000). *Experiencing Politics: A legislator's stories of government and health care.* Berkeley: University of California Press.

5. Paperback edition, Grove Press, 2002.

6. Reverby, S. (1999). Rethinking the Tuskegee syphilis study: Nurse Rivers, silence and the meaning of treatment. *Nursing History Review,* 7, 3–28.

7. *Ibid.,* p. 11.

8. *Ibid.,* p. 20.

9. Buresh, B., & Gordon, S. (2000). *From Silence to Voice.* Ottawa: Canadian Nurses Association.

10. Diers, D. (1984). To profess—to be a Professional. *Journal of the New York State Nurses Association 15*(4), 21–29. See the beginning of this section.

11. *Ibid.,* p. 28.

12. Czaplinski, C., & Diers, D. (1998). The effect of staff nurse specialization on length of stay and mortality. *Medical Care, 36*(12), 1626–1638.

13. Diers, D., & Potter, J. (1997). Understanding the unmanageable nursing unit with casemix data. *Journal of Nursing Administration, 27*(11), 27–32.

14. Diers, D., Bozzo, J., Blatt, L., & Roussel, M. (1998). Understanding nursing resources in intensive care: A case study. *American Journal of Critical Care, 7*(2), 143–148.

15. Aiken, L.H., & Mullinix, C.F. (1987). The nurse shortage: Myth or reality? *New England Journal of Medicine, 317*(10), 641–646.

16. Aiken, L.H., Clarke, S.P., Sloane, D.M., Sochalski, J.A., Hunt, J., Rafferty, A.M., & Shamian, J. (2001). Nurses' reports on hospital care in 5 countries. *Health Affairs, 20*(3), 43–53.

17. Reverby, 1999, *ibid.,* pp. 3–28.

SECOND THOUGHTS

I believe one of the functions—the duties—of leadership, is to say out loud the most obstreperous ideals and values of the discipline. One of the privileges of leadership when one is an academic is access to platforms from which to speak; another is a certain protection from negative sanctions, such as getting fired. That probably overly optimistic analysis comes from more than 40 years of experience in a liberal, private University that will surely terminate a tenured Professor for using University facilities to download child pornography and perform child sexual abuse, but it will tolerate outrageous public and private opinions as part of a commitment to diversity of thinking.

Speaking obstreperously probably suited my personality, although I think of myself as actually quite quiet, timid, and chicken. But with the responsibility to use a leadership position or role in the service of advancing others, I morph into a *Tyrannosaurus Rex*.

The papers here, especially the early ones, do not read as obstreperously as they did when they were delivered. Times change; we do actually make progress and issues that seemed mission critical in the 80's such as nurse practitioner/MD relationships, pass into nostalgia.

The danger in crafting a leadership role based on being out there on the edge is that one learns to love the challenge and eventually may find confrontation where there isn't any. I've seen that happen with some of my nursing colleagues who came to professional maturity before I did, and it made them unpopular, snickered at behind their backs. It is hard, though, to step back and let others keep the issues moving, in a different time, with a different style.

A public leadership role is different from a leadership/management role such as a Vice President for Nursing or a Dean because public leadership is dealing with strangers, faceless audiences whom one wishes to convert or at least inspire and whom one doesn't have to see again in the faculty meeting next week or the budget discussion tomorrow. I have believed that it is important for someone who has access to audiences of nurses and others to articulate our aspirations as well as our problems. *Never badmouth nursing in public.* Nursing is so huge that our knowledge touches on practically everything in health care and lots of things outside as well. I have tried to use nursing to speak to themes other than health care such as feminism, but that has had very limited success. Nursing is still, in 2004, not a discipline the public equates with insight, intelligence, or the kind of social status that gives us credibility. So we have to do it personally, person by person, encounter by encounter and gradually, oh so very gradually, things begin to change.

We're speaking of nursing and social change here, and social change takes a very long time. Recognizing that social change is the right label for many of nursing's struggles might give us a perspective that invokes patience and perseverance rather than anger and bitterness. But it's hard.

It is made infinitely easier by being in the company of others who are trying to do the same thing.

I started a paragraph here that would have named the "company," the people who have influenced the way I think about leadership and policy. The paragraph threatened to turn into a whole chapter. I love nurses and nursing and the people who do it and I am constantly amazed and astonished by the creativity and depth of nurses. I will find another way to thank and praise my idols, who include staff nurses, editors, faculty colleagues, physicians, University administrators, nurse practitioners, nurse managers, deans, directors of nursing, Chief Nurses in other countries, operations researchers and organizational behaviorists, and 40-plus years' worth of students in nursing and public health.

But you gotta' *listen.* From a presumption of respect for the work.

At the Tony Awards ceremony in 2001, one woman recipient gushed, "I want to thank everyone I've ever known!" That's more or less the way I feel.

WRITING NURSING

WRITING NURSING

I really am a very shy and private person. But given a chance to talk about nursing in public, I'm out there.[1] That was what I had to train myself to do when I became a Dean so young and in such an interesting time in nursing and health policy and politics.

I came to develop a writing and speaking style that are indistinguishable. I write as I speak and speak as I write. That gives me an odd presence in committee meetings and teaching.

The selections in this section are about writing in and about nursing. The first few come from work done when I was an Editor. The last few might be read as applying those lessons.

ENDNOTE

1. This is not an uncommon thing for people who are thrust into some kind of public arena. I especially like Anne Garrels' book, *Naked in Baghdad* (New York: Farrar, Straus and Giroux, 2003) on this theme. As an NPR reporter, she was trying to get the story of the Iraq "war" right and that transcended what is apparently her other wispy personality. A good friend told me that when I was Dean, I had several personalities. The Dean, the Professor, the Donna. It took me a long time to understand what she said, but she was right. I'm a stone killer when I think nursing is being undervalued or dismissed and I can be awfully terribly aggressive (oh, the stories I could tell...). Not a useful tactic and one I've worked to use only on very special occasions.

WHY WRITE, WHY PUBLISH?

This piece was written to pull together a light approach to inspiring nurses to write, especially about the work. I used it in writing workshops and eventually it became a staple handout. I still dig it out when I run across a colleague who has terrific ideas but who just can't seem to get them down. It was originally published in Image *(13(1), 3–8, 1981, used with permission).*

The answer to the question "why write" or "why publish" is just as simple as "why not?"

One writes or publishes because one wants to. Simply wanting to isn't enough, however, for there are all kinds of internal and external reasons why people don't write or publish or can't seem to get themselves together to do it. Over the years, I have amassed something of a collection of reasons why people don't. None of these, of course, applies to you.

The first one goes like this: "I want to write but I don't know how to write good." ...

This complaint from nurses is an all too real one. College English teachers, including the President of my University, have complained that secondary schools are not teaching students how to write, so that when they get to college, they have difficulty putting an English sentence together, to say nothing of making it say something clever. College English teachers gripe that college students can't even spell much less punctuate, or parse a sentence or tell the difference between a transitive and intransitive verb. Everything from grade inflation to transformational grammar to poorly trained high school teachers is blamed for this deplorable situation. Yet it is quite true that something bad has happened during the last 20 years in secondary schools and it is also true that when students reach college, they are too often woefully ignorant of common rules of writing.

In nursing, the problem is compounded by our peculiar educational system in which none of the three kinds of programs that prepare nurses emphasizes writing as a necessary skill or even a subject that might be interesting as an elective. Diploma and associate degree programs may not even require a writing course. Baccalaureate programs are not much better when college courses center on the sciences, or perhaps an ethics or philosophy course, and neglect the study of the language.

In clinical nursing education, evaluation of students is sometimes wholly pinned to multiple choice tests or short answer quizzes, leaving the student no opportunity to even use the written language, assuming she knows how. Nursing faculty are no less badly trained in writing, so falling back on other ways of student evaluation is natural. We now have in nursing several generations of nurses who have little training in writing, less experience in writing about their chosen field, who therefore approach the thought of putting pen to paper with anxiety that borders on antipathy.

While it is a fact that nurses are not even as well prepared for professional writing as everyday college students, that still isn't an excuse. The following is not an original thought at all: the best preparation for writing is *reading*. One learns to write not only in formal settings and classrooms, but by reading the work of others and paying attention to the way words are used. Reading does not have to be confined to either esoteric or professional literature. Any piece composed of words is fair game for learning about writing, the better the writing, the better the learning. But if one's taste doesn't run to Susan Sontag or John Updike or Hemingway or the *New Yorker* or *Evergreen,* there is still the daily newspaper, the incredible variety of slick magazines on the stand in the grocery store, the eternal continuing education flyers one gets in the mail, the backs of catsup bottles, the signs in store windows, or even letters from one's mother. At the very least, reading alerts one to words everywhere and how they work and how they can be made to work. Excellent writing crops up everywhere from children's books to science fiction, from nursing journals to advertisements, from hard-headed research through frothy fiction.

Television is said to have ruined many of us by turning us away from the printed word. But there's no reason to let a machine that has an "off" switch interfere with your desire to write. If you feel you can't use the language properly, there are solutions. Reading is one. Taking a course or workshop or studying on your own is another. Simply writing, anything, anywhere, any chance you get is yet another.

"Okay," you say. "So I can learn to write. But I can't get started."

It's awfully hard to get started writing if you don't have an idea. I like the story about the humorist, Robert Benchley. Every morning when he got up, he rolled a sheet of yellow paper into the typewriter, stared at it a moment, typed out the word "The," then waited for inspiration to strike. One morning he sat and stared longer than usual, finally sighed, and wrote, "The hell with it" and went back to bed.

Inspiration doesn't hit like a stroke of lightning, with an idea fully grown, a pithy topic sentence and a profound conclusion neatly formed in the frontal lobe, all ready to spring from fingers to typewriter. More than anything, writing takes discipline, including the discipline to sit in front of the infernal machine for however long it takes to squeeze out the first words from the constipation of the brain.[1]

Writing isn't easy for anybody, not even people who make their living doing it, and don't let anybody's prolific output convince you to the contrary. ... Yet the use of the language to describe is so important a task that the agony and the torture are not only worth it, they are necessary. To approach writing as if it is going to be easy will just lead to disappointment with slow progress. To approach writing as if it is going to be a complete pain is just as troublesome, especially if the fantasy of pain is so intricate that it makes one never start to write.

Assuming you have an idea, how do you start? Just start, that's all, in whatever style makes the most sense to you. Some people start with detailed outlines, some never outline. Some write the middle part first and leave the beginning and end until last. Some let an idea simmer in the back of the mind until it simply won't be contained any longer and presses on the finger tips to get to the keyboard. Some invent tricks to get along—when I have trouble starting a paper, I get a brand new pad of yellow lined paper, at least seven carefully sharpened pencils, sit at my dining room table and write in longhand until the words begin to flow too fast for that method. Some people have tried and true rituals to get started writing—put the cat out first (never second), wash the dishes, pile the papers on the desk *just so,* pour a glass of milk or a cup of coffee, take the phone off the hook, put on one's favorite disreputable old college sweatshirt, walk up and down the stairs three times, then sit down to write.

Writing is hard work and we need to have a sense of humor about it. Anything one can do to make it easier ought to be done, whether it's compulsive rituals or other ways of fooling oneself into comfort. But the best way to start writing is just to start and worry later about whether it's perfect (which it will not be). To wait for the perfect first sentence is to drive oneself mad with obsession, while if one just starts to write, one will trick oneself psychologically into perceiving progress and that in itself will make the writing easier.

"But," you say, "I don't want to contribute any more junk to the literature than is already there."

Terrific, but what makes you think you'll do that? To start with the thought that whatever one writes will be junk is a sure way never to start at all. On the other hand, if it truly turns out to be junk, no self-respecting editor will accept it for publication, so you don't have anything to worry about.

It is quite true that there is a lot of bad writing, some occasionally worse thinking in the literature, and not only in the nursing literature. The most common criticisms one can make of most of the professional literature in any field is that it is dry, dull, and ponderous when it isn't outright ungrammatical. Many nurses feel, with reason, that they don't want to write that way, yet they feel somehow they ought to, otherwise nobody will read it, or they'll be thought superficial or unintellectual.

There is an absolutely crucial need in nursing for writing about nursing, about patient care. That is the field we know best, those of us who practice, and nobody else can write about it as we can. There is no rule that says such writing has to be dull or pedantic or that it has to be cute and trivial either. For some reason, it seems very hard for nurses to think about writing what they know best, and know better than anyone else in the world, and that's patient care. Yet when you hear nurses talk, that's what we talk about, and the best of us describe the work with color and precisions, subtlety, flavor, and emotion— all of the qualities that make descriptive writing superior.

To write about nursing, or patient care, would not be to contribute more junk to the literature. We moan a good deal in nursing about how little we are understood by the public, or other professionals, or Congress, or somebody else. We won't be much better understood until and unless we put some energy into communicating in public form what our work is like, how it looks, how it feels, how it works or doesn't. ...

When nurses are stumped for a topic to write about, the best suggestion is to write about what nursing care is, using the latest patient as an example. It doesn't have to be an exotic case of syringomyelia or something—any nursing care will illustrate the process of thinking. Yet that thinking is so undervalued in the field, thought so intuitive, that the exercise of trying to write about it will serve two purposes: to make it conscious to the nurse writing and to make it visible to the audience. Either or both will be a contribution.

"Okay," you say, "but suppose I'm not quite up for that kind of writing yet. What can I write about?"

There's a legend floating around that writing is different from talking. You talk all the time, don't you?

If you're a faculty member, you must prepare a lecture from time to time. How do you go about it? By reading all that you can get your hands on that might help in thinking it through, then developing an outline or some notes or something to keep you from panicking in front of the class. Usually, you have to search a long time to find the right kinds of articles because nobody has written what you want, right? So why not write up a lecture as an article? You already have the references, you have the feedback from the class about which points are the important ones and which ones bored them to sleep. You have a beginning, a middle, and an end, you have notes or outlines or some framework. I am astonished by how infrequently faculty think of turning their lectures into articles or books. All that work in preparation and it's gone in the amount of breath it takes to talk for an hour or so. And if it really has taken a lot of work to track down the right references because they don't exist, that in itself is an argument for making your very own reference.

So you're not a faculty member. Do you do inservice education? Do you speak to garden clubs or Rotary or your church group or your jogging club about health or nursing? Do you write to your college roommate about the patient you've just cared for? Do you go to professional organization meetings, prepare testimony for public hearings, debate with a doctor? Do you read articles and criticize the foolish thinking? Do you even sit around and brood about the state of nursing, or the state of the world, or the rottenness of your administrator, or the nastiness of the med students?

Any occasion is grist for the writing mill. Any firmly held conviction, any thoughtful critique, any vested emotional energy is a potential spark for the writing fire. (And anybody who caught the mixed metaphors in those sentences is well on the way to becoming a writer!)

"But," you say, "I don't have time to write."

That is the most pitiful excuse there is. Parkinson's Law says, "Work expands to fill the time available." A corollary is the work contracts to fill the time available. Writing, like any other activity, is a choice and to choose to do one thing means something else will not be done, or at least will be postponed.

Perhaps that's a bit harsh. Writing is an activity that takes a different conception of time. There is no minute-to-minute decision making with writing, no drama, no frenetic hustling around, no short staffing, no irritations of others. Writing is a singular, contemplative chore, and thus needs to be learned, just as one once learned how to organize one's care for eight or ten patients on a shift. Writing makes nurses (and lots of others) nervous because it is so lonely and private and silent except for the clack of the keys or the scratch of the pen. Writing is slow, and not for the impatient.

Writing is not valued in most clinical institutions so it is hard to argue with one's supervisor that one should have time to do it on the job. Even in university settings, it is hard to find regular free time from student conferences, committee meetings, or lecture preparation to sit down with nothing else to do but write. Yet if one wants to write, there is no way to do it other than to take the time, whether it's weekends or evenings, sabbaticals or leaves, vacations or days off, coffee breaks or lunches, or rides on the bus to work. Writing won't make its own time; time has to be made for it and something else will have to go. It's the individual's own decision what that something will be, and the consequences of that choice are also the individual's. Nobody can make the time for writing but oneself.

People's styles of writing are different. I need a block of time, a few hours, to write, with nothing else pressing. A friend can write a few sentences now, a few tomorrow and not lose the train of thought. I wait until an idea is firm, or a deadline coming, before I sit down to write; another friend writes regularly and religiously every Friday in a time she carefully preserves. Still another friend writes her exquisite papers by dictating as she drives to and from work, a 40 minute commute each way. And yet a fourth friend sits and agonizes at the keyboard over each sentence, doing pushups when he gets stuck, and his carefully crafted articles show that attention. Figure out your own style, then arrange the time to do it. Or decide not to, but don't complain that there isn't time.

"But," you say, "I have nothing original to say, everything's already been written about."

This one deserves two responses. The first is this is pure balderdash. The other is, you're partly correct.

There is a myth that says if an infinite number of monkeys sat at an infinite number of typewriters, in an infinite amount of time they would produce all the written works of the world. That is the only circumstance in which I can imagine that everything would have been written about.

This comment comes most often, in my experience, from people who are not voracious readers. They sense correctly that there must be something in the literature that they don't know about and they would be embarrassed to write something that later turned out to be unoriginal. In certain academic spheres, that's a realistic worry. While originality is to be valued wherever it's found, in scientific writing at least, building on past work is the rule, not the exception, and ignorance of the literature is a sin. Yet the literature is always there; using ignorance of it as an excuse for not writing simply means one does not want to put in the work to do the reading before one can do the writing. That excuse is a killer in academic institutions. ...

What is the search, then, for originality and why is it thought to be an impossibility and therefore, an excuse for not writing?

It may be that nurses new to writing believe that only the perfection of pure originality is worth doing, and since that can't be done, forget it all. Perfect originality is thought to mean that nobody else has ever thought about a topic just this way, nobody has ever used exactly these words, nobody has done and published anything at all relevant to this cherished idea. Those thoughts are naïve. Nursing lies in the crossroads of so many bodies of knowledge, theories, attitudes, values, concepts, and descriptions that it is unlikely that there is absolutely nothing already written that could be relevant to one's own idea. It may even be true that somebody has already had the idea and studied it and published the findings (as frequently and depressingly happens in research, usually just as your own completed study is about to go to the binder).

This excuse may also reflect a state in the evolution of an idea. In the early stages (though one doesn't know it's early) one is half conscious that one has a new and original idea, but one isn't sure and since the idea isn't quite hatched yet, it seems better not to commit it to paper lest it be found to be embryonic by someone who has thought more about it. If one keeps thinking, however, and reading and thinking some more, the idea evolves and there comes a time when one knows that despite all that's in the literature, one really *is* onto something good, something original. So long as one keeps thinking and searching and refining, one has the chance of actually coming up with something original. The minute one decides that one can't, or that one's dandy little idea probably isn't, the mental processes just stop and so does the opportunity to make an original contribution.

"But," you say, "I can't do a whole article—I don't have enough to say."

From a standing start, a 3500-word article looks mighty intimidating. So does a 45-minute speech. Perhaps, then, an article isn't the way to start.

My first publishing effort was a long letter to the editor, written with two other people. It was so thrilling to see my words set in type that I was hooked forever. Letters to the editor are relatively easy to write and editors are undyingly grateful for thoughtful comments that begin to stimulate a dialogue. ...

Co-authorship is another good way to get started in publishing. The second thing I ever published, and the first article, was done with a psychiatrist colleague and it was so painless I couldn't believe it. We met to talk about the content and taped that meeting. His secretary transcribed it, he cut and pasted, I added and subtracted, and presto—an article! That's a very easy way to write since it leaps across the distance some people think there is between talking and writing.

In my experience with new writers, they tend to under-write rather than over-write. Wonderful, complicated ideas are buried in one sentence on the way to grand conclusions. Large thoughts are dropped in the middle of a paragraph without elaboration. So I suspect that the excuse that you don't have enough material for an article and thus won't even start turns out much of the time not to be true. But you will never know unless you try.

"But," you say, "you seem to assume that everybody ought to write and I'm just a (fill in the blank)"—staff nurse, instructor, new graduate, old retread, diploma nurse, clinic nurse, and so on and on.

Writing is for other people, hmmm? And criticism is for you?

It's all too easy to sit with this month's nursing journal in front of the fireplace and rail about the stupidity of one author or another, or toss aside the journal in disgust. Criticism is just fine, is even publishable. Put your money where your mouth is.

In nursing, the people we need to do the writing are the people for whom it's the hardest, the most foreign, the easiest to put off. We need to have nursing writing done by people who are close to patient care, and we need them to write about patient care. That is not to say that all others should be muzzled, I am only elaborating the earlier point that there is a crying need for writing about what nursing is, how nurses think about it, what it's like for both patients and nurses. That writing has to come from those who know it most clearly and daily, and they are the most qualified for that kind of writing. The perceptions of the new staff nurse and the clinical wisdom of the veteran must somehow get out of their heads and onto the paper, for we need their words so much.

You don't have to be a faculty member, professor, an academic, or an administrator to write. Those of us on tenure ladders have to, which may explain why some of the nursing literature is so awful. I wish for the day when staff nurses and others in direct patient care contact will find hospitals adding to their clinical ladder systems a way to count writing and publication toward merit increases or other internal reward systems. Wouldn't it be nice if nurses who wish to write were supported officially by the system, with library time, or secretarial help? Until that unlikely day, writing will continue

to be work on top of fulltime work for adtive nurses and nursing will continue to be the lesser.

"Okay," you sigh. "But I don't know how to write professional writing."

For heaven's sake, don't learn. Too much professional writing is slogging
and turgid when it isn't full of syntactical and semantic strangeness. Nursing
jargon is no worse than anybody else's jargon; it's just that we own it, so we
feel freer to criticize excesses like "Potential alteration in comfort" or "self
care deficits" or "knowledges, skills and competencies" or "holistic man." ...

The recent intellectual history of nursing has its roots in the teachers' colleges of the mid-century, and we suffer from the same kind of language abuse.
And we make up others. "Baby," for example, becomes "neonate"; "food"
becomes "diet"; "operation" becomes "surgery" and "pain" becomes "alteration in comfort."

Anybody who feels she can't write professional jargon ought to be
instantly canonized, applauded, and granted a permanent writing fellowship
on the spot.

"Okay, okay," you say. "The real problem I have, see, is writing and publishing are so, well...*public*."

Ah, now we get right down to it.

You're absolutely right, publishing is public, making public or available for
public consumption one's cherished words and ideas. That's downright scary,
especially if you've not done it before. What if you're wrong? Or stupid?

Shyness is not a good excuse for not writing. Writing *is* more public than
not writing, but a whole lot less public than appearing on television, speaking
in public, participating in a committee meeting, or taking care of patients.
Print is static and relatively non-participatory; the most feedback one can
expect is a letter or two and even the most critical letter will still be received
in private.

Writers forget that editors of books or journals have no less a desire not to
appear stupid than writers do, and a whole lot more experience and training
in protecting the pubic from ill-thought ideas or half-baked prose. Editors
must exist in part to protect authors from themselves, and to back up their
judgment to publish when that has been the decision. Submitting one's darling manuscript to an editor is in itself an act of public exposure, but even
when negative, the consequences are quite small.

Even academic types who are under the publish-or-perish gun forget why
universities are so insistent on writing and publication. It is, indeed, so that
ideas become public, become part of a dialogue that, when it works best, has
the effect of pushing forward the boundaries of thought, science, or understanding of the world. That is the mission of a university, and the mission of
a learned profession, which nursing is becoming. To publish is to enter into
public forums where ideas are challenged, adopted, criticized, applauded,
berated, accepted, or rejected and good, bad or indifferent, published ideas
make a dent in other people's thinking where private contemplation never

can. To publish is publicly to expose your thinking, to make public an aspect of your privacy. To write, to publish, is to make visible your thinking and your work, and in universities, only visible work can possibly be evaluated for promotion or tenure or appointment. It is the obligation of the professional to do more than simply *profess*. Students are willing captives for one's brilliance. One's professional colleagues, reached through publication, are not always so swept away.

So, yes, publishing is very public but there is no other way to develop and exchange ideas on such a scale.

"Alright, already," you say. "I've given you lots of reasons why *not* to write or publish. Now, you tell me why I *should*."

First, writing for publication gives you a chance to reach wider audiences than you ever could with individual contacts. Writing gives you a chance at fame, and what's wrong with that? Publishing gives you a shot at personal power and gives an outlet for personal ambition, though we're not supposed to feel that as women or as nurses. It's simply a fact that it's fun to have your name recognized for something you have written, even when the writing is criticized. It's also fun to enjoy tiny touches of fame, deserved, or not, to feed your eroded ego.

Writing for publication might make money for you, though don't hold out for early retirement unless you can come up with the great American textbook. Not many people make much money on writing, especially professional writing, and the people who do make significant amounts do it full time. But writing for publication can supplement an income and provide nice resources for present enjoyment or future plans.

If one is an academic type, writing for publication will get you promoted, even to tenure, and nothing else will in distinguished universities. The carrot and stick of publishing or perishing is real and it won't go away, and if we're honest about it, many of us wouldn't get around to putting pen to paper without the tenure push.

Those are all practical reasons.

There are other reasons to write and publish that vary more with personal style.

Some people write to fill the need for self-expression. Teaching, talking, speaking may not be enough outlets for very creative people, people with lots of ideas, so writing is another way of filling that need. Some people find it easier to write than to stand up in front of a group, be it students or a larger and more anonymous audience. Some few people have a truly burning *need* to write and publishing is almost the frosting on the cake.

Writing is a wonderful way of thinking something through. Being forced to put down on paper an idea, develop it in some kind of form that makes paragraphs and sentences, is excellent discipline and superior learning. The very act of writing is an act of scholarship if one aspect of scholarship is clarity and precision of thought, for writing gives one's amorphous notions structure. An idea held in the head will just be fluff until it begins to take form as words on paper. Exposing an idea to the eyes also exposes the holes in thinking, the leaps in logic, and unformed conclusions, so writing is a tool for thinking. Writing forces you to sharpen and hone, refine and polish thinking. Writing makes thinking real.

Finally, you might write simply for the love of words. To read beautiful combinations of words is one kind of treat; to think them up oneself is quite another, and is an esthetic experience available to even those who can't draw a straight line or play a note on the piano. Writing sends one back to read, to find compelling sentences, or sounds that speak to the heart. Writing makes one search for words and the meanings, and that search leads one into history and literature, and writing begins to cultivate the civilized mind.

Why write? Why publish? The best answer would be the answer Louis Armstrong gave when he was asked, "What is jazz?"

"If you have to ask, you'll never know."

ENDNOTE

1. As I was keying this in (in 2003), Paul Simon was singing, "want to be a writer, find a quiet space and grab a humble pen." Paul Simon, *Hurricane Eye,* **You're the One,** Warner Bros. #47844 10/00.

THE ROLE OF THE EDITOR

This is an "inside" piece.

There is an "organization" in nursing called the International Academy of Nursing Editors (INANE). Thelma Schorr, then Editor of the American Journal of Nursing, *thought up the acronym. Pamela Brink, Editor then and now of* Western Journal of Nursing Research, *and others created this thing. It has no dues, no officers, no headquarters, no newsletter, no website, no agenda, no public policy statements. It exists for nursing editors to gather and tell stories and work on common problems. Someone volunteers to host the meeting every year and it moves around the USA and internationally.*

Editors are a peculiar bunch. We are united because we love to read and we love the language. And we are mostly volunteers, not often paid unless we edit very large circulation journals that carry advertising. We are united by trying to make nursing better, and the way the outside world understands nursing even better.

This speech was the keynote address for the INANE meeting in 1992, in Sarasota, Florida. At the time, I was Editor of Image—Journal of Nursing Scholarship, *official journal of Sigma Theta Tau, International.*

This is one of the few occasions when we editors can legitimately whine in public. This is a private meeting and this paper is never going to be published because none of you would accept it for publication. It is an extended editorial and, as *we* know, but many of our budding authors don't, only editors get to write those. ...

John Hall Wheelock, an early editor for Scribner's, defined our job:

> The function of an editor...is to serve as a skilled objective
> outsider, a critical touchstone by recourse to which a writer
> is enabled to sense flaws in surface or structure, to grasp and
> solve the artistic or technical problems involved, and thus to
> realize completely his own work in his own way.[1]

279

We are the invisible hand (and eyes) and only those of us inside the fence know what we have done to make the printed version make sense. If we are acknowledged at all, it may be in a graceful footnote, and that only really happens with book publication. No one really knows what Pat Lewis did to make Pat Benner's first book fly, but a comparison between her first and second shows the difference. No one knows that the premier LPN textbook writer is dead and that each subsequent edition is done by an editor, Nancy Evans. Harrison of the giant internal medicine text, Gray of *Anatomy,* Williams of *Obstetrics* are all in the great word processor in the sky. Indeed, did you know that Virginia Henderson never even met Bertha Harmer, but produced several editions of Harmer and Henderson's *Principles and Practice of Nursing* entirely alone?

Journal editors are grey eminences behind our green eyeshades, shyly retiring behind the words of our authors and rarely invited to lunch at 21 as the commercial editors of renown were: Bennett Cerf, Woollcott Gibbs, Maxwell Perkins, and the like.

Thus when one reads Perkins or Gibbs or Bill Zinsser of the old *Life* magazine on what it is to be an editor, one must do it in the context of knowing that they had legions of unemployable BA's in English to screen manuscripts before they even saw them, and so Maxwell Perkins of Scribner's could luxuriate, as he did, in "concerning himself with talent,"[2] in his case Hemingway, F. Scott Fitzgerald, Thomas Wolfe, and Edna Ferber.

Commercial publishers and editors do not have to deal with what comes in over the transom, or in FedEx or regular mail. You and I, on the other hand, must deal with chaff like this:

- "At any given point in time, many is the expression of the totality of events present at that point in time."
- "Choosing meaning points to the birthings and dyings inherent in each decision."
- "Cotranscending with the possibles is powering unique ways of originating in the process of transforming."
- "The richness of nursing knowledge is illuminated when the structural themes are integral with the unified perspective of the discipline."
- "Intuition is the reflection and reverberation of transpersonal caring made manifest to the nurse."
- "Negative certainty signifies a foreboding illness situation with a downward trajectory."

I did not make these up.

Bill Zinsser, who once edited me, to my great pleasure, says, "The problem is to find the real man or woman behind all the tension...For ultimately the product that any writer has to sell is not his subject, but who he is."[3]

What editor can possibly find the author embedded in the negative certainty or cotranscending with the possibles?

Maxwell Perkins cut what became *Look Homeward, Angel* from 1100 pages to 800. And did it in person with Thomas Wolfe, from 8:30 at night or "whenever Tom can come to it"[4] until 11:00 or so. Perkins wrote to Hemingway that Wolfe "shrank from the sacrifices, which were really cruel often."[5] There are days when I would love to cut one-third of the pages of a manuscript. And days when I would like to nurture talent.

One of the best and funniest exegeses about editing is Woollcott Gibbs' "Theory and Practice of Editing *New Yorker* Articles," quoted in full in James Thurber's *The Years with Ross*[6] and published nowhere else.

Gibbs begins: "The average contributor to this magazine is semi-literate, that is, he is ornate to no purpose, full of senseless and elegant variations, and can be relied on to use three sentences where a word would do."[7]

I think of that when I get:

- "when a system's entropic forces exceed the evolutionary forces to the extent that the steady state is disrupted" (means "death" by the way)
- "altered sexual conception actions". (This is a real one, one of the suggested nursing diagnoses. What on earth does this mean? Artificial insemination? Withdrawal? Birth control? Oral sex? I don't know.)

Try this one:

"The unification of a multidimensional School of Nursing is a homeodynamic process involving a pleurality [sic] of interactions through exchanges of internal personal belief systems and those systems external to the self which influence internal adaptations."

Gibbs is worried about adverbs, clichés and funny names, drunkenness, and adultery. We don't have to worry too much about those.

But in his paragraph # 24 (of 31), he rails against the cosmic last line. "Suddenly Mr. Holtzmann felt tired" is his example.

In the years I have been an Editor, I have come to believe that it is possible to edit out entirely nearly every *first* sentence in every article, if not the entire first cosmic paragraph.

As a writer, I know I write myself clear, so the first paragraph is just a way to get oneself going. But really:

"The need for nursing care by hospitalized patients has long been recognized."

"Pain is not something that can be experienced by the nurse."

"The costs of health care have been skyrocketing."

"Nursing needs to get into the educational mainstream."

The Woollcott Gibbs' of the world were free to nurture talent and make subtle editorial suggestions because they had rooms full of fact-checkers and copy editors.

It happens that the deadline for my editorial is the same as the deadline for getting edited manuscripts to the publisher. I have learned that I should not write an editorial after having just edited six or eight or ten manuscripts because I just want to KILL.

Computer-assisted library searches, word processing, and NCNR funding have seriously interfered with editors' mental health. Authors ask librarians to do searches, not realizing that the computer-based library indices most often used only cover up to the last 8 years or so and will miss the germinal article published in 1970. I worry excessively sometimes at the misinterpretation of whole lines of inquiry because the present author has not read the original work. Florence Nightingale's life span is easy to remember so I tend to snarl when an author reports that Miss Nightingale favorably reviewed something Isabel Hampton Stewart wrote in 1920 because by then, Nightingale had been dead for 10 years.

Authors turn over manuscript drafts or disks to secretaries to fill in the blanks of references. Only once in my tenure as an editor have I had a manuscript that has every single citation correct, meaning matching the text and complete, if not accurate, which, except for those articles with which I am personally familiar, like the ones I write myself, I cannot possibly check. (As an aside, I was once reading speedily through a manuscript only to be brought up short by a strikingly familiar paragraph. It should have been familiar. I wrote it, but the author just lifted it. It is an interesting challenge to write a rejection letter in this circumstance.)

By the time I've gotten through all the manuscripts, I am surly beyond belief and not in good shape to write a colorful, even inspiring, editorial.

Many other editors, including Pat [Edith P.] Lewis, who edited *AJN, Nursing Research,* and *Nursing Outlook,* and Florence Downs have written about the term paper phenomenon. That is when faculty tell students that their paper is just brilliant and publishable and so send it to me. Or to you. And most of them are not because most faculty aren't published either so they cannot advise students correctly. What is sad is that, as you and I know because we get to see the cover letters, a fair number of these "term paper"-type articles are really doctoral dissertations.

The Maxwell Perkins' and Woollcott Gibbs' did not have to deal with cover letters.

How many have you had that essentially say, "Oh, how hard I have worked, see the sweat and blood on this page, please don't reject me"? Or how often do you get manuscripts with the author's entire c.v. enclosed? I once even had a manuscript submitted with the author's newborn baby's picture enclosed. Cute kid. Bad article.

And then, of course, there is the correspondence, and here I suspect all editors of all kinds of publications get strange things.

I am constantly amazed at what readers think is controversial. One reader asked Sigma Theta Tau to cancel her membership because we published an article about HIV seroprevalence which reported the fact that in San Francisco, free bleach with instructions in six languages was being given out by AIDS activists. Another reader asked to be removed from the list because we published an article on lesbian parenting. The most mail we have had on any article in my experience has been one we ran about a year ago on career-oriented women with tattoos.

I thought the piece was kind of fun and it came with interesting illustrations. But one reader swore she would never read *Image* again, and another was convinced she knew why I had rejected something she had once submitted; my taste must be really bad. Those letters prompted a little rivulet of letters; oddly enough from people who aren't nurses, supporting the content and the article was referenced in the *New England Journal of Medicine*. Never can tell.

The grand prize goes to a letter I got this year on heavily embossed legal stationery, the kind you know is going to be trouble when you open the envelope. It was from the lawyers for the Eastman Kodak company telling me to cease and desist from calling our publication *Image* because we were intruding on their own copyrighted publication of a similar name. Since I'm, thank heaven, just the Editor, not the publisher, I turfed that to Sigma Theta Tau, who turned loose their own embossed-stationery lawyers who eventually produced an absolutely hilarious document compiling about $3000 worth of legal research to the effect that Kodak could kindly pick somebody else to sue, since they proved that there were more than 12,000 publications with the word "image" or something like it in the title. And the first legal citation was to a case involving Polaroid, which I thought was a nice touch.

What is it to be an editor?

First before anything, I believe it is to preserve and protect truth, justice, fairness, and the English language. The preservation of the First Amendment extends to the professional literature as much as it does to the public press, and we have in place systems to assure that, whereas newspapers are after what Suzanne Gordon calls the four C's: "conflict, crisis, control and competition,"[8] and accuracy may be trod upon. ...

It has long interested me that the single blind system of review is the norm in medical scientific publications, justified, their editors say, because the name and institutional affiliation of the authors is one criterion of the quality of the research.

This has actually been studied in psychology.[9] Two young assistant professors began a study in which, with the permission of the original authors, they retyped already published manuscripts, altered the names and institutional affiliations of the authors and resubmitted them to the journals in which they were originally published. They also informed the journal editors about the study, but not, of course, about the particular manuscript. There were 13 journals involved. Only three of the editors recognized the manuscript. One of the remaining articles was accepted again, and eight either were resoundingly rejected (no action was apparently taken on one). The reasons for rejection were overwhelmingly methodological with additional criticisms of the poor writing style. There was no mention of the ideas being old or familiar in the literature.

The investigators found an unusually high level of inter-reviewer agreement; reviewers apparently are able to agree on institutional prestige.

The investigators debriefed the editors and there the fun began. Two of the three editors who saw through the deception responded with threats and insults. One of the enraged editors threatened legal action and professional censure, sent a copy of his irate letter to the investigators' department chairman, and said that other manuscripts received from that university might receive well-deserved rejection as well. Another editor not only wrote a threatening letter but passed the matter along to one of his associates who also fired off an insulting letter. The person who reports this case writes that she has seen these letters and they are "notable for their lack of subtlety, their overt bullying, their degree of over-reaction, and their angrily paternalistic style."[10]

The investigators were then informed by their department chair that they would no longer have access to xeroxing or postage, and when one of them came up for a tenure review, his tenure was denied. He appealed and eventually won. But a manuscript based on this study was rejected from the professional literature under what the reporter calls "highly atypical" review procedures.

Two other flamboyant cases, one is sociology, one in social work, are worth mentioning. In the former, pseudo-manuscripts were devised which reported on a study of the mental health of pro-activist students versus anti-activists. Findings in half the pseudo-manuscripts favored the activists, and in the other half, favored the anti-activists. Recommendations for acceptance or rejection were based on the reviewers' political orientations, and the original authors' report of the study also received atypical review and quite typical rejection by the professional journals.

In the social work study, a pseudo-manuscript describing the effectiveness of a social work intervention (in half the submissions) or the ineffectiveness (in the other half) was submitted to 101 social work journals and 32 journals in other fields. Thirty-three journals reviewed it, and acceptance was recommended for the positive version by eight, and for the negative version by four. But when the author tried to publish the results of the study of editorial policy, he was literally run out of the country and eventually ended up in Hong Kong.[11]

I believe the Editor's role and responsibility is, to the extent possible, to create the balance and also the tension between the popular and the good. Sometimes that means overriding reviewers when they are, charitably, having a bad day. It means making sure that the reviewers really understood the material. Sometimes it may mean going to some lengths to be sure the manuscript is treated fairly.

Sometimes it means either searching out or working with authors with original, if not exactly mainstream, ideas. And sometimes it means rejecting your colleagues, friends, and Governing Board members.

I won't bore you here today with the Editor's role in preserving the English language. We all do it, more or less well, although I too have been taken to task when I let the use of "contracept" as a verb slip through.

Oh surely, Editors must recruit reviewers, stroke board members, pay attention to the budget and the advertisers and the publisher.

But what the role of the Editor really is, and what keeps us doing it, is to immerse oneself in the field so that one knows the good stuff from the not-so-good, the trends from the idiosyncrasies, so that through our invisible work, we can really make a difference.

ENDNOTES

1. Wheelock, J.H. (1950). *Editor to Author*. New York: Scribner's.

2. Kuehl, J., & Bryer, J. (Eds), (1971). *Dear Scott, Dear Max—The Fitzgerald-Perkins Correspondence*. New York: Scribner's, p. 13.

3. Zinsser, W. (1976). *On Writing Well*. New York: Harper's, p. 5.

4. Kuehl & Bryer, *ibid.*, p. 9.

5. *Loc cit.*

6. Thurber, J. (1957). *The Years with Ross*. Boston: Little Brown, pp. 122–126.

7. *Ibid.*, p. 122.

8. Gordon, S. (1992). "That's what nurses do?" *Revolution—The Journal of Nurse Empowerment, 2*(1), 52–57.

9. Sieber, J.E. (1989). On studying the powerful (or fearing to do so): A vital role for IRBs. *IRB 11*(5), 1–6.

10. *Ibid.*, p. 4.

11. *Ibid.*

COLONIZING: A MEASUREMENT OF THE DEVELOPMENT OF A PROFESSION

Florence S. Downs, then Editor of Nursing Research, *and I had a running dialogue about academic pretension expressed in ponderous writing. Indeed, we continued that in the recent correspondence in which I asked for and she gave permission to reprint the co-authored article below.*

This is first and only satire I have ever written, and fiendishly difficult it is, to avoid being too arch on the one hand, and giving it all away on the other. This is a real study. I really did count up all the titles in the journals to produce the graphs. (Originally published as Diers and Downs in Nursing Research, *1994 43(5), 316–318, used with permission.) The penultimate line is mine; wait for it!*

The extent to which nursing can claim to be an intellectual discipline has flavored academic policy and political arguments for parity. The available structural measures of professional development—number of refereed journals in the field, dedicated research funding from NIH, number of doctorates and doctoral programs—all show remarkable progress. Whether nursing's intellectual work has achieved scholarly credibility is not well measured by these indices: structural variables do not tap process or product. We have tested a quick, easy, and replicable measure of scholarly complexity found in the nursing literature and compared our findings to scholarly complexity in other fields.

CONCEPTUAL FRAMEWORK

Dillon[1] proposed the measure: "titular colonicity is the primary correlate of scholarly quality."[2] "Titular colonicity" means the insertion of the colon (:) in titles of articles.

Dillon argued for the colon as the predominant characteristic of scholarly publication on the basis of a study in which the colon appeared in 72% of the titles of articles in "current journals in education, psychology and literary criticism: and in only 13% of articles published in 'nonscholarly journals'.[3] He thus reasoned that titular colonicity is an index of scholarly complexity, explaining that as the science and scholarship of a discipline advance, it becomes impossible to contain the ideas in a manuscript without a colon in the title. The colon separates the ideas and defines or calibrates them. As the discipline becomes more scholarly, the titles of articles reflect that complexity:

> By nature and function the colon divides long periods of prose endeavoring to articulate within a single utterance a series of mutually interrelated concepts and propositions, along with the chain of definitions and presuppositions thereby entailed and the network of connotations and deductions therein permissably implicated.[4]

Dillon tested this hypothesis empirically by surveying titles of manuscripts published in the major organs of their respective learned societies: in education, *Review of Educational Research* (RER), in psychology, *Psychological Bulletin* (PB), and in literary criticism, *PMLA* (Publication of the Modern Language Association). Selecting the first and every tenth volume thereafter, he calculated percentages of colonic titles ($N = 1,150$) through 1980. In a further expansion, he performed the same calculation on a sample of 30 additional journals in the same disciplines for 1980.[5]

The results, he reported, are "unequivocal," particularly for the period from 1950 on, when there was a pronounced and sudden ascent in colonicity. By 1979, about half of the titles were colonic; by 1980, three-quarters were colonic.

> How will it end? Soon, it can be predicated, 100 percent of titles will contain a colon. What then of the progress of the enterprise?—room for younger scholars, future configuration of the disciplines, and so forth...Alternative devices might be readied, perhaps journals of colonic research founded.[6]

The journals Dillon surveyed began publication in 1884 (PMLA), 1904 (PB), and 1931 (RER). While nursing scholarship is not that old, titular colonicity does seem to be creeping into the nursing literature.[7] The purpose of the present investigation was to replicate Dillon's studies in the scholarly nursing literature to examine the progress of scholarly complexity.

METHODS OF STUDY

In nursing, there is, regrettably, no equivalent to the journals Dillon studied in terms of the roles they play in their disciplines. But we used two of his other sampling criteria to select nursing journals for review, exacting standards and high rejection rates and a generalist, rather than specialist, audience of considerable devotion. Rejection rates and generalist focus of the journals were obtained from Swanson, McClosky, and Bodensteiner's review of nursing publications.[8] The term *devotion,* as defined by the journals, refers to those most often read and assigned in doctoral programs in nursing.[9] The journals selected were *Nursing Research, Advances in Nursing Science, Image, Research in Nursing and Health,* and the *Western Journal of Nursing Research. Nursing Research* began publication in 1952; *Image* in 1967[10]; *Advances* and *RINAH* debuted in 1978; and the *Western Journal of Nursing Research* in 1979.

Because nursing journals are younger than those in the other disciplines, all titles of all volumes of the five journals through June 1993 were surveyed. Editorials, news reports, book reviews, technical notes, and commentaries were excluded. Reliability for detection of colonic titles was 100%.

FINDINGS

The sample of journals with total percent colonicity is described in Table 1. The rise of the colon in nursing scholarship is shown in Figure 1. For this analysis, all titles in all five journals were combined by year. It can be seen that scholarly complexity was already in evidence when the younger journals entered the field. Titular colonicity has apparently stabilized since about 1980 to about 30%.

When colonicity is examined by journal by year, an intriguing pattern emerges. As Table 4.1 shows, *Advances in Nursing Science* has double the prevalence of titular colonicity, with the pattern established early in the journal's life span. In fact, the other four journals were heading in the same direction, but from about 1983 on, colonic titles dropped in all except *Advances* (Figure 2). In 1993, however, colonizing appeared to be rising again in the other four journals.

DISCUSSION

Nursing's scholarly complexity lags far behind education, psychology, and literary criticism. Even by 1993 (Dillon's data stop in 1980), nursing scholarship

TABLE 1 ARTICLES BY JOURNAL AND PERCENT COLONIC

Journal	N	N (%) Colonic
Nursing Research	1964	402 (20.5)
Image	576	137 (23.8)
Advances in Nursing Science	408	210 (51.5)
RINAH	499	117 (23.5)
Western Journal	420	81 (19.3)

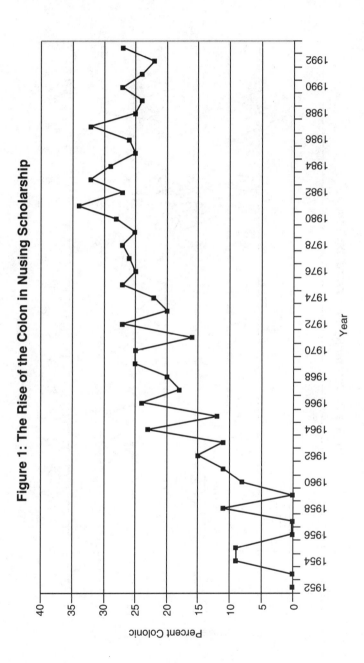

Figure 1: The Rise of the Colon in Nusing Scholarship

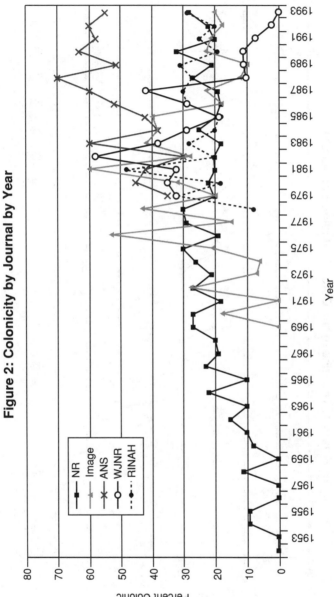

Figure 2: Colonicity by Journal by Year

was only about 33% colonic, while the fields Dillon studied were at three-quarters and rising. While nursing is a much younger intellectual discipline, this explanation may not be comforting. A further analysis of the data shows that it took literary criticism 50% of its life span (to 1980) to rise to about 10% colonicity; psychology and education took 40% of their respective life spans. Taking 1952 as the beginning, nursing achieved the 10% mark at 33% of its scholarly life span. Nursing's one-third, however, is only 10 years, while literary criticism's half is 50 years, psychology's 40% is 40 years and education's 40% is 20 years. Clearly, nursing's scholarly complexity is on the fast track.

There are, however, alternate interpretations of these data. Is it possible that titular colonicity is equivalent to grade inflation, now notorious in the liberal arts and science fields of which literary criticism and psychology are prominent, and of which education is derivative? Some support for this line of argument might logically be derived from the observation that newer nursing journals, which represent newer specialties, are pretenders to scholarship and indulge in titular colonicity to establish their scholarly standing.[11]

The difference among the five nursing journals studied suggests two new hypotheses that require further testing. Like any other form of punctuation, the colon has a particular use: "delivering the goods that have been invoiced in the preceding words."[12] Thus, the use of a colon when simply adding words ("Diapering and Diaper Rash: A Pilot Study") is not correct. Analyzing good or appropriate titular colonicity might offer prescriptions to carry forward nursing's scholarly agenda. The Modern Language Association publication has raised colonicity to an art form: "Rapping and Raping: An Analysis of Rhyme and Sexual Abuse in Elizabethan Prose."[13] Surely nurses could be equally creative, instead of tagging "A Literature Review," or "Summary of Findings," to perfectly understandable titles.

Another avenue for further research arises: examination of the contents of articles for colonicity. One of us (FSD) has noted that the humble comma has fallen into disuse, to be replaced by semi-colons, which in turn have been replaced by colonization. Perhaps the next stage of scholarly growth could be measured by the disappearance of the colon from titles and its proliferation in the body of the text.

An important underlying assumption must also be tested. Insertion of colons in article titles is assumed to be the work of the scholars (authors) writing. However, it is noted that titular colonicity was firmly and publicly controlled by at least one editor of one of the journals surveyed.[14] The extent of editorial complicity in colonizing the literature has not been examined. Are some editors inflating scholarly complexity by adding colons where they weren't before? Are some editors, perhaps unaware of the importance of titular colonicity in defining scholarship, undermining the field?

Finally, the present study simply cries out for replication among the scholarly journals in nursing specialties, nearly all of which are younger than the journals surveyed here. Perhaps some specialties are emerging (or pretending to emerge) as scholarly more quickly than others. Further studies of titular colonicity will expand our understanding of nursing's scholarly growth and potential, and the extent to which we aspire to the high colonic.[15]

ENDNOTES

1. Dillon was then an assistant professor of education at the University of California, Riverside. We do not know where he is now. We are grateful to Prof. Thomas R. Knapp of the Schools of Education and Nursing, University of Rochester, for bringing Dillon's work to our attention.

2. Dillon, J.T. (1982). In pursuit of the colon: A century of scholarly progress: 1880–1980. *Journal of Higher Education, 53,* 93–99.

3. *Ibid.,* p. 94.

4. *Ibid.*

5. Dillon, J.T. (1981). The emergence of the colon: An empirical correlate of scholarship. *American Psychologist, 36,* 879–884.

6. *Ibid.,* p. 96.

7. Diers, D. (1989). Letter to the Editor. *Nursing Research, 38,* 381; Downs, F. (1989). Response. *Nursing Research, 38,* 381.

8. Swanson, E.A., McClosky, J.C., & Bodensteiner, A. (1991). Publishing opportunities for nurses: A comparison of 92 US journals. *Image—Journal of Nursing Scholarship, 23*(3), 33–38.

9. Gay, J.T., Edgil, A.E., & Rozmus, C.A. (1989). Nursing journals read and assigned most often in doctoral programs. *Image—Journal of Nursing Scholarship, 21*(4), 246–250.

10. While *Image* began in 1967, publication was not regular until 1969.

11. Diers, 1989, *ibid.*

12. Fowler, H.W. (1965). *Modern English Usage.* (2nd Ed). Oxford, UK: Oxford University Press, p. 589.

13. Okay, so we made this one up. But something quite close to it is contained in *Murder at the MLA* (Jones, D.J.H. [1993] Athens, GA: University of Georgia Press) and the author was not kidding.

14. Information for Authors (1993). *Image—Journal of Nursing Scholarship, 25*(1), 35.

15. The authors gratefully acknowledge James F. Diers, MA, who gave important critical comments on an earlier draft of this article.

CONGRATULATIONS! YOU'RE THE WORST!

*Florence Downs declared a contest: produce a terrible opening sentence for a research report. This was irresistible. This is from the Editorial announcing the winners (*Nursing Research, *34 (2), 70, used with permission).*

The grand prize winner is Donna Diers of Yale University for a superbly dreadful sentence in the Parsonian mode of presentation. Note the magnificent redundancy, the carefree overdocumentation done with total disregard for the format required by *Nursing Research,* and the exquisite lack of punctuation that adds just the proper degree of confusion. Certainly, what follows is the height of failure.

> The interaction coefficient[1] in dyadic[2] helping[3] relationships[4] as occurs between nurses and patients[5] or nurse practitioners and patients[6] or clients[7] (for the distinction is characterized[8] by mutuality of duality as opposed to consensus of opporunity[9] correlates positively[10] with hierarchical but not dominance-performing distribution of rewards[11] (as occurs in balanced professional negotiations) and requires investigation beginning with taxonomical theoretically qualitative investigation but includes quasi-experimental derived hypothesis.[12] ...

If you can consciously write poorly, you know how to write well.

EDITORIALS

As before, the editorials here are from Image—Journal of Nursing Scholarship *(1986, 15(2), 30 and 1989 21(3), 122) used with permission. The first is early in my editorial tenure when the "nursing diagnosis" labeling movement was flowering. It drove me nuts. In my mind, the re-labeling of perfectly good words for diseases was an unfortunate response to organized medicine's claim that nurses could not diagnose disease, we could only diagnose responses to disease or "alterations" in processes. This is nonsense, especially in the world of advanced practice.*

This editorial is probably an overly subtle attack on this phenomenon. I could have been more...er...precise.

ON WORDS

A colleague passed the bowl of sour cream and chives for my baked potato and said, "Do you want to doctor it up?"

That started a line of thinking.

To "doctor" a cold is to take medicines. To "doctor" the confidential files is to adulterate them. To "doctor" the baked potato is to change its basic taste, consistency, and calorie count.

To "nurse" a cold is to go to bed with a good book, a box of tissues, a heating pad, and the phone off the hook. To "nurse" a car with a flat tire to the side of the road is to drive it slowly and carefully, making use of whatever steering control it has left. To "nurse" along a tray of herb seedlings is to water them often, cover them with plastic wrap in diffused light and, if you're really serious about it, sing to them.

We "doctor" *up* and "nurse" *along.*

One could conclude that these slang uses of nouns-turned-into-verbs connote that doctoring is changing the basic nature of things, while nursing is supporting the basic functions. An artificial separation at best. But we editor types get entranced with words.

A manuscript submitted to *Image* had the phrase, "they had a knowledge deficit" in it. The manuscript no longer has that phrase because it doesn't mean anything. Or more precisely, it doesn't mean anything very precise.

Oliver Sacks, a neurologist, has produced an exquisite book[1] in which he discusses what he calls "clinical tales." Neurology, he says, is a "mechanistic science, a system of capacities and connections. Deficit is neurology's favorite word. ... Either the function is normal or it is defective or faulty."[2] Thus in neurology, "deficit" has a precise meaning (which Sacks goes quite beyond, describing not only the pathology of symptoms but the experience of them). A "knowledge deficit" then is a defect.

That would mean a defect in knowledge, and knowledge is not among the things that can be broken. Or does the phrase mean that those in question did not have the information? The information was wrong? They could not understand it? They were ignorant? Stupid? Deluded? Untutored? Brain damaged?

What one decides to do to fix a knowledge deficit depends on what it is, precisely labeled. The language of anatomy or physiology is fine for describing parts of the body or processes of production and excretion. "Fractured femur" locates the problem; so does "trisomy 21" or "atrial ventricular fibrillation." As mapping the body and its process down to the cell level has become more particular, it has been possible to have more precise labels, precisely measured. And the vocabulary has grown.

The English language is full of subtle differences in etymology and meaning, just there for us to pick among in describing the behavior (including how the body behaves) to which we should pay attention. It is easy to settle on vague words and hope that operational definitions will name the properties. But when we are dealing with experiences of illness or disease, stress or joy, imprecise labeling understates the majesty of the phenomenon and the work in attending to it.

"Rude" behavior is different from "hostility"; "anxious" is different from "worried"; and "alteration" in anything is merely a change, with no sign of the direction of the change. The human body, the experience of living, the practice of professions deserves the kind of language that evokes the color and clarity of the work. Sacks' book is full of examples.

How about providing some of your own?

ON MODERN LANGUAGE

This editorial, 3 years later, speaks for itself both in terms of the theme of writing accurately, and clearly, and in revealing a certain political leaning. This is not a good editorial in the sense that there is too much going on. An Editorial ought to make one *point and move on. But still, I like it.*

For some years apparently, the Modern Language Association of America (MLA) has been debating, sometimes acrimoniously, various aspects of sexist or discriminatory language, toward creating new standards. The Commission on the Status of Women in the Profession of the Association has proposed new guidelines, contained in a book edited by Frank and Treichler, *Language, Gender and Professional Writing.*[3]

It raises one's consciousness about many issues, sexist language being only one of them.

I bought it thinking it would be helpful with some of the common problems manuscripts present, especially the "she" or "he" and generic "man" issues. It certainly is, with a thorough theoretical and sensitive discussion, eight alternatives and six guidelines. But the authors go on to deal with other troublesome issues, including another one that crops up often—the generic "they" as in "Nurses...they...". This construction seems to appear most often in non-clinical theory pieces, which may or may not mean something important. In clinical articles, authors tend to say, "Nurses...we...". The generic "they" makes the authors seem remote from the audience, which is strange if they are nurses. The rule, according to the MLA, should be to use the generic pronouns as little as possible, always making explicit the referents for "we," "our," "their," "us." The immediate consequence of reading this passage is a commitment on this page never to use the editorial "we" again, to conceal what are actually my very own thoughts and words. I promise.

A theme in the book is that the charming old ways of expressing things aren't so charming and probably never were. The editorial "we" is one of those. But even more important is the appeal to use words not only sensitively, but accurately, being mindful that sometimes the aim for utter neutrality obscures real and important ideas. For example, "domestic violence" is a gender-neutral term which hides the fact that most "domestic violence" is wife (woman) beating. "Incest" as a "family problem" spreads the guilt over however many family members there are, when the epidemiological fact is that most incest is father-daughter. The language scholar, Julia Penelope, says this usage "trivializes both the victimization of children and the male predation protected by the family."[4]

Neutral language, intended to remove prior sins of discrimination, may simply create the new sin of obfuscation. Perhaps there is a lesson for nursing here. In the early days of nursing diagnosis, an explicit agenda for the creation of new diagnoses was that they not be prejudicially worded. "Bad mother" (as if one would ever chart that anyway) was to be replaced by "alteration in parenting." Reminds me of the acronym sometimes used in newborn nurseries: FLK—funny looking kid, which turns out to be a useful stimulus for genetic or congenital problem workups). Neutrality is not always the highest priority.

We nurses care a lot about caring. Perhaps our modern language could use a review to see the extent to which it adequately expresses that central concept, or controverts it. For example, researchers write about the "subjects" of the study, by which they mean the people in the sample. Rarely, however, are the people really "subjected" to something not in their interest, and without their informed consent. If we are serious about caring, might it not be more accurate simply to say who the sample were: "participants," "couples," even "patients," or "clients," or "adolescent girls and boys" and turn them back into human beings? Do we really want to "intervene" instead of "comfort," "counsel," "talk," "change the dressing," "give the medicine," or even "nurse" (as a verb).

The MLA Committee extended its work into particular problems of scholarly writing, including citation practice, referencing, indexing, and the use of forms of address (Ms, Miss, Mrs.). On the last point, the threshold guideline for living persons is to use the form they prefer, including Professor or Dr. For historical figures, do not be anachronistic. Thus Miss Nightingale, not Ms (although she might well have preferred Ms!). The list of references is fascinating reading all by itself because not only are whole names used (Julia Penelope, William Safire) but where necessary, reference is made to other names under which the individual (usually the woman) might be known: see also Stanley, Julia Penelope, thus making it possible to recover the scholarship of women.

I think the book might have interest and impact not only in the small community of editors, but more generally to any community that aspires to justice in language and clarity in thought. And besides, sometimes it is just plain fun to read:

> ...in the 15th edition of the massive medical textbook *Williams Obstetrics*...which incidentally contains no pictures of women or babies, only parts, charts and organs, the index includes the entry "Chauvinism male, voluminous amounts, pp. 1–1190." Perhaps the indexing, done by the daughter of one of the editors, had some effect for the next edition lists only "Variable amounts."[5]

I checked the 18th edition—no listing for chauvinism. Perhaps it's been eliminated, or perhaps only the subversive feminist indexer has.

ENDNOTES

1. Sacks, O. (1986). *The Man Who Mistook His Wife for a Hat*. New York: Summit Books.

2. *Ibid.*, p. 81.

3. Frank, Francine Wattman, & Treichler, Paula A. (1989). *Language, Gender and Professional Writing*. New York: The Modern Language Association of America.

4. Penelope, Julia (1986). Lexicon of liberation. *Women's Review of Books, 3*(2), 9.

5. *Ibid.*, pp. 29–30.

THE ADVENTURE OF THOUGHT AND THE ADVENTURE OF ACTION

Speaking to an audience not composed of nurses is a different kind of challenge. One cannot use the professional shorthand we all use when we get together.

This speech was the welcoming address to the entering graduate and professional school students at Yale, September 23, 1983. Ordinarily, the President of the University would have given the welcoming speech but the late A. Bartlett Giamatti asked me to do it. I was by then the senior dean, rounding on 12 years in that role. I've always thought Bart just didn't want to have to give one more speech and this was an easy one to turf. I, on the other hand, took it as an occasion to demonstrate (if I could do it right) what nursing can do.

As I recall it, the speech was scheduled for a Wednesday afternoon. The previous weekend, I had been invited to dinner at Myrtle "Kitch" and Bill Aydelotte's summer home in Waterford, CT. The other guests included Florence and Henry Wald along with three other couples, including another nurse and a minister. Bill Aydelotte was a distinguished professor (his field was modern English history). Kitch is one of the early doctorally prepared nurses. She had done fundamentally important work on the working environment for nursing. Florence Wald brought hospice to the USA. She comes from a family of distinguished academics and is a fascinatingly complicated intellect. Her late husband, Henry, was an architect/engineer and their relationship, as Kitch's and Bill's, was lovely to watch.

After dinner, we were sitting in the living room of this cottage and somehow the topic of my assignment to do this speech came up. By then, I must have had a draft in mind, for Kitch remembers the conversation turning on the notion of "craft" I intended to use. As Kitch described it, "Our debate was very lively that evening. Everyone became involved. And since the group was comprised of an engineer, a minister, nurses, a historian, and a lawyer, many and varied points of view emerged. Very stimulating and energizing! Sam (the minister) said he was going to make use of the ideas for a sermon! The evening was a great success!"[1] The discussion was truly a salon *in the French sense of huge minds tossing ideas around. I remember driving home that night feeling as if my head was exploding. Their generosity and kindness were priceless.*

I found it immensely satisfying to use words about nursing to connect to a very mixed audience, and to craft a speech in both the High Church prose one must affect in these kinds of ceremonial events and the vernacular. People laughed in the right places. The speech surprised some of my University colleagues who only saw me in committee meetings. Battling over a budget or negotiating tenure appointments doesn't allow one to show how much I really love and understand This Place, Yale, warts and all.

And, of course, a major speech at Yale must include some reference to that other place up the road in Boston: Harvard.

Mr. President, Officers of the University, decanal colleagues, faculty, students of the graduate and professional schools of Yale:

It is reported that at an anonymous institution somewhere north of here, the dean of the law school annually greets incoming students with the instruction to look to the person on the left and the one on the right and realize that in a year, only one of the three of them will be left.

It is written that at a fictitious medical school, the dean greets the new students with the news that of their number, ten will fail the science courses, two will contract tuberculosis, one will die of hepatitis, and four will become schizophrenic.

A friend informs me that at a certain business school (also somewhat north of here), the dean's introductory remarks are an extended plea for generous gifts to the alumni fund.

I have resisted copying the law school approach, for it simply is not true, in law or any other school. I have discarded the proposed medical school orientation because it, too, is not true. And with great strength of character, I have put aside the temptation to plead for alumni fund gifts.

I have struggled, however, for a way to provide for all of you a shared picture of what this place is and alert you to examine your experience within it. For just as commencement addresses take one last shot at filling in the spaces in the graduates' learning, sealing in the resin as it were, orientation remarks should make the sap flow, not be just filler between two hymns.

One fact (perhaps the last true example of that endangered species you will encounter) I give you: by Yale's tradition, there is no commencement address. Thus, arduous as your time here may be you may look forward in 1984, or 5, or 6, or 7, or 8, or 9 (we do hope you are all gone by 1990) to a mercifully brief and moving commencement at which, by God's tradition, the sun almost always shines.

At first glance, nothing other than your simultaneous presence seems to provide common ground. Unlike undergraduates, you are not defined well by age or even generation. Some of you are already beyond basic professional education, for you are already musicians, foesters, actors, nurses, teachers, perhaps published poets. Some are entering a profession for the first time, and will emerge from here as physicians, lawyers, scholars, ministers, managers, scientists. Some will find the experience more contemplative than social; others will mine the human encounter whether the encounter is with audiences, juries, parishioners, or patients. Your tools will be pencils, protractors, or computers, or you will practice with your hands, voice, body, argument, or empathy.

A reading of the bulletins of the various professional schools, and the graduate school you now enter, reveals little consistency in requirements for the degree, course loads, curricular structure, advisor systems, grading practice, or for that matter, tuition. Yet every single catalog defines the student body by its unusual promise, demonstrated talent, and strong motivation, which is why you are here.

I, on the other hand, am here today to try to bring together, at least in abstraction, the various graduate and professional schools and students. And perhaps in the process, propose some ways of thinking about higher education that might make sense of your own experience as well as this event.

The literature in higher education is full of invidious dichotomies. "Art," is the opposite of "science" it is said; "science" is not "scholarship"; "pure" science is set against "applied" science; "science" or "scholarship" are contrasted with "performance" or "practice." The heuristic usefulness of such dichotomous divisions has become locked into educational policy and politics and, unfortunately, by labeling the core of disciplines, it may be thought that boundaries are also defined.

The words used to define are thought also to describe disciplines, which is not true. In all cases, the words understate the scope and majesty of what you enter here. "Art," for example does not completely describe the work of the musician, actor, painter, poet, or architect. "Science" does not contain the whole of biology, medicine, or physics. "Scholarship" is not all there is to history or French or political science.

If there is an important dichotomy to understand, it is not the ones I have set up as straw men. It is the difference between undergraduate education and graduate education. Among the many ways to think of that difference, I have chosen three.

The first is that graduate and professional students are older than undergraduates. A fairly obvious empirical observation, perhaps, but oddly one does not see much consideration of what that observation might portend. Undergraduates are most often 16 to 22 years old. Cognitive psychology, human development, and any number of other disciplines have helped us understand that people—16- to 22-year-old people—may look grown up but have had a very limited number of years in which their neurologic functions, hormonal balances, or social learning have prepared them to grasp the intricacies of both the "liberal arts" and late adolescent life development. It is something of a modern miracle that universities do as well as they do with a confusing societal mission of educating people whose synapses are less than fully functional, not only to grasp the subtleties of literary interpretation or research method, but to understand the world and make choices about living in it with civility, humor, and a personal sense of self and values. The students are to be congratulated for this accomplishment as well!

For the faculty of the graduate and professional schools, there is the unstated luxury of being able to depend on working with people with a level of life experience and maturity that allows collegiality impossible when students are younger. Whether as students you feel ready for it or not, the process of graduate and professional teaching is to draw out rather than to stuff in.

The newer intellectual disciplines rely heavily on the flashes of insight of those new to the field, for innovation and discovery are simply waiting to be made. The older fields rely on new people to question the very nature of historic truth, for understanding is advanced when we know more about the context of discovery and verification and we cannot know that until we have new contexts, which you bring, against which to test older ideas. The limits of human capacity—intellectual ability, sensitivity, experience, or intuition— keep being expanded and we depend upon you to push.

It happens in all fields. The flute is now not only a wind instrument; in the hands of some, it can also be a percussion instrument, thanks to the effort of one who did not take for granted the limits of the tool. Number theory is profoundly changed by someone who did not believe that the traditional way of thinking about prime numbers exhausted the possibilities. The social significance of drama and the theatre is intensified when public performance is used to teach us something about apartheid, or dying, or intimacy, or the use of silence, or the glory of language as it illuminates life. Forestry is no longer only the study of plants and trees and how they grow, but the relationship of that to human life and leisure, and then the consequences of human interventions upon nature. Law is not just logical argument, but increasingly ethics, tragic choices, standards for civilized existence.

The first theme, then, is that graduate education is interactive, for the clashing of minds and ideas is what moves knowing forward.

The second theme has to do with a part of what is to be learned: skill.

"Skill" is a much-abused notion, for it implies a mindlessness—a division of thought from physical action. There is something vaguely prepubertal about the notion of "skill," as if all the skills one would ever need to know are learned by the age of ten. "Skills" are the rudiments of more complicated things, it is thought, and therefore, rote, unchanging, mechanical.

The acquisition of skill is taken to distinguish graduate education in the humanities and social sciences from professional education, and advanced education from undergraduate. There is in all the graduate and professional disciplines important emphasis on development of skill—whether it is measurement calibration, listening to heart sounds, paint brush technique, or careful documentation of sources.

Advanced education must include skill development, but it is neither fair nor accurate to assume that the use of such skill is easy or automatic. What is to be accomplished in graduate and professional education is in part the absorption of learned skills so deep into the banks of memory and fibers of the nervous system that they can be called up and counted upon with instant reliability. Viewed from outside, excellent performance—whether it is acting or lecturing or writing or diagnosis—appears so effortless that it is therefore thought to be only skill. Carefully learned skill frees the mind for analysis, for decision-making, for innovation and choice, whether the choice is a tint or shade of color, a kind of breath control that makes the bass notes vibrate, a twist of meaning, or an original hypothesis.

Skill is thought to be static; once learned, it sticks and endures. Yet the importance of skill is that it is never taken for granted. The 200th time one plays a D minor scale, the 3000th *picea pungens* one sees, the 154th laboring woman one supports, the 72nd reference on a given topic all remain fresh to the educated person; for there is always an opportunity to learn more and to make understanding deeper through repeated experience. No matter how many times data collection is done, every occasion contains the possibility of creation, of discovery, and therefore of change.

Skill is application and thus connects the mind and intellect with the body, and both of those with the social contract. Learning skill is advanced beyond undergraduate education which does not require mastery, but at the same time, skill is not what defines graduate or professional education, for skill mastery is only the board from which it is possible to leap.

The third theme here is perhaps the most important characteristic of graduate and professional education. It is the element of passion that you bring to it because you have chosen a life of special devotion to a particular interest. What makes one choose to continue to pursue some line of inquiry, some discipline, science, art, or profession is passion—a love so deep that to express it fully requires immersion. More than a passion simply for learning, this passion inflames the spirit and forces one not just to learn or to practice but increasingly to *become*. One *is* a scientist, a minister, a scholar, an actor, a physician.

Passion is informed by wonder. Wonder is felt in recognizing endless possibilities in the chosen field. There is wonder in discovering the need to balance responsibility with liberty, discipline with license, containment with exploration. And there is wonder in realizing that the challenge of school is no longer purely intellectual, but rather is figuring out what you are, so as to use that ability, talent, intellect, experience, soul to both fuel and live up to the intensity of commitment passion requires. That realization does not happen until one has identified, on whatever grounds, one's choice of basket to put one's eggs in.

Along with passion and wonder goes another dimension of the intellectual work of specialization. That is the learning of generosity, for to feel wonder is to admire the work of others or the mystery of the unknown, which is an act of giving, of generosity. And that generosity is followed quickly by the pain of humility as one confronts the bottomless realization that there is always more to learn and feel and grasp than one possibly can.

The quality, then, that most distinguishes undergraduate from graduate education, no matter what the field, is specialization.

Now, commentary on higher education is full of hortatorical demands that students not become so specialized in particle physics or the novel of the 19th century, or law, or medicine that you can no longer appreciate Jackson Pollack, Don Shirley's jazz, or a walk in the park.

Specialization as intellectual effort is not so much narrowing as it is deepening; not so much removing one from thinking about other things beyond one's particular specialty choice as developing that part of the physiological brain in which analysis and synthesis, creativity, and imagination can be channeled.

To choose a field of study or professional practice is indeed to eliminate competing choices. But to choose to pursue law and not simultaneously follow philosophy, or to follow a passion for history and not composing, or medicine and not forestry is only a focus, not a decision to let atrophy other interests and talents. A liberal education gives one an appreciation, even a love, for bodies of knowledge or information or fields and therefore the capacity to admire the work of others. Choosing one field does eliminate an equivalent investment in another, but does not cancel enthusiasm. People of scope and brilliance, which is what you are, can easily accommodate more than one thought at a time, and more than one focus of energy. Further, a decision for specialization in training at one time does not preclude either a change of mind or a different decision at another time. What we worry about is that your passion for whatever field you have chosen not consume you entirely so that your other interests or enthusiasms or expressions of gifted amateurism go undeveloped.

Many otherwise sane writers have complained wistfully that the store of information in any field and any specialty is now too great to be comprehended by any single person.

It is not only the accumulation of knowledge that has made it impossible now for anybody to grasp the whole of any theory, whether it is the role of symbolism in Shakespeare, the ecology of the Sahel, sonata form from Mozart to Bernstein, constitutional law, or financial analysis. What has happened to knowledge is that the world has intruded upon it and now ideas that once could be considered in pristine isolation hold no validity without an understanding of their history and place and geography. Freud's views of libido, ego, and id are no longer possible to understand and appreciate for their historic significance, if not for the predictive value, without understanding the life of his time and place, his addiction to cocaine, his wish to appease his reading public by calling hysteria a female fantasy rather than a realistic reaction to incest. The study of the effect of acid rain on the ecology of New England is enlivened when the economics and politics of industrial and military development are added. Contemporary history, economics, literature, or art are fundamentally changed when alternative paths of explanation are provided by the increasing attention to information from those who did the work of battle rather than leading the charge, or those who saw the bombs dropped or their families led away, or those who care for people wasted physically or culturally when artificial drought claimed their land because the water was diverted elsewhere.

What links the graduate and professional schools or disciplines is not only their difference from undergraduate education but their shared values and the nature of the work. The notion that there is a real difference between "graduate school" and the University's "professional" schools implies a uselessness to the tradition of scholarship for its own sake that is fair neither to the humanities students nor to their colleagues in performance.

"Pure" or more generally "basic" science or scholarship (for the two are very much the same in a context of values) has been thought to be pure or basic because the content of the field and of the research or scholarship is untouched by values, which are thought to be corrupting. Values as biases are corrupting when they eliminate, consciously or otherwise, consideration of alternative hypotheses or points of view. Perhaps only number theory or theoretical physics are immune from a societal context, but even if they are, so what? Is there truly an important difference in either the science of the scientists, the scholarship or the scholar, between those fields which produce useable, applicable information more or less immediately, and those which do not? They are different, surely, in their methods, and perhaps in the psychology of their adherents. But doing mathematics or nuclear physics is neither harder nor easier than doing law, or medicine, or composing, land management, or nursing.

Scholarship or science are professions just as architecture is, or business, or stage design, pediatrics, or any of the other majors you have signed up for. There is no intellectual arena in which application or performance is either impossible or forbidden. Even in the most esoteric and least functional field the science or scholarship is used, and that means applied, to stimulate the person with the next theorem or hypothesis, the next set of equations, if not for building a better rocket launcher.

The distinction between those who think and those who do reminds me of an equally silly comparison between the University, withy its ivory or ivy-covered towers and the so-called "real world." As President Giamatti has pointed out, the life of the mind, the life of study and scholarship and science and performance is no less real than any other way of living. Thoughtless stereotyping assumes that science or scholarship is creative, uses the imagination, requires discipline that the performing arts or applied sciences do not. No one who has watched a student cellist work for precisely the right angle of the elbow to draw out the pianissimo required by the composer can believe that for long. No one who has watched actors rehearse, knowing that the study of the language, of movement, of the play writer's intentions, of psychology, has preceded the rehearsal, can doubt the complexity and intelligence of that particular kind of doing. No one who has sat through a case analysis in marketing and heard the use of economic theory, analysis of human behavior, and ethics can come away thinking business is simple.

Thus, in a search for ways to describe what is common to the experience of the kind of specialization and professional education that you are here for, one must discard the convenient labels and go for a commonality, really a community of meaning, bound together by some shared conception of the nature of the work, mutual identity, equality, and equity.

I spoke earlier about the influence of personal development upon the life of the mind, about passion, skill, wonder, and qualities of intellectual work. And I suggested that the words used to describe the field of graduate and professional study—art, science, applied science, performance, practice, scholarship—do not completely adumbrate the work.

Perhaps what we are about, in part then, is the teaching and learning of *craft*.

Crafts, it is thought, are minor art forms done by nimble-fingered natives or by women at home with time on their hands and a basket of yarn at their feet, so maybe you shudder at the notion that your art or science or profession might have something of craft in it.

Craft has the meaning of strength as well as skill, and surely the muscular leap of insight the scholar, the clinician, the lawyer feel (and "feel" is the operative word) when she or he suddenly *understands* it is a show of strength. In crafts, the esthetic is connected with the functional. The work of the mind in craft is holding a mental image of the finished product, then selecting material, tool, and technique to create. Such selection is very complicated and requires much more than mere practice or skill, for it takes knowing the structure—the theory, if you will—of the wood or metal or warp.

Craft requires more than simply understanding of the material, just as scientists and scholars and clinicians and performers cannot settle for simply knowing and keeping that knowledge confined in the head. Craft is what the delicate work of science and scholarship is, when the struggle for clarity and precision is going on. Craft implies beauty as value. The search for beauty is what motivates the clinician as much as it moves the performer, the scholar and scientist as much as the artist. Surely cure is more attractive than disease, and belief more beautiful than confusion; logic is prettier than irrationality, and order more decorative than chaos. Nature can produce art but only human beings can do craft.

"Craft" unlike "scholarship" or "science" implies visibility, a product of the hands. The work of hands is nearly always less valued than the work of the mind, but visible work is complicated because it is judged by others. Yet the work of all the graduate and professional fields is visible, always.

Scholarship is visible when it is published or taught and it requires exactly the same discipline of form and style, substance and clarity as service or professional practice. The craft of the lawyer, the minister, the physician brings together the parts of the discipline called art or science in the service of others, so the notion of craft as service is yet another way in which the work of the graduate and professional fields have a common base. In fact, all of the fields are not only crafts, but also have in them all art and science and scholarship as well as service, and all share a common purpose. And that purpose is, precisely and painfully, to change the world.

Some of us have a societal professional mandate for change, we physicians, nurses, lawyers, ministers. Some of us have a less explicit but equally compelling agenda: to make the world more beautiful through music, or art, or architecture, or writing, poetry, or their complex mix in theatre. Even the most arcane of the academic disciplines harbors this operational mission of production, whether the product is formulas, or gifts of graceful expression. All visible products, then, of graduate and professional school faculty and students change the world, for we cannot help but make change.

What is exciting about being in this place, in this blink of geological time, is that we are entering a period of the most profound change. Yes, there will be substantive discoveries of subatomic particles or explanations of autoimmune disease or socioeconomic trends or computer applications, and you will make some of them. But you will also participate in more ephemeral changes, as you inadvertently do today.

The President's choice to provide me the opportunity to greet you this afternoon is a symbolic event both for you and for me. I have chosen, therefore, to speak in metaphors of community, commonality, living, and connectedness which are rooted in my intellectual tradition as a woman and my conceptual base as a nurse.

There is one final way in which we are all connected. We are all part of the moving river of history and tradition, as your printed program makes clear. I am privileged today to wear the academic gown of Elizabeth BixlerTorrey, third Dean of the School of Nursing. Fortunately, it fits. The hood I wear is the academic hood of Annie Warburton Goodrich, first Dean of the School of Nursing, and it is over 60 years old. Its threadbareness is deserved.

I shall end then, by invoking my predecessor's words. Miss Goodrich was writing in 1933 about why nursing should be a university-based discipline, for Yale was the first university to accept nursing as a field worthy of the University's standards and name. Her words are about nursing, but I ask you to make a mental substitution of your own noun, for her truth transcends my beloved field.

She begins by quoting one Chancellor Lindley:

> A liberal education will lift any ordinary job from the level of task to the level of an art, and from the level of an art to the level of a religion—through the leadership of artists, not the merchants of art.

Miss Goodrich goes on in her own words:

> To be less than artists in this field of human engineering is to betray the greatest cause upon which man has yet embarked.

And she continues:

> ...the function of the college should be to stimulate, not appease the great hunger for life of mental satisfaction.

To the nurse... (she says, and here, substitute scholar, actor, musician, lawyer, whatever your profession)

> ...to the nurse, working in the different levels of the social structure, in touch with the fundamentals of human experience is given a unique opportunity to relate the adventure of thought to the adventure of action; this to the end that a new social order to which we are committed by our forefathers may be realized.[2]

ENDNOTES

1. Aydelotte to Diers, Email, August 18, 2003.
2. Goodrich, Annie Warburton. (1933). *The Social and Ethical Significance of Nursing.* New York: Macmillan, p. 14. Republished by permission on the occasion of the 50th Anniversary of the Yale University School of Nursing, 1973.

FINDING NURSING

I fell in love with Australia on the first trip and have returned as often as I am asked, at least annually. During the 20+ years I have been visiting, I have witnessed the stunning move of nursing into the universities, nearly overnight, the growth and development of nursing scholarship, the development of a particularly Australian brand of nursing politics and policy. The issues for nursing there are not different from those in other countries, including the USA. First always is the general invisibility of nursing in management, clinical, and policy contexts.

The College of Nursing of New South Wales has no equivalent in US terms. It is part honor society, like Sigma Theta Tau. It provides post-graduate certification courses in a large number of specialties. It engages in serious policy work. It has housed research including some of the most powerful policy-related studies in nursing in Australia: casemix (DRGs and nursing acuity), and nurse practitioners.

The College puts on an annual event, the Oration. It is held in the Great Hall of Sydney University, a cathedral. It is decorated with Australian native flowers in profusion; an organ processional escorts the officers and officials of as many organizations as have sent representatives. Like all public nursing events in Australia, it is inherently political.

I was invited to give the 2002 Oration, the first American in some years. I used the occasion to try to stretch myself, to develop ways to talk about nursing that were different from anything I'd ever done. (Used with permission.)

It was a gorgeous October evening, in Australian spring. The purple jacarandas were blooming, as were the Gymean lilies, an impossible plant that can grow nearly 30 feet tall with a huge complicated rose colored flower on a skinny, woody stalk. I wore my doctoral academic gown, which is scarlet with a white navy-style collar, and a black velvet hat. I look something like the guy on the Beefeater gin bottle.

An occasion like this requires not only a different style of writing, but a presentation that is close to preaching. They told me afterward this was truly an Oration.
I have left the Australian spelling intact.

The honour you have done me by inviting me to give this Oration is matched entirely by my terror at the thought of doing it. The deliberate solemnity of the occasion and the setting, the importance of using this brief time to fashion a "gathering," in the Quaker sense, of nurses on the 50th occasion of the Oration—I take this gift in this sunburned country, now a second home to me, with profound appreciation and humility.

My friend, the late Professor John D. Thompson, he of DRG fame, once received an award for that work with Professor Robert Fetter and was required to give an oration. He defined an oration as "a paper without slides which addresses a theme more cerebral than a research report."[1] And indeed, I feel naked without my PowerPoint and laser pointer, my line drawings and ClipArt.

For this occasion, I *will* attempt something different from the charts and graphs and data-driven presentations you might normally expect from me. Important as research and data-mining are, tonight I wish to suggest that there are also ways of finding nursing that reveal different facets of the work, giving us new ways of expressing our contribution to society.

For that's what it's all about, no?

Had I not been asked to give this Oration, I would not have exposed myself to the writing about nursing practice in Australia as I have done, and I am much the better for it. I hope you—the leadership in nursing here—appreciate...no *revel in, celebrate*...the incredible nursing practices and scholarship you have created. On your own terms, and on a very fast track, as Australians would always do.

When I talk about finding nursing then, it is not because nursing is lost. Nursing has existed as long as human kind. As nursing has evolved into professional practice with educational standards, our own science, politics, and policy issues, our literature has contained a fair amount of dithering as well as reasoned debate about what nursing *is*. There is something to be said for considering the various ways in which nursing can be found, and the purposes to which the exercise of finding can be put.

There is finding nursing in the grace of grinding daily practice of the profession whether on the ward or in the community or in the classroom or the metaphorical corridors of New South Wales Health [Department]. There is finding nursing to justify budgets and hospital expenditures. There is finding nursing to compete with other disciplines for university approbation and support. There is finding nursing to attract new lives into the profession. There is finding nursing's roots in our history to inform our present.

There is finding nursing in publication and presentation, in interdisciplinary circles.

"Finding nursing" really stands for finding ways to understand and then to portray the complexity of our work, whenever and wherever we need to do it, increasingly in public places and contexts.

I take my marching orders from your very own Agnes Mary Lion. In introducing the first Annual Oration of the NSW College of Nursing in 1953, she said that the purpose of conducting such orations was "to invite women...to present a word-picture of the lovely colour and pattern that is traced on the canvas of modern life by 'human kindness skilfully administered' which is nursing. To emphasise the value of every minute particle of pigment, every tiny brushmark so that each member of our profession will be further convinced of the community's need of her."[2]

So let me tell a tiny brushmark story of a mother's experience of nursing:

> When my son Colter was six years old, he was diagnosed with Hodgkins disease. I will never forget the day he was about to receive his first blood transfusion. We were all there in the room: three residents, a nurse, myself, and Colter. Everything had been prepared, and the procedure was just about to begin when Colter suddenly shrieked: "Wait a minute! Stop!" The doctors were taken aback.
>
> The nurse asked, "What's the matter, Colter?" Colter replied, in fear and trepidation, "Is this *girl* blood or *boy* blood?" The doctors were truly at a loss for words, but the nurse replied without missing a beat, "Well, of course it's *boy* blood, Colter! We wouldn't give you *girl* blood. That has *cooties*!"[3]

The community's need of her....

I start with this story to illustrate first, the power of anecdote to express something important about the practice of nursing and second, to draw out the fact that nursing's focus is not only on personal services but also on what science calls "operations." Not operations as surgery, but operations as making things work. That is the very hardest part of nursing to convey to others, to explain to the world, to make visible, to *find* in nursing. For capturing nursing as practice and operations, we might think about the methods and media that especially serve the living sense of action, surprise, rhythm, and crescendo, and particularly what it feels like to do this work.

Feels?

But isn't nursing about scientific performance?

I turn to your Megan-Jane Johnstone whose work in bioethics is astonishingly direct, which is a lovely characteristic of Australian nursing scholarship. In one part of her book, she discusses the way nurses felt about working in instances of spontaneous abortion (and other settings) studied by two

American psychiatrists. They (who were, of course, from Harvard, not Yale) concluded that the distress nurses reported in participating in this sort of situation was largely the product of nurses "over-identifying" with the fetus. These psychiatrists concluded that the nurses who over-identified the most were themselves adopted or had adopted children or had had difficulty conceiving—variables on which they had absolutely *no* data.[4]

Hear the words Johnstone uses to describe this:

> The quantum leap in logic...can only be marvelled at...What [the nurses] saw was a tiny and uniquely human form of life made vulnerable by medical intervention. This sight—as any delicate sight has the power to do—caused in the nurses...emotion. This feeling...is hardly startling and certainly hardly the basis for making a sound psychiatric diagnosis! The medicalisation of emotion is something which all caring, sensitive and feeling people need to be very aware of and ever vigilant to avoid.[5]

Megan-Jane Johnstone's analysis of this idiosyncratic medicalisation of emotion signals how difficult it is in nursing for us to live a professional life in which feelings—our own and others—are simultaneously so organically fundamental to the work and so hard for others to take comfortably. And so hard to capture and use in research and policy.

Claire Fagin and I said it this way when we wrote about the metaphors nursing holds for our many publics. One of the metaphors is intimacy:

> Nurses are involved in the most private aspects of people's lives, and [we] cannot hide behind technology or a veil of omniscience...Nurses do for others publicly what healthy persons do for themselves behind closed doors. Nurses, as trusted peers, are there to hear secrets, especially the ones born of vulnerability. Nurses are treasured when these interchanges are successful, but most often people do not wish to remember their vulnerability or loss of control, and nurses are indelibly identified with those terribly personal times.[6]

We are finding new ways to understand the emotional (and bioethical) contexts in which nurses work as painful contemporary decisions hit us.

There has been a fascinating series of articles recently in the USA evaluating the state of Oregon's controversial "Death with Dignity" act which made it legal in that state for physicians to prescribe and make available lethal drugs in amounts to assist patients to suicide. There is no provision in this law for any further participation of the physician in administering the drugs. Assisted suicide is a hard thing to think about. Two recent studies have examined the extent to which, in Oregon, physicians are actually participating in this activity and then, in hospice settings, the perceptions of nurses, not about participating in assisted suicide, but more interestingly, in what they have observed are the patient situations that occasion the wish to fashion care so as to die with dignity.

The data about physicians shows that they struggle with their own values (note: not feelings) to decide how to respond to a patient's request under the law, or at least that's the way the data is collected and reported.[7] Indeed, the subtitle for the article is "These are uncharted waters for both of us [physicians and patients]". The decision to assist with suicide or not tests the Hypocratic oath as well as perceptions of the law to the extreme. The writing (including letters to the Editors) is emotional but not *feeling*. It is on the level of morality—"yes," participating in assisted suicide is right or "no," it's not with whatever arguments the writer poses. There is a substitution of moral condition for the intimately personal *experience* of physician and patient. In contrast (and I am not setting this as superior reasoning) the study of nurses focuses on their work in helping patients come to their own decisions and then working to make that happen, sometimes in spite of their own moral opinions about physician-assisted suicide.[8] The title of this article is "*Experiences of...nurses...*" Interestingly, both studies come to the same epidemiological conclusion about the most frequent reason patients ask for assistance of this kind—a desire to control the circumstances of death—but what that means to either discipline is quite different. Nurses' experiences are not medicalised emotion here but their moral stances are not examined. In contrast, physicians are denied feelings and pressed to declare their moral positions.

When nursing moved into the university, in the USA or in Australia, we were pressed to look like other academic disciplines. That meant we had to have theories and hypotheses and research methods and explanations for our work. For a time, in the USA, we turned to social science to save us. I suppose that was because we needed to distinguish ourselves and our intellectual work from medicine. That was a political decision, to keep schools of nursing from being handmaidens to schools of medicine. ... In Australia, my observation would be that, rather than turning to social science, your early intellectual work (and early here means about 1986!) turned to more lonely philosophical turns of mind, perhaps making a connection with the traditions of scholarship of your own universities. Since you went from hospital school bases so quickly through the levels of education, you have not been as subject to the overarching political power of schools of medicine as we in the USA have been. That has produced, I think, interesting differences in the research and scholarship here from other countries, not only the USA.

Your scholarship, like ours, had to dig its roots into what I have called "finding nursing." Social scientists in the USA were asked to help us define nursing through research, and, of course, that is a silly question.[9] Some of us wrote that we already know what nursing is, now we were challenged—in the 1960s—to demonstrate the effects or impact of nursing practices. ...[10]

Here, listen to your leader, Judy Lumby:

> although many technological devises when first introduced were presented as time-saving, in reality the nurse has been left to ensure that, for example, the tracing leads are placed correctly..., the monitor is accurate, readouts are recorded...for the doctors and the patient is educated about the...technology. Unlike other workplaces where it seems that the introduction of technology has...changed the level of staff required, in health [care] the opposite has occurred. We needed better trained staff and more of them...While technological devices in hospitals provide more accurate data, they require skilled insertion, management and interpretation of results if the data are to be believed.
>
> Without such reassurance, the utility and safety of new technology is questionable.[11]

That is a clear piece of prose, aimed for an audience of lay persons and policy makers. It will make a difference.

Listen to another, this by my great friend, Mary Chiarella:

> Tonight patients will die in nursing homes and on wards and many of these cases nurses will not wake the doctors to confirm that the patient is dead, simply because there will be no need to do so. They will contact the relatives, lay out the patients and help the famil[ies] to grieve. Today or tomorrow or the next day, a nurse may or may not intervene to stop a doctor from making a mistake which might harm the patient. It will not depend on the law. It will depend on the courage of the nurse. Nurses operate inside (or outside) a legal framework which unsufficiently recognises their work and their presence. The developing body of jurisprudence which calls itself health law will not be complete until it addresses the problems and difficulties encountered by nurses...and recognises their central role in health care delivery.[12]

These examples are intended to not only to speak to difficult contemporary issues in nursing but also to show how powerful, pointed prose conveys the nature of our work to audiences outside the discipline so much better than high-flying conceptual paradiddles.

When nursing was struggling for our place in academe and in the professional worlds in which we operate, we needed to use the language of those settings. Now, I believe we might be also—not better—but *also* served by seizing upon an unnoticed benefit of the move of nursing to the university: the fact that we now have students and graduates who come from different educational strands than did our mothers and fathers and aunts and uncles. That means that there is building now a cadre of nurses who have new tools, new ways of talking, writing about the nature of the work. These people will force us to different ways of thinking about our science, and our art and our craft which will move nursing to places we need to go, in policy and practice.

We need to seek these new forms of expression to capture the intricate emotional intensity so decried by the psychiatrists about whom Megan-Jane Johnstone wrote. Nursing has in it always the uncompromising combination of horror and joy, of birthing and dying, pain and cure, and those are as real and as worthy of communicating as statistical significance, clinical pathway variances, the qualities of evidence, and cardiac monitoring. We are grown up enough as a discipline to find the sensibility to turn description to lyrical language.

Listen to my colleague, David Evans, as he writes about passion as a part of nursing excellence:

> Excellent nurses are inflamed by nursing. The flesh may fail. The spirit may momentarily sink. But in the inner reaches of ourselves as nurses, we hunger and thirst after nursing. ...A nurse cared for Amy, a 13-year-old girl with...scoliosis...He taught her about a spinal fusion with Harrington rod insertion. He medicated her. Both afraid, they comforted one another in the cool hallways of the OR: "You really didn't hurt me with the needles," she sobbed, filling the tremulous spaces in their talk...Later...the obligatory Demerol injected to calm the...pain, he stood beside the bed as her mother leaned over Amy, vulnerable and fragile in the half cast. He yearned to enter that twosome, to feel their pain and their unity. He saw only their profiles in the dim light, so alike and so close. But the communion was sacred. If there was a passion in his involvement with this family, there was also a passion in keeping his distance. Benevolently rejected, the nurse needed the humility to appreciate that. It took deep energy—passion—to do that.
>
> ...Passion unifies us and makes us spiritual and professional equals. Rubbing someone's skin with modulated strokes is as profound an experience as delivering a thunderous appeal for restitution before a Senate Sub-committee. If we think about this passion in nursing, then perhaps we can understand our own frustration at others' views that most of nursing is menial and often meaningless drudgery, as if it were some prison sentence we dutifully endure while we grope, pilgrim-like, toward the free air of teaching, administration or an expanded role. Nonsense. To be an excellent nurse is not to be serving time; it is more to be making love.[13]

David's lyrical powers are highly developed—he was an English teacher before he chose nursing. In this brief passage, he elevates the description of what Beverley Taylor,[14] and her inspiration, Alan Pearson[15] call the "ordinariness of nursing" to the level of art. It is important to note that Taylor's point of view is not only the experience of being a patient, but also the experience of doing nursing, doing "ordinary" things to and with strangers, which transforms the experience to from ordinary to extraordinary for both participants.

In a conversation with Professor Pearson, whom I had not met before, last July in Melbourne, I told him that while I was taken with the notion of "ordinariness," Beverley Taylor's book made me sad. "Sad" probably wasn't the most felicitous word. What I really meant was that the intricate notion of ordinariness as the social contract in nursing simply cried for forms of expression that could find the wonder, the glory, and majesty of nursing, that might require not so much description as scriptural prose or poetry.

Listen to this:

> Nursing puts us in touch with being human. Nurses are invited into the inner spaces of other people's existence without even asking, for where there is suffering, loneliness, the tolerable pain of cure or the solitary pain of permanent change, there is the need for the kind of human service we call nursing.
>
> The intimacy that is the core of nursing gives us a peculiar aura, and just as some people feel awkward in the presence of a visibly pregnant woman—so clear is the fact of her intimacy—some people are embarrassed in the company of nurses. We are supposed to be dignified over vomitus, uncringing at the sight of blood, calm as we debride the decubitus, pack the wound, give out the bad news. Nurses must hear, but never tell, the secrets of the dark side of the soul, the hates and jealousies, the anger and violence, the cursings at fate, the bargains with God. The terrors of psychosis, the joy of a peaceful and happy birth, the erosions of poverty and discrimination that turn a body thin and sour-smelling are part of the nurse's world, all day, every day.
>
> ...The nurse is in charge of all of the health-care system and must make it work in the service of those who need and want it. It is the nurse who must see that the room is warm and the ice is cold, the dinner is served properly and on time, the doctor is called and informed, the family is comforted, the lab gets its results back on time, x-ray pays attention, the floors are swept, and the costs—ah yes, always the costs—are kept down.[16]

That was a much younger me, writing for an educated lay audience. My experience in using this kind of writing—scriptural or not—is that it penetrates better than the judiciously balanced prose we usually use for professional communication.

But is such writing academically or politically credible?

Your own Kim Walker has given voice to this thought in a lovely essay.[17] Kim argues for the legitimacy of "poetics" and a narrative tradition as research, as scholarship, to build a space for "narrative rememberings", a permanent record of that "vast and messy thing called 'practice' available for reflection, analysis, theorizing." He particularly notes that "the ways in which we use language are utterly pivotal" and a couple of pages later, presents a poem by his school-friend, Janet Charman:

> i remember
> on afternoon shift
> how I stroked
> my own passion
> into some old lady's
> unsunned
> flabby back
> concentrating
> in the afterdinner
> hotwash
> on stupefying
> the sick old body
> into fragile
> comfort
> with these gentle
> insistent attentions[18]

Janet Charman is a professional poet. Kim writes that she never practiced long as a nurse, but clearly her memory of the work endures.

Hear a similar song from a young man in his first weeks of nursing:

> Name: CP
> Age: 34
> Sex: Male
> Race: Caucasian
> Admission Date: August 1, 1999
>
> I spoke with him
>   Or was it at him?
> "Just in case," I told myself.
> Just in case he was afraid.
> Just in case he was confused.
> Just in case he needed to hear his name.
> Just in case the cough when we suctioned him was more
>   than reflex.

Just in case he knew how fucked up he was.
Just in case there was someone behind the Duratear glazed
    eyes who was
Hovering
In my nightmare, unable to scream,
    Claw,
    Kick,
    Cry,
    Or reason his way out of it.
Just in case my voice or words could comfort him.[19]

In commenting on Janet's poem (and in words that apply equally to John Leopold's), Kim unites us in a moment we have all shared: "In these words is caught...such an elegantly simple chain of signifiers [which] vivify and incarnate the work we do, which is often dismissed and demeaned as trivial, ordinary and routine. But it is work only some care to do." Kim calls such expressions a "culturally creative act." In suggesting research as one way to retain and remember instances of nursing, he raises interesting possibilities that are available to more of us as nurses than is poetry, which requires different forms of narrative gifts. In making "poetics" intellectually credible, Kim may have given these deeply felt "signifiers" a conceptual legitimacy that comes with an analytic assignment. Which is, of course, the essence of scholarship.

To have access to story telling, lyric writing, to poetry as well as to other art forms I have not dealt with tonight opens new possibilities both for nursing self-expression, and for making our words reach out, for making our work visible in ways that traditional research, conventional political argument, and professional whingeing do not.

We do not yet have in nursing collections of writing and poetry that make themselves available for the kind of thematic analysis Kim Walker would like to see. But there are beginnings. Cortney Davis and Judy Schaefer in the United States have collected one volume, "Between the Heartbeats—Poetry and prose by nurses" that I find so powerful I have to put it down between essays.[20] There are scattered, mostly privately published volumes of nursing poetry. Occasionally, one can spot a nurse in the poetry page of the *Journal of the American Medical Association*.

I was thrilled to discover a former colleague from Yale, Jeanne LeVasseur, in those pages in one she called "The Lullaby":

You are holding the telephone
for a dying woman, right against her cheek
a woman near coma for weeks, now
her throat opened for breathing
and unable to speak.

You think this call hopeless,
the waterwheels softening,
slowly easing their rush and flood.

> Then she hears her daughter's voice,
> her eyes dilate, and her face,
> which looked puffy with drugs,
> takes on that soft, smudgy light of May,
> when women in mountain villages open their shutters
> and the early air tumbles in, gauzy and pink.
>
> I don't know what her daughter said.
> But it's as if this woman were surveying the blue
> alleys of the town below, mountains brightening
> in the east. She cradles the phone,
> makes clicking sounds with her tongue,
> tapping excitedly with one finger,
> the low drowning in her throat like reeds
> rushing in streams.
>
> What did her daughter understand?
> I write this for her:
>
> Your mother lay with the phone beside her ear.
> Those sounds you heard were a lullaby.
> You made all the difference.
> She died rocking a baby to sleep.[21]

Listening to poetry is its own fulfilment, but reading it and noticing where the poet has put the punctuation and the italics and the spacing is yet another experience. The tradition of this Oration is that it is published in hard copy so that you, too, can see what I've been reading.

We find nursing, therefore, not only in data and research and data mining and policy statements and White Papers, and Senatorial reports—I loved the title of your most recent one: "The Patient Profession," such a lovely double entendre.[22] We find nursing in capturing the experience of doing this work and putting it in words that sing and echo in our very souls.

The last example is the product from my favorite nurse-poet, Veneta Masson. Veneta was a nurse practitioner in an inner city clinic in Washington, DC when she wrote a series of poems that capture her patients and her work. This one is a whole cantata of nursing.

> Just
> who do you think you are, Maggie Jones
> following me home from work
> insinuating yourself into my evening
> shading my thoughts?
>
> Just
> who do you think you are
> lying flat as a pancake in the middle of your bed

your world ranged around you in brown paper bags?
(Rather like a dead Pharaoh in his tomb, I'd say
buried with all his treasure).

So you fell one day and had to be taken
    to the hospital.
You didn't break any bones, after all.
You came home in a taxi
climbed the steep flight of stairs to your room
took to your bed and stayed there.
That was three years ago, Maggie
three years with only one thing to look forward to—
    livin'.

I'm here by the hand of the Lord, you always say
    when I come.
Though the hand of the Lord didn't smite the rat
    that bit your foot
    that cold winter day last year
    as it foraged in your sheets for bread and jelly.
I guess it'll be all right
    you said in your genteel way
    looking up at me with soft doe eyes as I dress
    the wound that brought us together.

Why don't you go to a home? We ask, shocked
    to see the condition you're in
    (the church ladies, the social worker
    your niece, your nephew and I).
Because I still have my right mind
    you say simply.

A nursing home is no place
    for someone who still has their mind.

But it's not safe here, we say
    (the church ladies, the social worker
    your niece, your nephew and I).
Don't you know they shoot drugs
    and people in this neighborhood?
I've never been bothered
    you say, matter-of-factly.

What about fire? We say
    (the church ladies, the social worker
    your niece, your nephew and I).
There was a fire once, and the fireman carried me out.

I own my home and I own my grave plot
and I plan to go from one to the other
when the Lord calls me
you say quietly, clutching a packet
of long white envelopes.

But now your gas is cut off
until you come up with $700.
You're lucky it's not freezing and there's an electric
coffee maker we can use to heat water to wash you.
I guess the money will come from somewhere
you say, looking at me steadily.

And Meals on Wheels has cut you off because it's a bad
neighborhood to begin with and then
the front door fell off its hinges
onto the Meals on Wheels delivery lady
I guess there's enough food in the United States
to feed me
you say, looking at me knowingly.

And
they've taken away your homemaker because they say
you need more care
than the agency can give.
I guess things will work out
you say, looking at me trustingly.

How can you lie there and say, serenely, you guess
things will work out?

Your room is cold
your sheets are soaked with urine
your skin is bleeding from bedsores
you don't know where your next meal is coming from
you're a poor old lady
hidden away
in a falling-down house
in a no-good neighbourhood
And you have expectations?

You told your niece not to worry about you
the nurse was coming.
Hey, Maggie Jones, don't wait for me, don't count on me.
I'll bathe you
dress your wounds
treat your minor ailments

even do your laundry and bring you food
   once in a while.
But save you?
God alone—the hand of the Lord—can save you.

I see you now in my mind's eye and wonder
   as I sit
   after dinner
   in my warm house
   on a safe street
   in a good neighbourhood.

Just
   who do you think you are, Maggie Jones?[23]

ENDNOTES

1. Thompson, J.D. (1992). The privilege of making a difference. Oration on the occasion of the awarding of the Baxter Prize, Association of University Programs in Public Health, Washington, DC, March 21.

2. Lions, A.M. (1977). Introductory address. First annual oration. In: Annual Orations 1953–1976, NSW College of Nursing, Sydney, pp. 12–13.

3. Dziurgot, P. (2001). Without missing a beat. Annual Report, Yale New Haven Hospital, New Haven, CT, USA, p. 15.

4. Char, W.F., & McDermott, J.F. (1972). Abortions and acuity identity crisis in nurses. *American Journal of Psychiatry, 128*(8), 957–962.

5. Johnstone, M.J. (1989). *Bioethics: A nursing perspective.* Sydney: W.B. Saunders (pp. 232–233).

6. Fagin, C., & Diers, D. (1983, July 14). Nursing as metaphor. *New England Journal of Medicine,* 309:116–117.

7. Bascom, P.B., & Tolle, S.W. (2002, July 3). Responding to requests for physician-assisted suicide—"These are uncharted waters for both of us." *JAMA, 288*(1), 91–98.

8. Ganzini, L., Harvath, T.A., Jackson, A., Goy, E.R., Miller, L.L., & Delorit, M.A. (2002, August 22). Experiences of Oregon nurses and social workers with hospice patients who requested assistance with suicide. *New England Journal of Medicine, 347*(8), 582–588.

9. Ellison, M., Diers, D., & Leonard, R.C. (1965). The use of behavioral science in nursing: Further comment. *Nursing Research, 14*(1), 71–72.

10. Diers, D. (1970). This I believe...about nursing research. *Nursing Outlook, 18*(11), 50–54.

11. Lumby, J. (2001). *Who cares? The changing health care system.* Sydney: Allens & Unwin, p. 42.

12. Chiarella, M. (2002). *The legal and professional status of nursing.* Sydney: Churchill Livingstone, p. 262.

13. Diers, D., & Evans, D.L. (1980). Excellence in nursing. *Image, 12*(3), 27–30.

14. Taylor, B.J. (1994). *Being Human—Ordinariness in Nursing.* Melbourne: Churchill Livingstone.

15. Pearson, A. (1988). Unpublished graduation address, Lakeside, Quoted in Taylor, *op cit*, p. 5.

16. Diers, D. (1982). Between science and humanity: Nursing reclaims its role. *Yale Alumni Magazine, 45*(5), 8–12.

17. Walker, K. (1995). Nursing, narrativity and research: towards a poetics and politics of orality. Reprinted in Rolfe, G. *Research, Truth and Authority* (2000) (pp. 87–102). London: Macmillan.

18. Charman, J. (1987). *2 Deaths in 1 Night.* Auckland: New Women's Press.

19. Leopold, J.R. (2002). Chronic vegetative state. *Do you see what I see?* New Haven: Yale University School of Nursing. (p. 12).

20. Davis, C., & Schaefer, J. (1995). *Between the Heartbeats—Poetry and Prose by Nurses.* Iowa City: University of Iowa Press.

21. LeVasseur, J. (1995). The Lullaby. *JAMA.* Reprinted in Davis & Schaefer, *ibid.*, p. 104.

22. *The Patient Profession: Time for Action. Report on the Inquiry into Nursing.* (2002, June). Commonwealth of Australia Senate.

23. Masson, V. (1999). Just Who. *Rehab at the Florida Avenue Grill* (pp. 56–60). Washington, DC: Sage Femme Press.

THE POWER OF NARRATIVE

The distinguished health policy journal, Health Affairs *(sponsored by Project Hope) has a special section called "Narrative Matters" under the editorship of Fitzhugh Mullan, MD. The section is intended to showcase narratives— stories—that might matter to how policy makers think of things.*

The W.K. Kellogg Foundation had funded two conferences on writing narrative in health care, one for physicians and one for the media. In their second iteration of funding, they proposed a conference on nursing. Diana Mason, brilliant Editor of the American Journal of Nursing *worked with* Health Affairs *to plan a conference about how to connect nursing with policy through narrative writing. This is the keynote that began the conference, October 3, 2003.*

I was told that I was asked to do this in part because I could be witty.

Whatever comes out as wit and humor comes out of my writing the content and context. I can't be funny on command. The ability to do that in public speaking, well, that comes with practice. The gift of a happy childhood, with parents who loved to laugh and have fun, that gives me a reservoir.

The experience in this conference was an epiphany. A "company of nurses" as writers and poets, teaming with journalists, showcasing nursing writing and thinking in the context of policy, oh, I felt home. *The speech I constructed, and that's the right verb, worked. I really did throw papers around and they laughed in the right places. I had never done this kind of "performance" before and probably won't do it again.*

This occasion and the response to my work solidified where I want to grow next. The gift of having some more years ahead needs to be spent carefully.

This has got to be the scariest speaking engagement I ever accepted.

You've got my writing idols here and you want me to speak to *them?*

And I haven't actually ever even met some of them before?

Veneta Masson, whose poetry and narrative wiped me out from the first one I ever read and whose words I use (carefully attributed, of course) all the time, most recently in Australia where her poem, "Maggie Jones" stunned an audience of nursing leadership in Sydney.

And Echo Heron, whose books I buy in hardback and with whom I had a short but powerful correspondence. (Echo, I'm really sorry for the critique accusing *Mercy* of being "too California"—I didn't get it then. I do now.)

And Suzanne Gordon, for whom I was once chauffer on the book tour in Southern Connecticut during which I learned more than I wanted to know about how ungrateful nurses can be when our work is gracefully and publicly revealed, as Suzanne did it.

And Judy Schaefer, whose work both as writer and editor I admire.

And Diana Mason, for heaven's sake! You have fundamentally changed— let's say rescued—our USA professional journal. You are moving the *American Journal of Nursing* to a new space in health care publication in nursing, subtly and cleverly, and building a presence for nursing in the upper middle class public eye that we have long coveted.

You don't want me, you want Anna Quindlen.

She has perfected the form: start with a people story, analyze it pithily, conclude with the fast policy connection, in 800 words or less. (And write heartbreaking novels on the side, and give public speeches that seamlessly stitch together her person, profession, values, humor, and narrative talent.)

But you've got me.

There's this park a couple of blocks from where I live in New Haven where I walk as often as I can, early in the morning. As I rounded the corner between the sundial fountain and the dog walker gathering place on a hot morning in August, the form if not the content of what has become this...event...struck me.

Drat.

Who cares about how I got these ideas?

THROW THIS AWAY

Start again.

I'm an unregenerate professor person.

So what IS narrative, look it up, gotta start there. I think of it as story-telling but is that right?

Okay: narrative is "story" or "account."

Well, that doesn't differentiate it from a research report, which is actually a story, other than there are arcane and silly style rules for how to put together a research report and God forbid it should have any people in it. That would violate HIPAA rules.

So much for *this* theme.

THROW THIS AWAY

Try this:

There is a tendency among nurses and not just academics to think that the only things worth writing and speaking about are the political forces, or the forays into obscurantic conceptual fog. We are faintly embarrassed to read the testimony of a patient who credits her nurse with saving her life, or making him comfortable, as if we were suddenly outed. Our work with patients is not well described in formalistic jargon, so patients tend to talk about our contribution in simple words: "The nurse (rarely named) was so nice to me," and that seems unprofessional to we who have studied psychology and communication and everything else to make that niceness professional.

When we are interviewed by reporters, we get tongue-tied because we don't know what the media want other than juicy stories about death or disability or pain or trauma or cancer. Anna Q says that's not right. There is no "the media." The print media and the electronic media work by different rules. From our point of view, they're the same: laypersons. And they can be conduits for our stories. Reporters, journalists write for the public who might be touched by stories that we find trivial and who trivialize the stories we'd really like to tell. The half-life of most reportage is about two days, so why should we bother?

Not long ago, the Hartford *Courant* placed a reporter on a nursing unit at Yale-New Haven Hospital for several weeks to prepare what turned out to be a long story about nursing today. The reporter came to really like the unit and the unit staff to like her. She began her article, which ran on the front page, with a story about how the nursing staff had dealt with a patient with the wandering of Alzheimer's. Instead of restraining him, they made a small sign that they placed on the back of his bathrobe that said, "please return me to 7-7." Of course, that's not *all* they did. But the nurses on 7-7 were horrified and felt betrayed when they read this, as were some who wrote letters to the Editor. I rather thought this was clever, creative nursing practice. So far as I know, no lay newspaper reader wrote in to say this was cruel or insensitive.

Another story: the major problem nursing has in a policy context is invisibility. Especially financial invisibility, since rarely can one discover nursing on a patient's bill (if the patient ever even saw the bill) or in the costing and forecasting systems in hospitals. Nursing unit/ward managers are managing small businesses, often with budgets in the millions of dollars, and their budgets are set on a somebody's pie-in-the-sky guesstimate of next year's patient days counted by the midnight census this year. They must supply braces, scalpels, gowns and gloves, and Podus boots from their budget, but they never get reimbursed when the patient's bill is paid. This is madness, from the point of view of sensible business administration. But this story makes people's eyes cross and slumber set in.

Nobody wants to read or hear about how hard nursing's work is; everybody's work is hard in one way or another. Nor do they really want to hear about the downside of the contexts of practice—the difficulty getting anything done, the idiot administrative commitments, the "elephant in the middle of the table" political discussions, the sometimes bitter interdisciplinary relationships. Everybody has those.

They want to hear our secrets and we don't want to tell them.

Well, so much for that thought.

THROW THIS AWAY

Where and when and how and why does narrative matter?

Here's a narrative about a narrative:

The statue of women veterans, who are, of course, nurses, in Washington DC, has a beautifully complex history. The sculptor, Glenda Goodacre, has caught both the horror of war and the triumph of succor. I know just a slice of this story and I participated in a tiny fraction of that serving.

Linda Spoonster Schwartz, now the Commissioner of Veterans Affairs for the State of Connecticut, was a graduate student in psychiatric nursing at Yale when, as a reserve Air Force flight nurse on a training flight over Pennsylvania, the hatch door blew off at 30,000 feet and Linda and her crew went into rapid descent. She suffered permanent neurological damage which you would never know unless she tells you.

Linda is a tiger as an advocate for patients and nurses and especially the veterans who are both. When the idea surfaced for a statue in DC, she and others turned to the tools of politics because that's how you get a statue done. I encouraged Linda to write an article for *Image*, as I was then the editor, because when something is in print, it can be used for all kinds of purposes. Besides, the story of women and nurses in Vietnam hadn't then been told in the general nursing literature.

Linda did, I edited just a tiny bit—Linda has literally kissed the Blarney Stone hanging by her feet in her strong husband's hands, she's a short person—and, after selected peer review, I caused it to be printed in *Image*. She started the article this way:

> The war in Vietnam was the longest war in the history of the United States—a war that redefined war. There were no discernable front lines, no safe places, no rules. Enemy soldiers wore what looked like black pajamas and rode bicycles; children threw bombs and progress was marked by body counts. ... When one thinks of Vietnam, pictures of combat soldiers, helicopters, burning flags and prisoners of war in Hanoi come easily to mind. Rarely do the images include women. ...
>
> The values that many women brought with them to Vietnam—to help, to heal and to serve humanity—were incongruent with the objects of war—death, destruction and devastation...Women devalued their own contributions as being "part of the job" or as being less important than fighting because they had it so much better than did the men.[1]

Linda also describes the complex circumstances of nursing in war:

> The seriously wounded or ill could be airlifted out of Vietnam to hospitals in Japan or the Philippines within hours of their injury. ...The flight from Vietnam to Japan

took between four and six hours, during which time the flight nurses were the senior medical authority. The environmental and physiological changes of altitude could completely alter a patients' condition, and complications could quickly set in. ...At one time there was a great push to move casualties out of Vietnam as quickly as possible so that, should they died in Japan or the Philippines, their deaths would not be included in the official "body count."

Well, my goodness, what a response we got. For nurses who served in Vietnam, it was the first time someone had validated their experience in mainstream nursing print. And I caused a number of the letters to the Editor to be printed in *Image*.

In this article, Linda does not delve into what became her passion later: Agent Orange. Agent Orange (dioxin) was a powerful defoliant used in Vietnam to get rid of the foliage and underbrush so that the enemy could not hide. It was sprayed from low-flying planes. But more than sometimes, the planes would return to base, which is where the hospitals and living quarters were, with too much load to land, so they would spray around the base: high tech lawn mowing. The metal drums that delivered Agent Orange were often cut in half to become barbecue pits for American troops.

Linda went on to do her doctoral work on the epidemiology of the effects of Agent Orange on women. Her presentation of these data, with narratives, buttressed with slides and figures, have created VA benefits for women as well as men for the cancers they suffer and for the birth defects of their children. And a recent reanalysis of the official data has put the Air Force on notice that their denials of the health effects of dioxin (which has its own policy context, of course) cannot endure.

Linda's article in *Image*, xeroxed a million times in flagrantly welcome violation of copyright law, got into the hands of senators and representatives. And when it came time to dedicate the statue, many grinding hard years later, Gen. Colin Powell (who ought to have known before) said that until he had read the narratives of nurses who served in Vietnam, he hadn't known the extent of women's presence in the war.

Linda's article used powerful rhetoric about service and sacrifice. When targeted at the patriotic heartstrings of Senators and Representatives and recalcitrant members of statue committees who didn't believe a statue of women would fit their standards for statues—their line was, "what's next, a statue of a dog?"—the narratives made a difference.

Okay, not too bad but not good enough.

PUT THIS ASIDE

Another story.

I asked Diana Mason to tell me why I am standing here instead of Anna Quindlen.

Actually, that's not the way I said it.

"Why *me*?"

Diana recalled that the *NY Times* had published in Nurses Week 2002 excerpts from a paper Claire Fagin and I had done some long years before, called "Nursing as Metaphor." Now there's a story.

Claire and I, as Deans for our respective schools of nursing at Penn and Yale, often found ourselves at the same meetings. Once we talked about how hard it was to convey the sense of what nursing is when we were in cocktail parties with University types, or on airplanes in Business Class, when your seat partner, usually a man, says, "And what do you do?"

So we wrote a piece about the metaphors of nursing. It was a sweet piece. We tried to get it into the *NY Times* and the *Philadelphia Inquirer,* and several other places without success. Claire finally turned to the PR people at Penn and a journalist revised it for us.

In moment of characteristic audacity, Claire submitted it to the *New England Journal of Medicine,* who took it, and she called me in triumph and suggested we go for simultaneous publication in the *American Journal of Nursing.* I called Mary Mallison and we worked it out. The timing of publications meant that it wasn't actually simultaneous, but we tried. Probably the one and only time that simultaneous publication has been attempted in the premier medical and nursing journals.

The essay started this way:

> For some time now we have been curious about the reactions
> of people we meet socially to being told, "I am a nurse."
> First reactions to this statement include the comment, "I
> never met a nurse socially before"; stories about the person's
> latest hospitalization, surgery or childbearing experience;
> the question, "How can you bear handling bedpans (vomit,
> blood)"; or the remark, "I think I need another drink."[2]

The shock of seeing something about nursing published in the *New England Journal* in 1983 is probably the explanation for the blizzard of responses we got, mostly from nurses. Interestingly, we got no responses at all from the *AJN* iteration.

This little piece has been reprinted in a whole bunch of other places, including state Medical Society journals, and every once in a while we still get a comment or a letter. Nurses have told me they keep it in a file of things to read when the work gets them down.

And the point is, this piece didn't work until it got put into a form of narrative that fit the purpose. What was different? I don't have it anymore, but I remember the original as being somewhat more whingeing, a very useful verb in British and Australian political vocabulary, not in ours, more is the pity. The journalist cut and pasted the order as well so that the point that would hook the reader—that is, that we as nurses are uncomfortable when we make others uncomfortable by announcing our profession—came sooner.

But I don't like to read it myself anymore. It doesn't sound like me.

Oh, get over it. Move on.

THROW THIS AWAY

As I was typing this out on my wonderful new laptop with the newest Microsoft software, I realized that the newest version (and all the old versions) of Word do not treat "nursing" as an adjectival noun. (Isn't that just a cute little bit of pedantry?) That means that when you write a sentence that says "Nursing's work," or "nursing's agenda," the little red wavy lines come up and when you go to the Tools, Spelling and Grammar menu, what you get as a correction choice is "nurslings"—young animals being cared for by a nurse.

Do we need to work on the Microsoft programmers? Or on the dictionary people who feed the Microsoft programs?

THROW THIS AWAY

Try this thought: writing for the audience.

Many thousand years ago, 1972, to be precise, I was appointed Dean of the Yale School of Nursing. I was 34 (and if you want to do the math to now, feel free...)

I might have been young, but I wasn't stupid.

Yale's PR folks wanted to publicize the appointment. It was ... er ... sexier, in, of course, a journalistic sense, than other academic appointment they had to write about. They even got the society page reporter of the local newspaper to interview me. One look and she knew I was not going to be a good source for beauty tips. Nevertheless, they took pictures of me in a borrowed lab coat under the hospital sign that said "Emergency Entrance," which I thought an apt metaphor.

I didn't know from nothing but I did know that this was a chance to make nursing visible and since that was going to be a large part of my new job, I'd try to make it work.

The Yale Alumni Magazine went free to all 90,000 or so living Yale Alumni including, as we know now to our sorrow or joy, depending on your politics, candidates for President, Supreme Court Justices or failed Supreme Court Justice nominees, AIDS activists, people who do crazy right-wing Web sites, people who support opera and art, and Gerry Trudeau of *Doonesbury.* The Editor of YAM at the time was William Zinsser, who had edited the old *Life* magazine. I liked his work. He wanted to do an article on "modern nursing" and suggested he interview me or have one of his staff do it. I demurred (isn't that a fun word?); I don't demure very well.

I'm maybe two months into this incredible position, feeling my way. Bill and I are in a Chinese restaurant a couple of blocks from the medical center,

having lunch. We have a conversation that is for me, an out-of-body experience: HE'S WILLIAM ZINSSER—FAMOUS EDITOR PERSON! I'm little
kid from Wyoming. I think he liked the way I talked and by then I had learned
that the way to write narrative was to write the way you talk. So I proposed
that I actually write an article and if he didn't like it, he could turn someone
on to interview me. I was very sure at that time that if I didn't do it, nobody
would get nursing right.

I wrote the thing. Bill changed one word and it went into the Yale Alumni
Magazine as the cover story with a picture of one of our graduate students in
a cap—had to have a cap—and a turtleneck sweater (!), along with pictures
of Dicken's evil nurse, Sairy Gamp, and Florence Nightingale.

This narrative mattered. Oh, not in a great big public policy sense. The
context is everything. The Dean of the Medical School at Yale whose term
started the same day mine did was Lewis Thomas, he of *Lives of a Cell, The
Youngest Science* and many graceful essays. That I entered into Yale's publications with a not-bad piece of advocacy prose made me more credible to this
very old, very male, very ignorant-about-nursing place in ways that made the
decanal job easier. I became one of them, surely not as high profile as Lew
Thomas, but one of them nevertheless. I learned the value of writing in this
publication as Yale Alumni hospitalized somewhere handed the magazine to
a nurse and said, "you might want to read this." Several of those nurses came
to us as graduate students.

Years pass and nursing again gets headlines as nurse practitioners start
having local and national visibility. A new Editor of YAM calls me, this is
now 1982, 10 years later, and asks for maybe 500 words on what's happening
at Yale with NPs.

I tell him it is not possible to capture nursing in small word counts, the
issues are so interesting, so I will write him a whole article, maybe 3000 words.
The article was called "Between Science and Humanity" and it began this way:

> The meticulous reader of the *Yale Weekly Bulletin and
> Calendar* of November 29, 1981 might have noticed, in
> between announcements of colloquia on immunobiology,
> Sanskrit and vector transformations, a lecture on Florence
> Nightingale. The truly obsessive reader would have noticed
> something odd: the lecture was sponsored not only by the
> School of Nursing, which might make sense, but also by
> the department of History, the Section of the History of
> Medicine, and the Department of Epidemiology and Public
> Health. If the reader hungrily followed University politics,
> he might have chuckled at the coincidence, for just the day
> before the lecture on Nightingale, the Yale College faculty
> approved a major in women's studies.
>
> It does not stretch the synapses too much to make these
> random observations fit. Florence Nightingale—founder of

modern nursing, statistician, sanitarian, Victorian anomaly, brilliant and devious woman—is a figure in not only the history of nursing and medicine, but the intellectual history of the nineteenth century, and lately she has been rediscovered as an important figure in the study of women. As the attention of scholars and historians turns to Miss Nightingale, so is public attention turning now to nurses as more than simply an occupational group who dress quaintly. Nursing might even (*mirabile dictu*) be the key to the reform of an obese and inhumane health-care system.[3]

By now I'm not trying to win a place at Yale, I'm wanting to use Yale to get the word out there. So I throw in a gratuitous Latin phrase, some insider allusions to University politics. He likes the article—I still do too—including these lines:

Nursing puts us in touch with being human. Nurses are invited into the inner spaces of other people's existence without even asking, for where there is suffering, loneliness, the tolerable pain of cure or the solitary pain of permanent change, there is the need for the kind of human service we call nursing.

The intimacy that is the core of nursing gives us a peculiar aura, and just as some people feel awkward in the presence of a visibly pregnant woman—so clear is the fact of her intimacy—some people are embarrassed in the company of nurses. We are supposed to be dignified over vomitus, uncringing at the sight of blood, calm as we debride the decubitus, pack the wound, give out the bad news. Nurses must hear, but never tell, the secrets of the dark side of the soul, the hates and jealousies, the anger and violence, the cursings at fate, the bargains with God. The terrors of psychosis, the joy of a peaceful and happy birth, the erosions of poverty and discrimination that turn a body thin and sour smelling are part of the nurse's world, all day, every day.

And this time I controlled the illustrations, which were pictures of nurse practitioners working. The journal even interviewed some of our graduates, carefully selected by me, so that they included Yale College men who had become nurses, and interesting stories of alumni connections.

Okay, sweetheart, nice stories.
Where are you going?

PUT THIS ASIDE

Is making narrative matter about rhetoric?
Claire Fagin and Linda Aiken are masterful at choosing and using rhetorical strategies to make their research and policy points. And they do it by

making equally exquisite use of existing agendas, which are not always clear and they change fast.

Linda's redefinition of the nursing shortage in the mid-'80s is one example. Her words and those of others, especially John Thompson's, turned that nursing shortage away from being a problem of nursing itself, to being the consequence of oligopsony in the employment market, and the general economics of society which govern when women who are also wives and mothers decide to work or not. And, in hospitals, to the effect of decreasing length of stay created by the DRG-based Prospective Payment System for Medicare, of which Prof. Thompson was one of the inventors, on increasing nursing care requirements. This point is still not understood well, partly because of another rhetorical device: "quicker and sicker." There isn't actually any good evidence that patients are leaving hospitals in worse condition. The point that hasn't been grasped is that when length of stay is decreased, it concentrates the needs for nursing on whatever days are left, and they are the "sick" days. The "quicker and sicker" language came from hospital associations as a way to focus blame on the DRG-based payment system.

But Linda and John (who was also a nurse) redefined it forever, I thought then. And then managed care, which is neither management nor care, came in and there were too many nurses and we had to cut, slash, burn in the rhetoric of "reengineering" which has now been thoroughly discredited, but that doesn't ease the pain of all of us who went through it.

And then along comes Claire Fagin again in 2001, hooking her monograph for the Milbank folks, "When care becomes a burden: Diminishing access to adequate nursing" to what was then building as policy focus: patient safety. A nursing shortage is arguably a *public* policy issue, in a country in which health care is privately funded for the most part, and nearly entirely privately managed. Claire's brilliance translated the present nursing shortage into a deficiency in "access to *adequate* nursing care"—which turns the issue on its head. Access to care is definitely a public policy issue and one guaranteed to grab constituents of elected representatives who can't get Grandpa into home care, or who worry about whether the person caring for the wife with breast cancer is a nurse or not.

I do a lot of work in Australia and now, New Zealand. My best friend in New Zealand is the Chief Nurse—isn't that a wonderful concept, the Chief Nurse of a whole country? We don't have such a position here and we could use one. The Chief Nurse of New Zealand is Dr. Frances Hughes, perhaps the best nurse politician I have ever known. Frances, and I suspect all Chief Nurses in the world, are masters at linking nursing issues to the rhetoric of the "government of the day," as they say.

I used to think that was duplicity, to change one's perfect words and concepts to match a political agenda.

But that was naïve. When governments are elected on the basis of their policy positions which, it is hoped, are not simply rhetorical, it simply makes sense to associate nursing's issue where we can. But that's a talent, a skill, not taught in Nursing 10b, or 348, nor even 1164, a cross-listed course with the Political Science Department. What *we* need is operational understanding of how the world works in the media and policy context that seem so ephemeral to us.

As I was polishing this presentation, I was reading Anne Garrels' book on her experience as an NPR reporter in Iraq before and during and now after the "war." She built it from transcripts of her NPR reporting, as well as her husband's emails to what must be a fascinating group of friends who worry about her. She captured for me the nuances of policy and politics and history and globalization and especially the human experience of Iraqis on all sides of their political divides, and the experience of the international business of media (sorry Anna Q) reporting. She did it through description, linked to stories of those whom she could interview, and careful observation—the physical reality of the Saddam palaces, the whoosh of a missile passing by her hotel window, the mood of the barber or the maitre' d in her hotel, her driver-slash-"minder."

This has possibilities.

PUT THIS ASIDE

Why should nursing especially be the focus for a conference on writing narrative that matters?

The gift of nursing is that we have the capacity to *witness,* in the old camp meeting sense of that word—to testify, to translate, to do more than simply watch. We are *there* in the experience of health care, in the first person.

We are first persons singular and collective.

Policy is about persuasion. Nursing is at the intersection of policy and reality. What we need to learn how to do is to turn the appreciation—the apprehending—we have of what it is to do the work of nursing, in the contexts of practice into a style and content of prose that speaks the language of policy.

We live in practice with those upon whom all the policy and political decisions eventually roll down. We must help give them voice.

And ourselves too.

Nursing is two things: the care of the sick (or the potentially sick) and the tending of the entire environment within which care happens. Policy is part of the environment.

Oh, dear...

TOSS THIS

I'm supposed to talk about the "Power of Narrative".

So I'm walking in my park on a trail through the woods and it hits me: how do we ever *know* that narrative matters?

Matterness isn't captured in conventional statistical analysis with probability figures. Although I was instructed to learn from a citation search that the things that I've written that are most cited are the more intra-professional, inspirational, pieces. They are not "stories". ...or maybe they are, now that I think about it.

Whatever.

TOSS THIS

Get it together, fool; you're supposed to do something about the power of narrative.

Actually, I think I have.

ENDNOTES

1. Schwartz, L.S. (1987). Women and the Vietnam Experience. *Image, 19*(4), 168–173.

2. Fagin, C.M., & Diers, D. (1983). Nursing as metaphor. *New England Journal of Medicine, 309*(2), 116–117.

3. See the previous section in this book.

KNOWING WHAT I KNOW NOW, WOULD I DO IT AGAIN?

This essay appeared in the Yale Nursing Matters *(3[2] p. 32, 2002, used with permission), a publication of the Yale School of Nursing. That issue featured a story on my retirement from the School, and this was the endnote.*

Would I choose nursing over, say, journalism or miniature-making, teaching English, or playing cocktail piano in smoky bars? Or even professional basketball? Tall women now have interesting career choices.

Would I choose again the terror of caring for my first patient?

Her name was Mrs. Gibson and she was in Room 108 on the south wing of Presbyterian Hospital in Denver and she was facing surgery to remove one of her very large breasts and I was 19 years old and nearly breastless in my spanking new uniform and cap. I was supposed to bathe her and be comforting.

Would I choose the same first job again? Even before I had passed State Boards (now NCLEX) I was to be the Chief Nurse at a Campfire Girls camp in the mountains above Denver. My first case was tick removal, which I knew how to do with a lighted cigarette. My second was acute homesickness, easily cured with a phone call to Mom. My third was to hold the head of the handsomest wrangler as I removed a bit of something from his eye in full view of 60 pre-teen girls.

I've never been so popular before or since.

Would I again choose psychiatric nursing? Would I succumb to the intricacies of how the mind and person works, from my first experience as a student nurse in a huge state hospital in Colorado on a men's ward where the treatments were either electric or insulin shock?

Would I choose again to emigrate across half the country to the Yale Psychiatric Institute (YPI) to study psychiatric nursing and practice it at a world-class hospital then changing the way it thought about nursing? Would I even recognize that I was in a world-class environment with psychiatrists who wrote definitive books and nurses who got federal research grants?

And then as a faculty member, would I choose again to mine my own and other's experience to begin to build a science of practice? Would I even have known back then that's what we were trying to do?

Would I have chosen to try to speak about the personal experience it is to care? Would I have chosen to live in the vast range of scientific, political, and policy issues, the issues of the rights and privileges and obligations of women professionals? Would I have chosen nursing if I had known how deep the sexism and nursism and public discrimination and invisibility are? And how much fun it would be to fight those monsters?

Would I have chosen nursing if I had known the excitement of pushing forward the boundaries of human service and participating in changing the health care system, shaping it?

Would I have chosen nursing if I could have anticipated the experience of being in the company of those who do this work?

You betcha.

And if I had it to do once more knowing what I know now, I would fall in love with nursing all over again.

SECOND THOUGHTS

Writing about nursing within the field is a piece of cake. All I have to do is capture the words of nurses who do the work. All I have to do is listen.

Writing about nursing for outside the field is very hard.

There's about to be a sea change and about time. I think we in nursing have gotten a grip on our internal issues (the many ways to become a nurse, the industrial issues) to allow us to talk about the nature of the work and the environments for practice without being defensive. There is so much more in nursing to unite us than to divide us. When we are united on description and understanding of the work and of those who do it, including all of us— licensed as RN or LPN/LVN and people who do not hold licenses but who give of themselves every day, evening, and night to patients—do we not call all of that "nursing"?

Not long ago, I was meeting with the nursing staff on a certain nursing unit (all who could come that Thursday at 3 PM). I'd done some analysis of the work on the unit with the Nurse Manager because this unit was thought to be "troubled." This is a unit designed to be an HIV unit, but with the changes in the science, HIV patients no longer fill the rooms, all of which are single, and half of which are negative pressure rooms. So the unit fills up with patients who require these accommodations, including a good lot of what we euphemistically call "behavior problems" and "pain management." Toward the end of the conversation, I asked them to tell me how they describe their work to their families. Nearly uniformly, nodding to the one nurse who articulated it, they said: "I can't describe it; they wouldn't understand."

How can we write and talk about nursing so others understand?

First, we have to understand our own language and claim the right to talk about nursing and patient care as if we own a big chunk of it. It is ours, thank you very much, including outcomes such as length of stay and mortality. *The reason for the existence of the modern hospital (home care, nursing home) is to provide nursing.* I'm serious.

We will honour our sensitivity to patient privacy and dignity while crafting our stories to reach a public.

Then, we need to understand the demands of the language of others. The media wants spicy stories; we have a million of them. The policy types want something to hang their work on; we can supply the hooks. We need to target our stories; they aren't just sentimental fluff. We can use them for management change, for policy change, and for political advantage.

Some 300 pages ago, I began this exercise with the notion that *nursing is two things: care of the sick (or the potentially sick) and the tending of the entire environment within which care happens.* "Tending" is a muscular commitment that extends us into politics and policy and management and operations and journalism and advocacy.

And speaking of nursing.

Index

A

Accountability
definition of, 166
of intensive care nurses, 206
of primary care nurses, 115
responsibility, authority and,
205–206, 220
Advanced practice nursing. *See also*
Nurse practitioners
development of, 99
educational funding for, 194–195
primary care. *See* Primary
care nursing
Agent Orange, 256
AIDS epidemic, nursing demand
and, 230, 231
American health care system
contemporary observations,
248–249
previous predictions, 248
vs. Australian health care system,
252–253
American Nursing Foundation project
grants, 24
Analytic non-experimental studies, 59
ANA *Social Policy Statement,* 74, 76,
114–115
Annual Review of Nursing Research,
74–75

APACHE scale, for intensive care, 206
Applied science, *vs.* science of
application, 249–250
"At risk" groups, studies of, 69, 72
Australia
casemix management, nursing and,
243–246
ecology of, 252–253
health care in, 252–253
immigration policy of, 253
scientific research in, 253–254
Authority
accountability and, 205–206, 220
of intensive care nurses, 206
lack of, 224
prescriptive, 123–124, 126, 136
responsibility and, 169–170,
205–206, 220
Authors, editors and, 276
Autoimmune disorders, in female
Vietnam veterans, 256
Autonomy, lack of, 224

B

Background research, 20
Backlash, 171
Basic research, in health services, 58
Budget Reconciliation Act, 222–223
Burn-out, 145

C

Cancer rates, in female Vietnam
veterans, 256
Capitation funds, 193–194
Caring, 158–159
Case management, 231, 250–252
Case managers, role of, 118, 252
Casemix
definition of, 252
funding, *vs.* management, 244
nursing, 210
Case mix index, 259
CEUs (continuing education units), for
nursing practice research, 36
Charting, 196
Classical experimental design, 107
Clinical abstracts, 207
Clinical experimentation, as
unethical/impossible, 107
Clinical institutions, educational
institutions and, 238
Clinical judgment studies, 74
Clinical nurse specialists, 229
Clinical nursing research, 54–55, 58
Clinical practice. *See* Nursing practice
Clinical scholarship
background of, 79–81
benefits from, 91–92
comparisons in, 86
"concepts by intellection" and, 87
definition of, 90–91, 92
maturity of practice and, 87
observation and, 81–85
qualities of, 83
re-examination of conventional
wisdom and, 86, 91
research and, 86
thought process for, 91
vs. research, 91
writing/documenting, 92–93
Co-authorship, 275
Collaboration, in primary care nursing,
118–119
Commitments, personal, support from,
170–171
Community care, 251

Co-morbidity, 251
Comparisons
in clinical scholarship, 86
in research, 59–60, 86
Competition
between advanced practice nurses
and physicians, 127
economic, 117–118
health care industry, 146
in medical specialties, 127
Computer-assisted library
searches, 282
Computerization, in nursing, 239
Consciousness raising, 86
Continuing education
as nontraditional, 32
opportunities for, 235
politics of, 31–32
in promoting research
of patient care, 34–35
by practicing nurses, 36–37
through research knowledge
translation, 33–34
on research process, 35–36
translation of research knowledge
and, 33–34
Continuing education units (CEUs),
for nursing practice
research, 36
Contraction stress testing,
non-invasive, 56
Control, 232
Coordination of care, case managers
and, 252
Cost-effectiveness, of nurses, 61
Costs, health care
containment of, 49
for nursing services, 225–226
DRGs and, 162–163
in hospital bills, 145–146, 208
short staffing and, 222
unbundling of, 239
research knowledge on
containment, 47
Credentialling law, 207
Credit, for nursing work, 207–208, 212

D

Data mining, 258
Data systems, 235–236
Data usage, for nurse practitioner
    issues, 135
Death/dying studies, 71
Definition of nursing, 8
Dependent variable, developing
    measures of, 108
Descriptive/correlational studies,
    71–72
Descriptive studies, 59
Developmental research, in health
    services, 58–59
Diabetes case management, 250–252
Diagnosis Related Groups (DRGs),
    214, 218
  casemix and, 252
  casemix management *vs.* funding,
      243–246
  costs of nursing care and, 162–163
  disease classification and, 57
  health services research and, 58
  length of stay and, 257–259
  nursing allocations in, 212
  nursing cost weights for, 243
  nursing intensity and, 209–211,
      235–236
  nursing time deployment and, 209
  nursing under, 209
  psychiatric services and, 61
  purpose of, 162, 208–209, 244
  reimbursement money and, 227
  reimbursement rates and, 60
Dialysis, comparison studies, 60
Discharge planning, 231
Discharge summary, 207
Discovery process, 84–85
Discrepancies, as research problems,
    9, 18–19, 30–31, 103
Disease classification, 57
Disease management protocol, 251
Dissatisfaction, with nursing field, 229
Distrust, clinical scholarship and, 81
Diversity, value of, 49
Divisiveness, of nursing, 201

Doctoral degree nurses, research
    activity of, 24, 75
Documentation, 135, 207
DRGs. *See* Diagnosis Related Groups

E

Economic cycles, nursing shortages
    and, 259
Economic issues. *See also* Costs,
    health care
  competition, 117–118
  nurse employment and, 215
  for nurses in expanded roles, 200
  in nursing shortages, 220
Editors
  authors and, 276
  citation checking and, 282
  computer-assisted library searches
      and, 282
  controversial issues and, 282–283
  function of, 280–282
  job description for, 279
  legal issues for, 283
  letters to, 282–283
  single blind system of review
      and, 283–284
Education, nursing
  accelerated, 237
  BSNs, 234
  capitation funds, 193–194
  changes in, 195–196, 219
  competence testing, 237
  continuing. *See* Continuing education
  costs, as R&D costs for
      hospitals, 239
  diploma graduates, 234
  federal funding of, 179
  joint degree options for, 237
  liberal, 160
  movement into university
      setting, 130
  for nurse practitioners, 114
  nursing, preparation for writing
      and, 269–270
  nursing practice and, 95, 161,
      236–238

Education, nursing *(continued)*
　for nursing research
　　participation, 75
　primary care movement in, 114
　research issues in, 24–25, 45
　resources, 237–238
　science in, 160–161
　student recruitment, 232–233
　in university, 147–148
　university-based programs, 94
Educational institutions, clinical
　　institutions and, 238
Education/training, for nurse
　　practitioners, 123
Empathic resonance, 85
Empirical research, theory-testing, 85
Environment, for nursing work
　entire, tending of, 219–220
　improving, 237
　as research target, 60
Ethical issues
　privacy *vs.* silence, 254–255
　research standards, 26
Evaluation research
　design of, 104
　for expanded role movement,
　　103–104
　methods for, 104
　nurse-midwives, 105–106
　problems with, 104
Evidence-based practice, 95
Expanded nursing roles. *See also*
　　specific expanded nursing roles
　evaluation research, 103–104
　malpractice insurance and, 182
　resistance to, 198–199
　studies, experimental design for, 107
Experimental study design, 59, 107
Experimentation, clinical, 70, 71
Expert witnesses, 125
Eyewitness testimony, of nurses, 182

F
Factor searching, 71
Federal funds
　for nursing, 198

　for nursing education, 179, 198,
　　237–238
　for nursing research, 211–212
First Amendment rights, 283
Foreign medical graduates, 231
Functional nursing, 205
Funding
　for advanced practice nursing
　　education, 194–195
　governmental. *See* Federal funds
　for nursing practice research, 45
　for research, 49
Future of nursing, 161–162

G
Gossiping, 168–169
Graduate Medical Education National
　　Advisory Committee report
　　(GMENAC report), 126,
　　199, 230

H
Health care costs. *See* Costs,
　　health care
Health care system
　ineffectiveness, nursing shortage
　　and, 240
　problems, real reasons for,
　　178–180
　provision of nursing care
　　and, 217
　purpose of, 60
Health insurance, competition in, 146
Health law, nurse practitioners and,
　　124–125
Health maintenance organizations
　　(HMOs), 116
Health policy research. *See* Policy-
　　related research
Health services research
　classification of
　　by design, 59
　　by purpose, 58–59
　　by time frame, 57–58
　definition of, 56–57
　development of, 57

Health Systems Agencies legislation
(H.S.A. legislation), 173–174
High-tech care, in Australia *vs.* United
States, 253
HMOs (health maintenance
organizations), 116
Home health care, nursing care
demand and, 231
Hospital administrators, 188
Hospital bills
costs of nursing care in, 145–146,
208, 211–212, 224–225
items in, 208
Hospitals
budgets, nursing costs in, 225
decentralized management of, 226
existence, nursing as purpose for,
197, 217–218, 221, 257
invisibility of nurses in, 260
liability for acts by employees, 228
outcomes, nursing effects on,
257–258
R&D, nursing education costs
as, 239
reimbursement, 162–163
short staffing, effects of, 221–222
"sick days," number of, 216
H.S.A. legislation (Health Systems
Agencies legislation), 173–174

I
ICD codes, 257
ICUs, nurse staffing and, 259
Identity as nurse, *vs.* identification,
177–178
Image—The Journal of Nursing
Scholarship, 90
Income, generated by nursing, 210
Industry relationships, 95
Influence, in health care, 166, 174
Information, informal passage
of, 168–169
Insurance laws, 117
Intellectual discipline of nursing, 286
Intensive care, 55, 205–206,
218–219, 259

Interdisciplinary education/activity,
252–254
Intimacy, of nursing, 143, 201–202
Invisibility of nurses
change in care systems and, 203
economic, 208
feminism and, 260
politics and, 176
reasons for, 207
solutions for, 256–257
vs. being a problem, 180–183

J
"Johns Hopkins" management
structure, 244–246

K
Knowledge, nursing
building through research, 94
future practice of nursing
and, 161
lay public and, 183–184
practice-based, 10, 49, 184–187
responsibility and, 183, 184

L
Labeling, diagnostic, 184–187
Language
knowledge, for clinical
scholarship, 81
used in observations, 82–85
Lawsuits
hospital liability and, 228
against nurse practitioners, 199
Leadership
ambiguity of, 172
awareness of real reasons for
problems, 178–180
definition of, 165–166
financial problems and, 167–168
information access and, 168–169
lack of, in nursing profession, 176
laws for, 177–192
non-randomness of universe
and, 166–167
public, 262–263

Leadership *(continued)*
responsibility/authority and, 169–170
seeking, 174
social responsibility of, 173–174
softer aspects of, 166
sources of, 184
visibility and, 171–172
vision and, 172–173
Legal issues
for editors, 283
responsibilities of nurses, 181–182
Legislation, 228
Length of stay
DRGs and, 214, 257–259
nursing effects on, 257–258
short staffing and, 221–222
Letters, to editors, 282–283
Letter-writing campaigns, 194
Liability insurance, 200
Liberal education, for nurses, 160

M
Malpractice
insurance coverage, 125, 200
issues for nurse-midwives, 147
legal aspects of, 181–182
Managed care, 230, 231
Management
case, 231, 250–252
decentralized, 226
decision making, informal information-passing systems and, 168–169
"Johns Hopkins" structure for, 244–246
operational, 257–258
Market power, in constraining physician practices/incomes, 248
Matrix management structure, 244–246
MDS (Minimum Data Set), 239
Measurements, good, lack of, 20–21
Measures, invalid, 108–109
Media coverage, public policy and, 255

Medical education funds, capitation funds and, 194
Medical practice acts, 131, 234
Medical specialization, competition in, 127
Medicare. *See* Prospective Payment System (PPS)
Medicine
boundaries of, 234
internal politics of, 188
specialist focus of, 118
Mental health system
nursing shortages and, 223
patient-centered research, 13–22
Minimum Data Set (MDS), 239
Modern nursing, description of, 142–143
Money, 167–168
Mortality rates, nursing effects on, 55, 257–258
MUGA, pre-scan orders, 56
Multiple-entry system, for nurses, 234

N
National Institutes of Health, Division of Nursing, project grants, 24
Nipple stimulation, for contraction stress testing, 56
Non-nurses, capitation funds for, 194
Non-patient studies, 67–68
Non-speciality nursing units, hospitalization outcomes and, 257–258
Nurse employment, nurse/patient ratios, 215
Nurse leaders
definition of, 165–166
informal sources of support for, 170
problem analysis by, 166–168
social contributions of, 173–174
Nurse managers
budget control for, 210–211
need for, 237
Nurse-midwives
competition issues for, 127, 146–147

documentation for, 207
  seniority, new physicians and, 116
  student research, 105
  third-party reimbursement, 135
  use of technology and, 204
effectiveness of, 58
evaluation research, 105–106
legal recognition, 135
physician presence for, 230
practice restrictions for, 230–231
research, 104–105
Nurse-patient interaction, 15–17, 202
Nurse-physician relationship, 114
Nurse practice acts, 131
Nurse practitioners
  acceptance of, 114
  attitudes/values of, 117, 129
  caseloads, 115–116
  challenges for, 112
  comparative studies of, 59–60
  competition issues for, 127, 147, 199
  complementary *vs.* substitutable,
    132–133
  consumers and, 136
  criticisms of, 102, 130
  definition of, 133
  educational programs for, 114
  education/training for, 123
  effectiveness of, evidence for,
    139–140
  formal training programs for, 130
  health care consumers and, 134–135
  historical aspects, 121–123
  in HMO settings, 116
  house staff training and, 128–129
  international role of, 120
  legal status of, 124–126, 131, 134
  licensure laws, 198–199
  nurse educators and, 131
  nurse-physician relationship
    and, 114
  in nursing practice research, 37–38
  physician oversupply and, 199
  physicians and, 99–100
  political issues for, 134
  preparation of, 102
  prescriptive authority for,
    123–124, 126
  in primary care, 46
  professional problems of, 134
  referrals, importance of, 127
  reimbursement obstacles, 120
  relationship with physicians,
    114, 130
  research on, 106–107, 109, 111
  role, development of, 99
  safety of, 199–200
  scope of practice, 115–116
  seniority, new physicians
    and, 116
  staying in work force, 132
  strategies for, 135–136
  visibility of, 136
Nurse researchers
  education level of, 36–37, 75
  ethereal nature of, 37
  intellectual elitism of, 49
  nurses in practice as, 36–37
  practicing nurses and, 9–10
  without doctorates, 94–95
Nurse-run programs, 48
Nurses. *See also specific types
    of nurses*
  activity in research, 24. *See also*
    Nurse researchers
  clinical wisdom of, 203
  conflict between, 114–115
  decisions for testing and, 55–56
  early criticisms of, 130
  functions/duties of, 196, 217
  identity of, 177–178
  intuition of, 54
  personal characteristics for, 144
  powerlessness of, 176, 187–188
  praise/bragging, 183–184
  professional growth of, 41–42
  quality of care and, 190
  responsibilities of, 169–170
  salaries of. *See* Salaries, nursing
  shortages of. *See* Nursing shortages
  as specialists, 218
  undervaluation of, 176

Nursing budget, 225
Nursing care. *See* Patient care
Nursing care plans, nursing diagnoses
   and, 184–185
Nursing casemix, 210
Nursing diagnoses, 54, 184–187
Nursing education. *See* Education,
   nursing
Nursing functions, 143–144
Nursing homes
  licensed personnel for, 222–223
  nurse shortages and, 229
Nursing intensity, DRGs and, 209,
   210–211, 235
Nursing literature. *See* Professional
   nursing literature
Nursing practice. *See also* Nursing
   practice research; Patient care
  analytical approach to, 34–36
  bridge with policy, 260
  changes in, non-research related, 46
  clinical work, 80
  definition of, 248
  effect of research knowledge on,
   53–54
  historical changes/trends, 195–197
  improvement, research role in, 53
  individualized patient care and,
   25–26
  nursing education and, 236–238
  performance studies, 74
  physician supervision of, 196
  policy and, 249–260
  research applications, 23–28
  restrictions, 230–231
  scope of. *See* Scope of practice
  studies on, 94
Nursing practice research, 79–80
  CEUs for, 36
  definition of, 30
  development, benchmark for, 42
  difficulty of, 36, 38
  directed at knowledge building,
   46–47
  on direct effects of nursing on
   patient variables, 48

  discrepancies as research problems,
   30–31
  environment as target for, 60
  ephemeral considerations, 37–38
  funding for, 45
  in future, 42, 44–45
  generations of nurses in, 41–42
  growth of, 31
  involvement of nurses in studies
   done by others, 37–38
  as nontraditional, 32
  political benefits of, 46–47
  progress in, 42–45
  promoting, continuing education
   and, 32–39
  on public policy decision-
   making, 48
  purpose of, 45–46
  supporting evidence for, 8
Nursing profession
  as "applied science," 7, 9
  as art *vs.* science, 189
  attitudes, in primary care, 117, 129
  boundaries, 233–234
  central role for, 212
  components of, 158–159
  contemporary, 217–220
  as craft, 189–190
  dangerousness of, 190–191
  definition of, 130, 133,
   156–158, 248
  effect, measures of, 108–109
  expanded role of, 102–103,
   114–115
  financial contributions to hospital,
   224–225
  future predictions for, 256–258
  invisibility of, 256–257
  issues, political *vs.* professional,
   200–201
  jobs. *See* Work of nursing
  lack of leadership in, 192
  leadership. *See* Leadership
  liabilities of, 220–221
  metaphors for, 156–157
  outdated views of, 155–156

patient-related activities, 144–145
as personal service, 201–202
phenomena, 184
powerlessness of, 227–228
process of, 189–190
as profession, 196
research. *See* Research; *specific
    types of nursing research*
resources
    data on, 239
    in nursing research literature, 74
role of, 141–148
salaries. *See* Salaries, nursing
services
    costs, operational barriers and,
        227–228
    financial accountability for, 257
    patient requirements for, 225, 226
shortages of nurses. *See* Nursing
    shortages
social contract of, 191–192
territorial problems, 183–184,
    188–189
as women's profession, 32
Nursing Research journal, history of,
    42–44
Nursing shortages
    auxiliary staff and, 197
    barriers for nurses and, 224–228
    feminist views of, 259–260
    health care system ineffectiveness
        and, 240
    hospitals and, 232
    implications of, 236–240
    increased nursing work and, 219
    long-term solution, 238–240
    money and, 225–227
    new, 220–221
    nursing demand and, 215–216
    as policy issue, 221–224
    problems of, 179
    Prospective Payment System and,
        214–215
    public policy and, 61, 146
    reasons for, 220–221
    redefinition of problem, 215–217

science and, 198
scope of practice and, 222
solutions for, 216–217
team or functional nursing and, 205
wider view of, 228–231
Nursing Studies Index, 66
Nursing theory, 67, 161
Nursing time, 225–226
Nursing work. *See* Work of nursing

O
Observation
    on bedtime behavior, 81–83
    in clinical scholarship, 81
    clinical scholarship and, 81–85
    initial, in developing research
        studies, 19–20
    language usage in, 82, 83–84, 85
    nurse-patient interaction and, 17–18
Occupational socialization, women
        physicians and, 248
Occupational therapists, 189
Oligopsony, 214–215, 259
Operational management, 257–258
Orientation, 15
Originality, writing and, 273–274
Outcomes research, 95
Outpatients, coordination of care for,
    251–252
Oxytocin injections, alternatives
    for, 56

P
Pain management, patient-centered
    nursing for, 19–20
Parkinsonism, L-dopa for, 84–85
Patient behavior, data sources, 21
Patient care
    demand for, 215–216, 231
    determining amount of, 210
    direct, as human service, 184
    as hospital purpose, 257
    individualized, 109
    in nursing literature, 183–184
    nursing practice and, 22, 143
    routine, demand for, 215–216

Patient care *(continued)*
 studies, 26–27
  difficulties with, 72–73
  nurse practitioner work and, 103
  promotion through continuing
   education, 34–35
  quality of care, 108
  rules for, 73
Patient-centered nursing
 definition of, 16
 effectiveness of, 16–18
 for pain management, 19–20
 for patient problems, 18
 research, interaction studies, 13–17
Patient characteristics, effect on
  illness/treatment, 110
Patient contact, first, 127
Patient health education, 108
Patient studies, categories of, 68
Pediatric nurse practitioner, 109
Personal contact, nurses and, 142–143
Personal popularity, leadership and,
  171–172
Phenomena of interest to nursing,
  74–75
Philosophy of nursing, *vs.* nursing
  theory, 108
Physical therapists, 189
Physician-nurse collaboration,
  239–240
Physician-nurse practitioner
  relationship, 99–100
Physicians
 as budget holders, 244–246
 competition with APNs, 127
 new, seniority of nurse practitioners
   and, 116
 oversupply of, 188, 199, 230
 relationship with nurse practitioners,
   116
 vs. primary care nurses, 119
Physician's assistants, 188–189
Policy
 bridge with practice, 260
 practice and, 249–260
 public *vs.* private, 248

Policy agendas, 135, 153
Policy-making process, 153
Policy-related research, 60
Politics
 agendas, 135
 backlash, 171
 benefits of nursing practice
   research, 46–47
 of interprofessional relationships,
   131–132
 nurse practitioner evaluation
   research and, 104
 nursing research priorities and,
   75–76
 vs. professional issues, 201
Power
 in health care, 166
 information access/control and,
   168–169
 not reaching for, 174
 of nurses, 181, 232
 sources of, 184
 of women, 171
PPS. *See* Prospective Payment System
  (PPS)
Prenatal care, neonatal outcome and,
  57–58
Preoperative instruction, 21–22
Prescriptive authority, 123–124,
  126, 136
Primary care nursing, 113. *See also*
  Nurse practitioners
 ANA *Social Policy Statement* and,
   114–115
 collaboration in, 118–119
 definition of, 116–117
 development of, 118
 efficacy of, 56
 function of, 118
 growth of, 46
 need for, 230
 research on, 48, 59
 role of, 203
 scope of practice, 205
 systems
  capabilities, basic, 117

case manager, 118
collaboration among nurses and, 118–119
traditional nursing service structures and, 115, 260
values in, 117, 129
vs. physicians, 119
Privacy, *vs.* silence, 254–255
Problems
anticipation of, 181
being part of, clarity from, 180–182
conception as nursing problems, 27
real reasons for, 178–180
research. *See* Research, problems
theoretical essence of, 25–26
Profession, nursing as, 155–158
Professional corporations, 125
Professional development, nursing journal articles on, 67
Professional identity, 177–178
Professionalization of nursing, 159
Professional nursing literature
changes in, 202–203
criticisms of, 271
journal articles, 69, 74
historical/biographical, 69–70
mainstream nursing research and, 69–70
methodological, 69
on research, 66–68, 69
public access to, 183
rediscovery of nursing work in, 206–207
writing. *See* Writing, about nursing
Professional policy issues, 208
Professional recognition, lack of, 224
Prospective Payment System (PPS)
case mix index and, 259
creation of, 214, 257
DRGs. *See* Diagnosis Related Groups
length of stay and, 259
nursing shortages and, 219
nursing under, 209
testing, 250

Prospective studies, in health services research, 58
Psychiatric therapy, public funding of, 188
Public image problem, of nursing, 236, 240
Public policy, 227–228
decision-making, 48
issues, 208
media coverage and, 255
nursing shortages and, 221–224
testing, 250–252
Publishing
reasons for, 269–278
of research, 110–111
university publish-or-perish mission and, 276–277

Q

Qualitative research
descriptive, 67
experimental, 67
merits of, 70
non-patient studies, 67–68
patient studies, 68
studies, non-publication of, 71
Quality of care
nurse practitioners and, 108
for nursing homes, 222–223
Quantitative research, 70, 71

R

Racism, 254–255
R and D projects, 58–59
Randomized controlled clinical trials (RCCTs), 7
Reading, as preparation for writing, 270
Recruitment, of nursing students, 236
Reform, health care system, 147
Registered nurses (RNs)
in dialysis units, 60
in nursing homes, 222
versatility of, 219

Reimbursement, 207
hospital, 162–163
third-party. *See* Third-party
reimbursement
Reimbursement money, 227
Replication of research, 110
Research. *See also specific types of
nursing research*
in Australia, 253–254
clinical, 54–55, 58
comparisons in, 86
contributions, for nurse
practitioners, 106–107
conventional thought and, 86
funding, 10
future directions for, 61
growth of, 66
as health services research, 58
history of, 66, 107
in improving nursing practice, 53
integrative reviews of, 86–87
knowledge, 46–47, 52
application to nursing practice,
23–28
effect on nursing practice,
53–54
on health care cost
containment, 47
quality of, 33
translation, continuing education
and, 33–34
lessons that should be learned from,
103–112
on nurse practitioner practice, 102,
106–107
in nursing education, 24–25
nursing significance of, 20–21, 27
in ongoing clinical situations, 21–22
priorities, 75–77
problems, 9
clinical insight for, 44–45, 48–49
descriptive/correlational design
for, 71–72
discrepancies as, 9, 18–19,
30–31, 103
as discrepancy, 103

qualities of, 18–19
source of, 19
process
abstraction of problem, 26
continuing education on, 35–36
in nursing, 25
purpose of, 52
replication of, 110
scope/variety of, 49–50
theoretical essence of problems,
25–26
vs. clinical scholarship, 91
Research-driven techniques, for
evaluation research, 104
Research studies, nursing journal
articles on, 66–68
Research subjects, 67–68, 73–74
Resource Information System (RIMS),
257
Respiratory therapists, 189
Respondeat superior doctrine, 228
Responsibility
accountability and, 205–206, 220
authority and, 169–170,
205–206, 220
nursing diagnoses and, 184–187
nursing knowledge and, 183, 184
Retrospective studies, in health
services research, 57–58
Revenue centers, spending authority
of, 210
RIMS (Resource Information
System), 257
Ritualistic behavior, 82–83
RNs. *See* Registered nurses
Routine nursing care, demand for,
215–216

S
Safety, 199–200
Salaries, nursing
ceilings for, 235
dissatisfaction with, 229
nursing shortages and, 238
range of, 224
vs. physician salaries, 145

Scholarship
  clinical. *See* Clinical scholarship
  definition of, 80
  qualities of, 81
  vs. science, 80–81
Schools of nursing, research program
    development, 7
Science
  of application, *vs.* applied science,
    249–250
  in Australia, 253–254
  connection with nursing service,
    249–250
  nursing knowledge and, 160
  vs. scholarship, 80–81
Scope of practice, 184, 206
  for nurse practitioners, 115–116
  nursing shortages and, 222
  for primary care nurses, 205
Second opinions of nurses, 203
Service delivery, in nursing research
    literature, 74
Sex discrimination, 145
Sexism, 255
Short staffing, effects of, 221–222
Shyness, as excuse for not writing, 276
Silence, *vs.* privacy, 254–255
Silence of nursing, feminism and, 260
Silencing, as survival technique, 260
Social change, nursing and, 263
Social responsibility, leadership and,
    173–174
Social scientists, in nursing research,
    7–9
Social workers, 188–189
Specialist nurses
  competition issues for, 146, 147
  knowledge of, 218
  shortages of, 146, 228–229
Specialized nursing units,
    hospitalization outcomes
    and, 257–258
State government, resistance to
    expanded roles for nurses,
    198–199
Strength, for nurse leadership, 171

Support
  informal, for nurse leaders, 170
  from religious beliefs, 171
Surgical procedures, in Australia, 253
Survival rates, for degrees of illness,
    110
Systems of care, 48, 58

T
Task discrimination, 233
Teaching hospitals, nurses in, 188
Team nursing, 205
Technology
  alternatives, 56
  assessment of, 76–77
  nursing and, 55–56
  use of, 203–205
Term paper phenomenon, 262
Theory, 85, 108
Third-party reimbursement
  for nurse-midwives, 135
  for nursing services, 126, 199
  for primary nursing care, 117–118
Thoughtful nursing, 184
Thought process, for clinical
    scholarship, 91
Time factors
  in defining nursing, 225
  in writing about nursing, 273
Transitions, community-hospital, 252
Translation of research knowledge,
    33–34
Treatments
  criteria for, 14
  definition of, 17
Trust, clinical scholarship and, 81
Truth, clinical scholarship and, 81
Turnover, nurse, 220–221
Tuskegee experiment, 254–255

U
Ultrasound, obstetrical, 55, 204–205
Universities
  accessibility of, 250
  publish-or-perish mission of,
    276–277

Universities *(continued)*
  science-service connection and,
    249–250
  social role of, 250
University of Technology—Sydney
  (UTS), 95

V
Values of nursing, in primary care,
  117, 129
Variables
  independent, refining definition
    of, 107
  wrong, selection of, 106
Vietnam veterans, female, 255–256
Visibility, leadership and, 171–172
Vision, leadership and, 172–173

W
Wellness care, 127–128
Women
  intellectual history of, 184
  physicians, occupational
    socialization and, 248
  Vietnam veterans, health problems
    of, 255–256
Work of nursing
  in future, 161–162
  general medical surgical
    position, 218
  increased, nursing shortages
    and, 219

nature of, 206–207
paucity of studies on, 74
task discrimination, 233
Writing, about nursing
  co-authorship and, 275
  credentials/background for,
    275–276
  criticism and, 271, 275
  difficulty of, 270–271
  editor's role in. *See* Editors
  excuses for not writing, 276
  inspirational sources for, 270–271
  jargon in, 276
  length of article and, 274–275
  making contacts from, 277
  money from, 277
  need for, 272, 275
  originality and, 273–274
  preparation for, 269–270
  reading and, 270
  reasons for, 269–278
  scholarship and, 277–278
  self-expression and, 277
  speaking/talking and, 267, 272
  starting, 271
  style and, 273
  term paper phenomenon and, 262
  time factors for, 273
  topic selection for, 272–273